Epidemiology *for* Advanced Nursing Practice

Edited by

Kiran Macha, MBBS, MPH

Adjunct Faculty and Research Coordinator
School of Nursing, Brooks College of Health
University of North Florida
Jacksonville, Florida

John P. McDonough, EdD, CRNA, ARNP

Professor
Associate Director for Graduate Studies
School of Nursing, Brooks College of Health
University of North Florida
Jacksonville, Florida

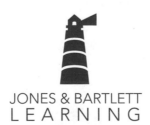

JONES & BARTLETT
L E A R N I N G

World Headquarters

Jones & Bartlett Learning
40 Tall Pine Drive
Sudbury, MA 01776
978-443-5000
info@jblearning.com
www.jblearning.com

Jones & Bartlett Learning
Canada
6339 Ormindale Way
Mississauga, Ontario L5V 1J2
Canada

Jones & Bartlett Learning
International
Barb House, Barb Mews
London W6 7PA
United Kingdom

Jones & Bartlett Learning books and products are available through most bookstores and online booksellers. To contact Jones & Bartlett Learning directly, call 800-832-0034, fax 978-443-8000, or visit our website, www.jblearning.com.

Substantial discounts on bulk quantities of Jones & Bartlett Learning publications are available to corporations, professional associations, and other qualified organizations. For details and specific discount information, contact the special sales department at Jones & Bartlett Learning via the above contact information or send an email to specialsales@jblearning.com.

Production Credits

Publisher: Kevin Sullivan
Editorial Assistant: Rachel Shuster
Production Editor: Amanda Clerkin
Marketing Manager: Meagan Norlund
Associate Marketing Manager: Katie Hennessy
V.P., Manufacturing and Inventory Control:
    Therese Connell

Composition: DataStream Content Solutions, LLC
Cover Design: Scott Moden
Cover Image: © carlos castilla/ShutterStock, Inc.
Printing and Binding: Malloy, Inc.
Cover Printing: Malloy, Inc.

Library of Congress Cataloging-in-Publication Data
Macha, Kiran.
    Epidemiology for advanced nursing practice / [edited by] Kiran Macha, John P. McDonough.
        p. ; cm.
    Includes bibliographical references and index.
    ISBN 978-0-7637-8996-1 (alk. paper)
    1. Epidemiology. 2. Nursing. I. McDonough, John P. II. Title.
    [DNLM: 1. Epidemiologic Methods   Nurses' Instruction. WA 950]
    RA652.M33 2012
    614.4--dc22
                                                              2010040780

6048

Printed in the United States of America
15 14 13   10 9 8 7 6 5 4

Contents

Preface

In ancient days meditation was used as a tool to search for answers within. In the modern world we use science to discover facts. In this Internet age we used Web search engines and personal experiences to develop *Epidemiology for Advanced Nursing Practice*.

My rural community impressions, exposure to World Health Organization Third World programs, graduate education in public health, and global experiences from India, the United Kingdom, Canada, and the U.S. healthcare systems have laid the foundation for this book. Authors of individual chapters have an immense working experience in the community in the topic in which they have chosen to contribute. Many are native to countries throughout the world but earned experience in the United States. I hope this global background will enrich this effort.

Epidemiology for Advanced Nursing Practice has integrated epidemiology and clinical nursing concepts to enhance decision-making skills for advanced nursing practice. Available epidemiological resources have been introduced to assist students in their research. Examples are provided to explain and simplify statistics. Current epidemiological practices have been well documented.

Experience comes through continuous application of epidemiological concepts in the community. Epidemiological topics expand with new and different challenges in response to continuously occurring global events. Although the future remains a mystery, we will hold on to the truth that is present.

Editors

Kiran Macha, MBBS, MPH
Adjunct Faculty and Research Coordinator
School of Nursing, Brooks College of Health
University of North Florida
Jacksonville, Florida

John P. McDonough, EdD, CRNA, ARNP
Professor
Associate Director for Graduate Studies
School of Nursing, Brooks College of Health
University of North Florida
Jacksonville, Florida

Authors

Michele S. Bednarzyk, DNP, FNP, BC
Assistant Professor
Director, Nurse Practitioner and Clinical Nurse Specialist Programs
School of Nursing, Brooks College of Health
University of North Florida
Jacksonville, Florida

Margaret A. Holder, PhD, FNP, BC
Assistant Professor
School of Nursing, Brooks College of Health
University of North Florida
Jacksonville, Florida

Carol A. Ledbetter, PhD, FNP, BC, FAAN
Professor
Director, Doctor of Nursing Practice Program
School of Nursing, Brooks College of Health
University of North Florida
Jacksonville, Florida

Lillia M. Loriz, PhD, GNP, BC
Associate Professor and Director
School of Nursing, Brooks College of Health
University of North Florida
Jacksonville, Florida

Jan Meires, EdD, FNP, BC
Associate Professor
School of Nursing, Brooks College of Health
University of North Florida
Jacksonville, Florida

Jürgen Osterbrink, PhD, DHL(hc), RGN
Professor
Director, Institute for Nursing Sciences
Paracelsus Medizinische Privatuniversität
Salzburg, Austria

Peter Wludyka, PhD
Professor
Director of UNF Center for Research & Consulting in Statistics
Consulting Biostatistician
School of Nursing, Brooks College of Health
University of North Florida
Jacksonville, Florida

CHAPTER 1

Epidemiology and Its Progress

"What we think, we become."
—Gautama Buddha

Kiran Macha
John P. McDonough

OBJECTIVES

- Describe epidemiology and the role played by nurses in this field of health care.
- Discuss epidemiological studies that have led to the discovery of various microorganisms.
- Explain the importance of statistics in epidemiology.
- Compare and contrast the terms "endemic," "epidemic," and "pandemic."
- Evaluate the types of prevention that are most cost-effective for the community.
- Integrate the components of epidemiological research.

EPIDEMIOLOGY AND ITS CHANGING DEFINITIONS

Scholars have defined epidemiology in various ways. Morris (2007) refers to epidemiology as the "study of health and populations in relation to their environment and ways of living." (p. 1165). Frost (1936) considers epidemiology to be "something more than the total of its established facts ..." and to include the "... orderly arrangement of facts into chains of inference which extend more or less beyond the bounds of direct observation." The most acceptable definition is "the study of the distribution and determinants of health related status or events in specified populations" (Last, 1988, p. 159).

Epidemiology is a branch of science that investigates the risk factors responsible for the causation of diseases through retrospective and prospective observations, a complete history of disease, and the frequency of occurrence or transmission mechanisms of disease in populations and explores preventive and therapeutic control measures. A responsible public health approach does not end at the level of investigation and planning for the solution of a particular disease. Public health professionals advance study conclusions and use these data to formulate public health policy and law.

Specific public health organizations in the United States implement public health regulations and policies in focused areas of expertise for the protection and benefit of the public. For example, the U.S. Food and Drug Administration regulates drug and medical equipment safety and usage. The ultimate goal of epidemiology is to eliminate or reduce the influence of risk factors that cause disease and promote health in the community.

In the 19th century most scientists believed the cause of disease was infection (Germ Theory). We now know that diseases are caused not only by infection, but also through other factors related to nutrition, environment, and trauma. Most of the epidemiological studies in the past were observational. Our current ability to integrate technology into studies for the investigation of disease causation has proved to be advantageous in preventing the spread of disease. The availability of advanced microbiological, chemical, and drug testing devices as well as our ability to communicate instantaneously have had a tremendous positive effect on our efforts toward prevention and planning. Both scientific and technological advances have permitted conclusions to be reached in less time while conserving resources and operating in a fully ethical manner.

ROLE OF ADVANCED PRACTICE NURSING IN PUBLIC HEALTH

The concept of public health has a long and distinguished history within the nursing profession. In 1893 Lillian Wald coined the term "public health nursing" to describe the teams of nurses who worked outside the hospital (Reverby, 1993). The main idea behind public health nursing was prevention of diseases for those who did not have access to medical care. Florence Nightingale (**Figure 1-1**) was instrumental in the creation of the position of "district nurse" whose primary responsibility was to promote health and prevent diseases through nursing care and education (Monteiro, 1985). According to the Association of Community Health Nursing Educators (1991), the goals of public health nursing are to promote, protect, and restore the health of populations as well as to prevent disease and disability.

Advanced practice nurses must be familiar with epidemiology, statistics, health promotion, disease surveillance, community health assessment, and current health policy to effectively deal with illness that transcends individuals. Nurses have been participating in providing health education, vaccination programs, and screening procedures in the community as part of primary prevention practices. Specialized educational programs have been encouraged by public health departments and universities across the country to enable nurses to become public health nurses. Although it is clear that all advanced practice nurses do not specialize in public health, it is essential

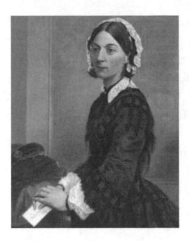

FIGURE 1-1   Florence Nightingale.
Source: National Library of Medicine; URL: http://ihm.nlm.nih.gov/luna/servlet/view/search?q=
B020487; Accessed April 5, 2010.

that all nurses engaged in advanced practice regardless of specialty have a working knowledge of the concepts of the wellness–illness continuum from a community or population perspective.

Nurses have taken a leading role in public health administrative activities and also in responding to public health emergencies. To counter acts of biological terrorism, there is a great need to understand and report the unexplained illness to the responsible agencies (Mondy, Cardenas, & Avila, 2003). Nurses are often the first health professional contacts in such emergencies, when critical information needs to be identified and reported promptly. They have clinical expertise and are also capable of functioning within the community and influencing and evaluating health policy changes. Nurses continue to face challenges as they work to educate the community on specific health needs, mobilize resources, and effectively implement public health policy guidelines. Because nurses have access to families, they often have opportunities to establish beneficial relationships with those in the community. Beyond communicating only with individual patients, exposure to families may be especially useful in identifying such issues as chemical abuse, domestic violence, harmful lifestyles, emotional problems, and other issues arising that may be related to socioeconomic conditions. When health problems are detected early, intervention may be more effective and the expenditure of scarce healthcare resources reduced.

Through the U.S. Department of Health and Human Services Healthy People 2010 project, 10 essential public health services were established for public health professionals to focus effectively on community priorities (see http://www.healthy people.gov/). The leading health indicators in a community are preventable risk factors that are responsible for the top 10 leading causes of death in the United States. Healthy People 2010 also offers resources to health professionals in association with each health indicator.

Nurses play a vital role in public health because of growing opportunities for the expansion of nursing roles in public health, the need for nurses in ongoing community assessment, planning for emergency responses, and community education (Plews, Billingham, & Rowe, 2000).

HISTORICAL EPIDEMIOLOGICAL STUDIES

In 1798 Edward Jenner (**Figure 1-2**) introduced the practice of vaccination. He carried out experiments by inoculating material infected with cowpox virus into incisions made on the upper left arm of human subjects (Baxby, 1999). Jenner described the disease's transmission as making "its progress from the horse to the nipple of the cow, and from cow to the human subject" (Dudgeon, 1980, p. 582). Those who were infected with the cowpox virus also were immune to infection with the smallpox virus. An infected individual previously living with other family members exposed to smallpox showed no signs of infection. This observation of immunity to smallpox in an individual who has been infected with the cowpox virus led Jenner to further experiment, finding that all patients inoculated with cowpox virus were no longer susceptible to smallpox. It was thought that the cowpox virus and smallpox virus shared the same antigens, resulting in cross-immunity.

Although current smallpox vaccines are completely different from Jenner's original vaccination material, the experiments of Jenner and others led to the development of vaccines that have been successful in combating smallpox and many other infectious diseases. Each of these discoveries involved the detailed study of the disease history, identification of mode of transmission, cross-immunity observations, and the courage to experiment.

John Snow (**Figure 1-3**) is considered a pioneer in modern epidemiology. He became famous for his study on the mode of transmission of the deadly cholera disease caused by the bacterium, *Vibrio cholerae*. Cholera is believed to have originated in India, spreading to other countries in Asia over time. The disease was believed to be a deadly, untreatable disease, infecting a larger number of individuals than the plague. Snow hypothesized that cholera was transmitted through water. He created a map

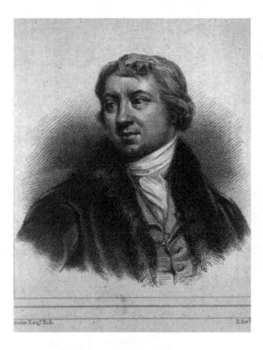

FIGURE 1-2 Edward Jenner.
Source: National Library of Medicine; URL: http://ihm.nlm.nih.gov/luna/servlet/view/search?q=B015691, Accessed April 5, 2010.

showing streets and water pumps to track the incidence of disease. He discovered that people drinking water originating from the upper regions of the Thames River did not suffer as high an incidence of cholera as those who were drinking water from the lower regions contaminated with sewage. He removed the handle of the Broad Street pump located in the lower region of the Thames River, and the number of cases decreased gradually.

Snow was instrumental in the application of epidemiological methods such as identifying common symptoms (case definition), creating maps showing the incidence and prevalence of disease, recording incidence data with time and place, testing water sources, communicating with local politicians, scientifically integrating the chain of events, proposing the mode of transmission of disease (water), and then taking effective public health action by pulling out the handle of the pump that he suspected to be involved in disease transmission (Snow, 1991).

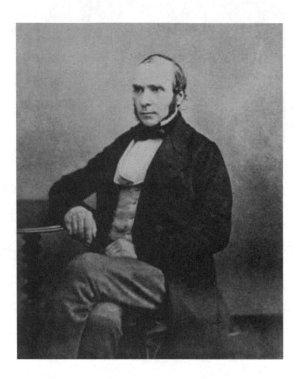

FIGURE 1-3   John Snow.
Source: National Library of Medicine;   URL: http://ihm.nlm.nih.gov/luna/servlet/view/search?q=
B08304; Accessed April 5, 2010.

Sir Richard Doll studied the incidence of cardiac and lung disorders in workers exposed to asbestos. He compared incidences of heart failure, pulmonary tuberculosis, lung cancer, and other respiratory diseases between workers who were exposed to asbestos and those who were not. Doll found that the risk of developing lung cancer was 10 times greater in the population exposed to asbestos as compared with those not exposed and that the incidence of chest malignancies decreased with a decrease in duration of exposure.

Smith and Spalding (1959), working as temporary advisers to the World Health Organization (WHO), investigated an outbreak of paralysis in Morocco. Local health authorities had been efficient in collecting incidence data. The advisers further investigated the outbreak, drawing conclusions from clinical and laboratory evidence, the geographical distribution of cases, socioeconomic factors, and case follow-ups. The clinical signs and symptoms of those affected were muscle weakness and loss of superficial sensations in the hands and legs. The affected were diagnosed with acute peripheral neuritis. Even though some patients suffered from fever and diarrhea, no trace of infection was detected. All routine blood tests and cerebrospinal fluid tests were negative. The role of infection as a cause of the epidemic was ruled out, because the culture of secretions from those affected yielded no growth of any microorganisms. The advisers suspected that poisoning caused the neuritis, which primarily affected those in living in poverty. One affected family suspected the olive oil they used for cooking was responsible for the paralysis. They fed the dog food cooked with the dark oil and then they also ate it. After several days the family and dog developed paralytic signs and other symptoms. On further investigation, the dark olive oil sold in the lower socioeconomic communities was found to be contaminated with orthocresyl phosphate, a synthetic oil used to lubricate jet engines. Similar outbreaks were reported in Switzerland, Germany, and the United States. The prognosis of the disease depended on the extent to which individuals were affected. Those who had spinal damage were permanently disabled; those whose distal muscles only were affected recovered within a year. This study, conducted by Smith and Spalding, shows that epidemiological investigations can take long periods of time and demand teamwork, a background in the clinical sciences, and knowledge of similar past incidents.

Goldberger (**Figure 1-4**), Waring, and Tanner studied the mode of transmission of pellagra, conducting an important classic experimental study in 1914. Pellagra is characterized by diarrhea, dermatitis, dementia, psychomotor disturbances, and sensitivity to light and can be fatal. Pellagra was initially believed to be a communicable disease because of the high incidence and prevalence rates noted in the United States. Despite treatment, there was no improvement in disease symptomology. The growing spread of this disease was identified as a public health emergency, with quarantine and isolation implemented for those affected or exposed. However, isolation and quarantine of such a large number of individuals began to drain public health resources, also impacting the nation's economic productivity.

U.S. Public Health Service officials conducted a study at both an orphanage and a sanatorium to better understand the disease and identify prevention strategies. The subjects' diets were slightly modified to replace grits (maize or corn) with protein products such as milk and meat. Within a year researchers noticed that the signs and symptoms associated with pellagra disappeared completely. The subjects were followed for second and third year, with the disease recurring only in those who reverted

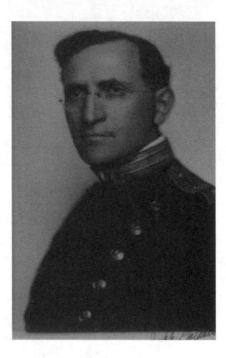

FIGURE 1-4   Joseph Goldberger.
Source: National Library of Medicine; URL: http://ihm.nlm.nih.gov/luna/servlet/view/search?q=
B012870; Accessed April 5, 2010.

to eating corn products. In those who continued to consume a diet high in protein, pellagra was not noted again. Sanitation, isolation, and other preventive measures did not help the subjects (Laguna & Carpenter, 1951).

In this example, successful investigations were carried out during the peak incidence of a disease in a situation where public health action was necessary to conserve public health resources, resulting in identification of the cause and transmission of disease that led to a decrease in mortality and morbidity. Other lessons learned were that dietary deficiencies can result in disease and that a balanced diet is essential to good health.

The summer is a perfect time in New York for mosquitoes to breed and spread disease. In 1946 an outbreak of an unclassified disease was reported in epidemic numbers, with both the New York City Department of Health and the U.S. Public Health Service investigating (Greenberg, 1947). The causative agent was unknown, but signs and symptoms were similar to chickenpox (fever, chills, sweats, backache, headache, and a maculopapular and papulovesicular rash). A black eschar (necrotic tissue) was also noted at the site of a bite and was assumed to be due to mites. An in-depth investigation was carried out in the apartment where the outbreak was believed to occur in an attempt to determine the cause of the disease. Using a step-by-step approach, clinicians, epidemiologists, and laboratory personnel were together able to solve the mystery after 3 months. Blood samples from the infected patients were collected and tested. Blood from mice was tested and found to contain an antigen similar to that found in human blood samples. Mites (*Allodermanyssus sanguineus*) were detected as ectoparasites on the rodents. Even though *Culex pipiens* mosquitoes were found in the basement of the apartment, laboratory investigations ruled out their involvement in the disease's transmission. Mice (*Mus musculus*) were surviving on garbage left in the incinerator. The signs and symptoms of the disease were grouped under "rickettsial pox" with the identified strain named *Rickettsia akari* based on the unique complement-fixation reactions of the serum antigens. This investigation involved keen exploration of the environment; the collection and laboratory testing of blood samples from humans, mites, mosquitoes, and rodents; and extraordinary teamwork.

Clarke and Anderson (1979) worked to identify whether the Papanicolaou (Pap) smear was an effective screening procedure for invasive cervical cancer. They conducted a case-control study in the city of Toronto. Interviewing the subjects helped identify the risk factors for cervical cancer. Higher education, higher age, lower annual income, and unemployment contributed to higher relative risk of cervical cancer in those who failed to have a Pap smear. Pap smear was considered to be less effective in those with adenocarcinoma because it arises from the mucous glands located in the endocervix in contrast to the squamous cell carcinoma that occurs at the squamocolumnar junction. The researchers concluded that "the Pap smear itself has no preventive value, and there must be appropriate follow-up and treatment of abnormal smears."

In 1976 an outbreak occurred as a result of an unknown agent that resulted in the hospitalization of 147 patients and 29 deaths. Patients all had signs and symptoms of pneumonia and a common history of attending the American Legion Convention at a Philadelphia hotel. During the epidemiological investigation, clinical, epidemiological, and laboratory criteria were clearly defined to identify the place, person, and time factors and cause of the disease. Clinical criteria included cough, fever, and signs of pneumonia in chest x-rays. Epidemiological criteria included patient attendance at the American Legion Convention in the period from July 21 to 24, 1976, in Philadelphia. A person was considered seropositive if he or she had a titer of 1:128 or greater by indirect fluorescent antibody assay used to detect unknown gram-negative microorganisms. The well-defined criteria, preparation of a quality survey questionnaire, interviewing skills, the ability to conduct a multistate study, systematic tracking of data, microbiological assistance, and resources for autopsy led to the study's successful conclusions. The newly identified pathogen was named *Legionella pneumophila*, with the signs and symptoms caused by it grouped under "Legionnaires' disease." Although the source was not identified, it was concluded that the pathogen was airborne and that air conditioners contributed to its spread. This is typical of an epidemiological investigation that led to the discovery of a previously unknown pathogen (Fraser et al., 1977).

Global efforts were carried out to eradicate smallpox, including mass vaccination campaigns conducted on a large scale in numerous countries. WHO experts initially believed the most effective way to eradicate smallpox was mass vaccination. The experts focused least on an epidemiological approach such as interrupting the transmission of the virus. Known to kill 400,000 Europeans a year in the 18th century, smallpox is transmitted by an airborne virus (Behbehani, 1983). Smallpox spreads slowly, with a lower transmission rate and incidence during September. In contrast, high incidence was noted in the month of April, but the seasonal relationship of virus incidence could not be explained.

An epidemiological approach called "eradication escalation" was implemented in 20 countries within west and central Africa during September 1968, a low incidence period. In this effort, four principal methods were used: (1) active surveillance, (2) outbreak investigation, (3) outbreak control, and (4) rapid communication of disease intelligence. Active surveillance included identification of the cases that were not otherwise reported through a disease-reporting system and through outreach involving newspapers, radio, and public alerting systems.

Outbreaks were actively investigated and efforts were made to identify and describe such events. The close contacts of those affected were vaccinated, and various epidemiological measures were taken to interrupt transmission of the virus. Incidence data from several locations within Africa were reported to the Centers for Disease Control and Prevention (CDC) in the United States. Weekly update from CDC was circulated to all active surveillance sites in Africa so that rapid prevention measures could be taken. With the same staff involved in both the active surveillance and mass vaccination programs, the effect of these combined actions had a positive impact on disease transmission. The incidence rate not only decreased drastically, but the seasonal variation also decreased, with the WHO certifying the eradication of smallpox in 1980 (WHO, 2010b). The effects of these epidemiological control efforts on a mass scale are noted in "West and Central Africa Small Pox Eradication Program" (Foege, Millar, & Lane, 1971).

Even with an appropriate plan, longitudinal epidemiological studies pose additional challenges for the researcher. These studies typically involve many participants, effective distribution of resources, a lengthy duration of time, implementation phase obstacles, extensive data collection, the training of interviewers, follow-up, participant intervention compliance, and participant access to study locations.

One such study in the 1940s involved an investigation of the effect of vitamin supplementation in the diet of pregnant women on children's intelligence (Harrell, Woodyard, & Gates, 1956). The study was conducted at two maternity clinics, one in Norfolk, Virginia, and one in Leslie County, Kentucky. The characteristics of the women attending these clinics were the same. Participants were divided into four groups, with each group receiving a dietary supplement (group A, 200 mg ascorbic acid; group B, 2 mg thiamine, 4 mg riboflavin, 20 mg niacin amide, and 15 mg iron; group C, placebo; and group D, 2 mg thiamine). The study started with 1,200 pregnant women in each clinic. By the end of the study, attrition reduced the sample size of participating women to almost half, and the numbers of children of participants who were tested for their intelligence had also declined. (The Terman-Merrill Revised Stanford-Binet Scale for 3 and 4 year olds was used to test intelligence levels.) Results showed that the intelligence level of participating 3- and 4-year-old children in Norfolk and Leslie County was higher than those of the placebo group. The intelligence level of children in Leslie County was found to be higher than that of children in Norfolk, with the higher intelligence attributed to the diets of pregnant women who had taken a combination of vitamins such as thiamine, riboflavin, ascorbic acid, and iron (mineral) as compared with women who had taken only thiamine or ascorbic acid. This study, conducted between 1945 and 1948, passed through many hurdles, with a high attrition rate for participants and their children, yet the success of the research was evident.

The effects of nuclear radiation on the human body were not well known before World War II. Even though animal studies were done to study the side effects of nuclear radiation, the difference in genetic structure makes comparison highly complicated. Moreover, studies have also shown that the outcomes of radiation differ depending on the age of the individual affected. The cities of Hiroshima and Nagasaki were destroyed with nuclear bombs at the end of World War II without considering the outcomes of such actions.

The Atomic Bomb Casualty Commission was established in the United States to monitor the effects of nuclear radiation on the survivors of Hiroshima and Nagasaki after survivors of the bombing reported a high incidence of leukemia (Lindee, 1994). The Commission's observations were based on incidence data for leukemia by age, distance of exposure, and type of leukemia. High leukemia incidence was reported near the nuclear bombing site, and as the distance from the bomb site increased, the incidence decreased. A higher incidence of acute leukemia was detected in victims younger than age 30 years, and chronic leukemia appeared at a young age in the individuals near the bombing site (<1,500 meters). Granulocytic leukemia was most common in the chronic leukemia group. The incidence rate of both acute and chronic leukemia decreased with time (Bizzozero, Johnson, & Ciocco, 1966). These observations have allowed us to understand the effects of nuclear radiation and the extent of its influence over time.

DISEASE TRANSMISSION DYNAMICS

Based on the mode of transmission, diseases are classified as communicable or non-communicable diseases. Communicable diseases are transmitted from human to animal, animal to animal, animal to human, and vice versa. The evolution of a microorganism to the degree that it can survive in a different species or genetic environment is a sign of an emergency. Pathogens can be directly transmitted through inhalation or wounds and can be indirectly transmitted when a vector is involved in the transmission process. Some pathogens produce free-living infective stages, and when taken up by a susceptible host, they further grow using the host's resources. The results of studies involving the identification of mode of transmission of a disease can significantly impact the action plan to contain the spread of disease. Such studies not only predict the probable response of the disease to control efforts but can also lead to further research on what happens when a pathogen is introduced in a system in which it does not currently exist.

Social and environmental factors affect the transmission dynamics of a disease (Weiss, 2004). Incidences of many diseases in the past were controlled through extensive public health initiatives, the use of antibiotics and vaccinations, insecticides targeting vectors, and improved surveillance. With globalization, climate changes, dietary preferences, deforestation, political decisions, misuse of and microbial resistance to antibiotics, and conflicts that disrupt a nation's economy influence the emergence and reemergence of disease. Other factors affecting transmission include modern technology, research on biological material, increasing nuclear radiation, and harmful gas emissions. Recently, the human immunodeficiency virus (HIV), Legionnaires' disease, swine flu (H_1N_1), and many other diseases have been newly discovered because of the availability of technology and planned epidemiological research studies. The containment of such diseases calls for collective human commitment and public health action.

The mode of transmission of a disease is dynamic, and patterns can change with time. Avian influenza initially was thought to be restricted to birds, and fears were expressed that it may spread to humans. Studies revealed that the glycoprotein virus receptor (Hemagglutinin) carried by the avian influenza virus attaches to sialic acid alpha-2,3-galactose receptors present on the alveolar cells in contrast to sialic acid alpha-2,6-galactose receptors present on the bronchial epithelial cells (Shinya & Kawaoka, 2006). The location of receptors makes it difficult for the avian influenza virus to spread from human to human. The human influenza virus attaches to sialic acid alpha-2,3-galactose receptors, which are present on bronchi and alveolar type II epithelial cells, thus easily transmitted through respiratory channels (Ma, 2007; Smith & Bazini-Barakat, 2003). Successful interspecies transmission and adaptation to a new genetic environment is possible through antigenic drift and antigenic shift processes. The 2009 pandemic swine flu has succeeded in this interspecies transmission.

Changing Patterns of Disease Incidence

WHO disease incidence data collected across the world are analyzed based on income. In high-income countries, coronary heart disease is the leading cause of death followed by cerebrovascular diseases, lung cancers, and lower respiratory infections (Mokdad, Marks, Stroup, & Gerberding, 2004) (**Table 1-1**). In contrast, infections cause the most deaths in low-income countries. This disparity is not just a result of income differentials but also many other factors. In the United States modifiable behavioral factors, such as tobacco smoking, physical inactivity, alcohol and drug use, unsafe sexual practices, use of firearms, and unsafe motor vehicle driving practices, contribute greatly to higher disease incidence rates among low socioeconomic status populations (Jemal, Ward, Hao, & Thun, 2005). Federal and state governments in the United States offer educational intervention programs to encourage behavior change to conserve the nation's health resources. WHO conducts preventive, educational, and immunization programs in developing countries to reduce mortality caused by infectious disease (WHO, 2010a).

Health Data Collection and Interpretation

John Graunt is considered the first epidemiologist (Rothman, 1996). In the 17th century he published a book, entitled *Natural and Political Observations Mentioned in a Following Index, and Made upon the Bills of Mortality* (Graunt, 1665), and also produced a weekly report, *Bills of Mortality*. He first described the relationship between population size and disease and was able to provide an estimate of the population of the city

Table 1-1   Leading Causes of Death in the United States in 2000

Cause of Death	No. of Deaths	Death Rate per 100,000 Population
Heart disease	710,760	258.2
Malignant neoplasm	553,091	200.9
Cerebrovascular disease	167,661	60.9
Chronic lower respiratory tract disease	122,009	44.3
Unintentional injuries	97,900	35.6
Diabetes mellitus	69,301	25.2
Influenza and pneumonia	65,313	23.7
Alzheimer disease	49,558	18
Nephritis, nephritic syndrome, and nephrosis	37,251	13.5
Septicemia	31,224	11.3
Other	499,283	181.4
Total	2,403,351	873.1

Source: Mokdad, A. H., Marks, J. S., Stroup, D. F., & Gerberding, J. L. (2004). Actual causes of death in the United States, 2000. Journal of the American Medical Association, 291(10), 1238–1245.

of London. William Farr and Rowe Edmonds developed the idea of vital statistics, and, using Graunt's data, they interpreted the health and welfare of the people (Eyler, 2002; Farr, 1852). In recent years the Framingham heart study, the community intervention trials of fluoride supplementation in water, and the Surgeon General's report on smoking and health have been recognized for their contributions, signifying the importance of health statistics.

PUBLIC HEALTH SURVEILLANCE

If a foreign army had landed on the coast of England, seized all the seaports, . . . ravaged the population through the summer and . . . in the year it held possession of the country slain fifty-three thousand two hundred and ninety-three men, women and children, . . . the task of registering the dead would be inexpressibly painful; and the pain is not greatly diminished by the circumstance that in the calamity to be described the minister of destruction was a pestilence.
—William Farr (**Figure 1-5**)

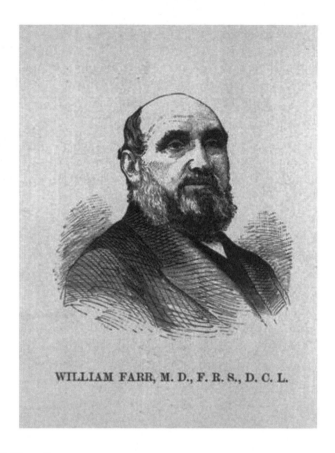

FIGURE 1-5   William Farr.
Source: National Library of Medicine; URL: http://ihm.nlm.nih.gov/luna/servlet/view/search?q= B06814; Accessed April 5, 2010.

Langmuir (1963) defined surveillance in its early days as "close observation of persons exposed to a communicable disease to detect early symptoms and institute prompt isolation and control measures." CDC has defined public health surveillance as "ongoing, systematic collection, analysis, and interpretation of data that is then disseminated to those responsible for preventing diseases and other health conditions." The monitoring of health status in the community had its beginnings in Italy, where isolation and quarantine were used as a means to control the spread of infectious diseases (Gensini, 2004). In 1935 the first national health survey was conducted in the United States. The establishment of the Epidemiological Surveillance Unit at WHO headquarters, Geneva, initiated global public health surveillance efforts (Declich & Carter, 1994). The main objectives of surveillance activity include detecting changes in the patterns of the disease across the world, recording the natural history and epidemiology of a disease (essential in formulating a control action plan), and providing information to healthcare professionals. Health data are collected by various methods.

Passive surveillance includes data collection through various data notification systems established by health departments as part of mandatory health law. Hospitals, physicians, and laboratories report these data to local health departments. The CDC issues yearly updates on notifiable diseases, with all resource agencies reporting on either case diagnosis or suspicion.

Active surveillance includes actively searching for cases and inquiring directly with individuals for signs and symptoms during epidemics or in a situation where an epidemic is anticipated. Surveys are conducted to collect these types of data in the community. The collected data are then analyzed and interpreted, with results disseminated to professionals so that prompt action can be taken. Because infectious diseases do not recognize any political border, an effective integrated and global public health surveillance system is needed to counteract the potential evolution of an endemic to an epidemic in this current world of globalization.

Epidemiological Triangle

Epidemiological studies on infectious diseases have helped epidemiologists identify the core factors involved in the disease process. Agent, host, and environment (as well as time) are most important in a disease's transmission (**Figure 1-6**). The agent is a microorganism that has the ability to cause disease. The host is generally either a human or animal infected by the agent. The agent survives on the resources of the host or is attacked by the host's immune system. Environmental factors such as air, water, soil, chemicals, diet, and genetics influence the disease transmission process. The time taken for the appearance of signs and symptoms caused by an agent in the host is the *incubation period*. The study of the epidemiological triad components of a disease helps the epidemiologist plan for an effective intervention to interrupt the transmission process and stop further evolution of the disease.

Epidemic

An epidemic is defined as the "occurrence in a community or region of cases of an illness, specified health behavior, or other health related events clearly in excess of

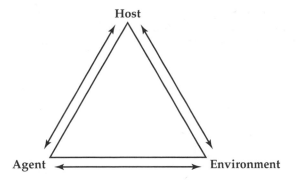

FIGURE 1-6   Epidemiological triangle.

normal expectancy; the community or region, and the time period in which cases occur, are specified precisely" (WHO). Epidemics are limited in space and time. Gradually they end and incidence rates decline with time because of recovery, secondary complications, or death. Immunity plays an important role in the recovery process. If there is only a minor change in the antigen, the exposed and unaffected may be vaccinated, the infected may be treated with drugs, drug prophylaxis can be offered to the exposed, and secondary complications arising as a result of the disease can be addressed. For example, individuals infected with influenza virus generally present with upper respiratory tract signs and symptoms such as sneezing and coughing and constitutional symptoms including fever, muscle aches, and fatigue. Acute respiratory distress syndrome can result, and the patient may die. Effective healthcare communication and timely action can stop the progression of disease, saving thousands of lives.

Epidemic Curve

The graphic representation of new cases originating because of the rapid transmission of a disease in an area during an interval of time is called an epidemic curve, or epicurve. Assimilating data to produce this graphic is time consuming on the part of epidemiologists. When retrospectively analyzed, the curve provides valuable information. For example, the incubation period of a disease can be calculated if the time of exposure is approximately known. The planning of responses to epidemics depends on the magnitude of the situation and may be associated with the number of cases that can be tracked on the graph. Looking at the pattern of the curve, one may be able to determine whether individuals were exposed to the source at one time or continuously

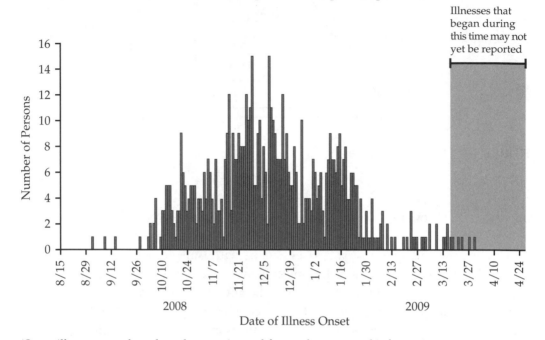

*Some illness onset dates have been estimated from other reported information

FIGURE 1-7   Salmonella outbreak.
Source: From Centers for Disease Control and Prevention. Retrieved March 21, 2010, from http://www.cdc.gov/salmonella/typhimurium/epi_curve.html

exposed or whether the pathogen was transmitted from person to person or individuals were intermittently exposed. The CDC offers Epi Info software for practice and understanding at its website (see http://www.cdc.gov/epiinfo/downloads.htm). **Figure 1-7** is an example of an epidemic curve.

Pandemic

A pandemic is an epidemic where the incidence of disease extends to a whole country or large part of the world. Pandemics are generally the result of the antigenic shift process in which new antigens are produced by the microorganism (Cinti, 2005). It can take several weeks for the immune system to develop a primary response to such situations. During this period the severity of complications in such infected populations will be worse. The key public health response to such pandemic challenges includes the development of a vaccine, which can also take some time. The strategies adopted in an epidemic are different from that of pandemics because vaccines are not readily available. Chemoprophylaxis and infection control practices such as hand washing, isolation, and quarantine are the immediate measures taken. When the vaccine is made available, mass vaccination is preferred. A strong political commitment is needed for such public health actions to meet the challenge. Long-term commitment and strategy depend on the information gathered from public health surveillance (Osterholm, 2005).

Endemic Disease

A disease that is prevalent in a population in a certain area for a long period of time is defined as an endemic. The risk factors for endemic diseases can include lack of personal hygiene, malnutrition, poor sanitation, contaminated water or food, unclean surroundings, low socioeconomic status, climatic conditions, the presence of other diseases, and an unresponsive political climate.

Herd Immunity

The inherent or acquired immune resistance offered by populations to the prevalence of a disease in a community is referred to as herd immunity. Vaccinations of populations play an important role in the development of immunological barriers toward the entry of a disease into the community (John, 2000; Paul, 2004). This immune resistance effectively reduces the efficiency of the microbe to transmit from person to person. Generally, 83% to 94% of the population needs to be vaccinated to achieve herd immunity to a given disease. Immune levels also depend on the virulence of the disease. The protection offered by herd immunity to those unimmunized because of the break in transmission process is called herd protection. Herd immunity and herd protection are two different terms. The oral polio vaccine offers both herd immunity and herd protection (because live virus is excreted in stools and can spread in the community), whereas the inactivated polio vaccine offers only herd protection. Tetanus vaccination does not provide any additional benefits to the unimmunized.

PREVENTION

"Prevention is better than cure."
—Desiderius Erasmus

When medical science was developing, there was no treatment to limit the spread of infectious diseases, and prevention was an effective tool. In the modern world we tend to believe we have gained relative dominance over infectious diseases with the discovery of antibiotics. However, the prevalence of noncommunicable diseases in developed countries is higher than the prevalence of infectious diseases. The only cost-effective way to reduce the incidence of diseases in the community is prevention. Prevention is divided into three levels.

1. *Primary prevention:* Actions taken to promote one's health that prevent disease and disability in an individual are referred to as primary prevention. Examples of primary prevention include vaccinations, the addition of fluoride to water and toothpaste, the use of a seat belt to prevent accident injuries, exercise, and folic acid supplementation in pregnancy.
2. *Secondary prevention:* Actions leading to the early identification, diagnosis, and treatment of a disease to limit the consequences of such exposure and to interfere with disease transmission are referred to as secondary prevention. Examples include screening procedures such as the Pap smear for cervical cancer detection, sigmoidoscopy for detecting colon cancer, blood pressure and serum cholesterol level measurements to prevent coronary heart disease, and oral intake of calcium supplements for those at risk of osteoporosis.
3. *Tertiary prevention:* Actions that promote activities of daily living to limit the progression of disease and complications in people suffering from both communicable and noncommunicable diseases are referred to as tertiary prevention. Rehabilitation is a primary approach comprising this level of prevention. Examples include avoidance of allergens in asthmatic patients; eye, renal, and foot screening procedures for diabetics; and treatments to reduce the severity of disease.

Quarantine and Isolation

In many situations involving public health emergencies, quarantine and isolation have been viewed as the immediate solutions to contain a disease. Quarantine and isolation are two different terms. The word *quarante* means 40 in Italian. During the days of the plague, ships were forced to anchor for 40 days at the port of Venice. "Quarantine" means physical separation of healthy individuals who have been exposed to a contagious disease. "Isolation" is defined as segregation and confinement of infected individuals from others who are known to be suffering from disease. Cholera, the plague, and other diseases that caused deaths on a large scale led to the idea of such preventive action. These actions can effectively interrupt the disease transmission chain, also offering the opportunity to treat infected individuals. From the information obtained from quarantined individuals, contact tracing can also be initiated. In Cuba from 1986 to 1994, HIV-positive individuals were quarantined. Quarantine does not work to reduce the incidence of a disease not transmitted through regular contact.

Not so long ago, sanatoria were set up for patients with tuberculosis, known as the "great white plague." The number of sanatoria declined with time as the incidence of tuberculosis declined. However, because of the reemergence of other diseases, the need for special facilities dedicated to housing those infected with one disease is growing. In Canada during the epidemic period of severe acute respiratory syndrome (aka SARS), almost 14,000 individuals were isolated. Such isolations can cause frustration in healthcare workers and also in quarantined individuals, restricting the movement of an individual, affecting one's employment status, and potentially imposing a psychosocial burden on society (Cava, 2005). To deal with such issues, strategies for emotional responses should be designed. Isolation can, however, save money and lives.

Epidemiological Research

Once the need for research on a topic has been identified, epidemiological research involves understanding the concepts of epidemiology, planning an appropriate study design, data collection, statistical analysis, and interpretation of findings toward conclusions to improve health. A study can be planned with or without human participants. Data reported by hospitals and laboratories to health departments can also be used. Genetic and molecular tools have increased the chances of identifying the source of disease in less time. The research techniques and lessons learned in the research of infectious diseases have been applied most recently to studying chronic diseases. An interdisciplinary collaboration is almost always essential for the completion of a successful study. Consent, ethics, and data privacy are other important components to consider in epidemiological research.

Outbreak Investigation

An unexpected rise in the number of cases of a particular identified or unidentified disease alerts public health officials to respond to the situation through focused investigation. Public health departments record patterns of diseases all year as part of their surveillance. Epidemiological investigations conducted to identify the causes of outbreak have led to the discovery of many new microorganisms. Epidemiological studies on influenza have helped us to understand whether or not vaccination programs are effective. Designated preventive measures to contain a disease need to be reviewed continuously because of the changing patterns of some diseases. The outcomes of such outbreak investigations should be communicated to both the public and healthcare professionals throughout the world.

Because of rising fears of pandemics among healthcare professionals, the incidences of cases are sometimes over-reported. The epidemiologist role in such situations is a difficult one, because he or she has to collaborate with other teams to identify the most common symptoms that the disease presents. Laboratory, genetic, and molecular tools help to identify the disease-causing organism from various specimens obtained from infected individuals. The accurate description of cases and identification of a specific diagnostic tool can result in confirmation of the disease. Surveys can then be designed to gather information from infected and exposed individuals. These data are used to construct an epidemic curve from which the incubation period can be calculated. Descriptive data can define certain characteristics of the disease (e.g., age group and gender affected). The patterns of exposure to the source (continuous, propagated, or intermittent) can be identified. After preliminary investigation, the next step is to identify the source and transmission methods of the disease. A hypothesis is then constructed and tested in the field by designing an appropriate study (case-control, cohort, or survey study) to identify the source of infection. An environmental investigation is also an important component to identify disease transmission pathways. (Outbreak investigation involves the epidemiological triad: the study of host, agent, and environment.) Preventive and therapeutic measures are designed to treat infected individuals and also to break the transmission pathways. The information is disseminated to healthcare professionals, and diagnostic tools are made available on a large scale. Prevention measures involving vaccination involve complex research studies and surveillance for any adverse effects of the vaccination.

After disease numbers are controlled, an effective public health surveillance system should be placed into action to monitor the situation. The success of an outbreak investigation lies in effective communication. The information is not only shared with public health professionals but is also communicated to the public through the media.

KEY POINTS

- Nurses play an important role in the field of epidemiology with their background in nursing science as well as skills for working in the community. With additional training on epidemiological concepts, nurses can be easily integrated into epidemiological fields—an opportunity that can expand the limits of their profession.

- Epidemiology is a science that deals with the determinants of health. Health data are collected from various sources such as hospitals, laboratories, and mandatory reporting systems in the community.

- Methods for gathering and interpreting health data were first attempted in London, England. Past endeavors have led to present-day data collection systems, monitoring systems, surveillance systems, and new roles for biostatisticians. Graduate nursing education programs in the United States have integrated a statistics component into their curricula and have encouraged nurses to learn and interpret health data. These skills enable nurses to conduct research studies and to interpret data and come to conclusions to plan further actions.

- John Snow and other epidemiologists who conducted historical studies laid foundations for contemporary epidemiological studies and research. The creation of maps, basic statistics, accurate event recordings, and retrospective event analyses were the simple steps followed. Current studies involve larger populations with multiple variables and use of advanced genetic and molecular tools for accurate diagnoses.

- Epidemiological concepts used for the study of infectious diseases are now applied to chronic diseases. Large-scale studies on chronic diseases have led to the identification of risk factors that form the basis of comprehensive screening and preventive measures implemented by health agencies worldwide. Nurses are involved in vaccination and other prevention programs in several countries.

- The epidemiological triad explains the transmission pathway of a communicable disease involving an infectious organism and noncommunicable diseases. By understanding how the host, agent, and environment are involved in the disease process, epidemiologists can design strategies to break the links involved in transmission pathways. Noncommunicable disease risk factors are communicated to the public, with responsibility for adopting behavioral change resting with the individual. The knowledge and skills of nurses can be used in this communication process toward the reduction of risk factors in a community.

- The importance of primary prevention is growing in the community because it promotes health and conserves healthcare resources. A nurse's participation is encouraged in such preventive actions.
- The incubation period for an infectious disease is an important piece of information that determines the time limit for epidemiologists in responding to an outbreak situation.
- The epidemic curve provides incubation period information and can help us determine the source of infection and patterns of exposure.
- Deaths in developed countries are primarily associated with noncommunicable diseases, whereas in developing countries communicable diseases are responsible for most deaths. The resurgence/reemergence of infectious diseases is a major concern because we are less aware of the new behavior of a changing microorganism.

CRITICAL QUESTIONS

1. What is the importance of epidemiology in the field of science?
2. Describe the role of nursing in the field of epidemiology.
3. Describe lessons learned from select historical epidemiological studies.
4. Describe the importance of statistics in epidemiology.
5. How can prevention activities lessen the burden of disease in communities?
6. Discuss the ethical, psychosocial, and other issues involved in isolation and quarantine.
7. Describe the steps involved in planning an epidemiological research study.
8. Describe the steps involved in the management of an outbreak situation and, by using Web resources, describe an outbreak investigation conducted by the CDC.

REFERENCES

Association of Community Health Nursing Educators. (1991). *Essentials of master's level nursing education for advanced community health nursing practice*. Louisville, KY: Author.

Baxby, D. (1999). Edward Jenner's inquiry: A bicentenary analysis. *Vaccine, 17*(4), 301.

Behbehani, A. M. (1983). The smallpox story: Life and death of an old disease. *Microbiology Review, 47*(4), 455–509.

Bizzozero, O. J., Johnson, G. K., & Ciocco, A. (1966). Radiation-related leukemia in Hiroshima and Nagasaki, 1946–1964. *New England Journal of Medicine, 274*(20), 1095, 1101.

Cava, M. A. (2005). The experience of quarantine for individuals affected by SARS in Toronto. *Public Health Nursing, 22*(5), 398.

Cinti, S. (2005). Pandemic influenza: Are we ready? *Disaster Management & Response, 3*(3), 61–67.

Clarke, E. A., & Anderson, T. W. (1979). Does screening by "pap" smears help prevent cervical cancer? A case-control study. *Lancet, 2*(8132), 1–4.

Declich, S., & Carter, A. O. (1994). Public health surveillance: Historical origins, methods and evaluation. *Bulletin of the World Health Organization, 72*(2), 285.

Dudgeon, J. A. (1980). Immunization in times ancient and modern. *Journal of the Royal Society of Medicine, 73*(8), 581–586.

Eyler, J. J. M. (2002). Constructing vital statistics: Thomas Rowe Edmonds and William Farr, 1835–1845. *Sozial-Und Präventivmedizin, 47*(1), 6–13.

Farr, W. W. (1852). Influence of elevation on the fatality of cholera. *Journal of the Statistical Society of London, 15*(2), 155.

Foege, H. W., Millar, D. J., & Lane, M. J. (1971). Selective epidemiologic control in smallpox eradication. *American Journal of Epidemiology, 94*(1), 311–315.

Fraser, D. W., Tsai, T. R., Orenstein, W., Parkin, W. E., Beecham, H. J., Sharrar, R. G., et al. (1977). Legionnaires' disease: Description of an epidemic of pneumonia. *New England Journal of Medicine, 297*(22), 1189–1197.

Frost, W. H. (1936). Introduction. In J. Snow (Ed.), *Snow on cholera* (reprint, pp. 11–39). New York: The Commonwealth Fund.

Gensini, G. G. F. (2004). The concept of quarantine in history: From plague to SARS. *Journal of Infection, 49*(4), 257–261.

Graunt, J. (1665). *Natural and political observations mentioned in a following index, and made upon the bills of mortality.* London: Martyn & Allestry.

Greenberg, M. (1947). Rickettsial pox—a newly recognized rickettsial disease. *American Journal of Public Health and the Nation's Health, 37*(7), 860.

Harrell, R. F., Woodyard, E. R., & Gates, A. I. (1956). The influence of vitamin supplementation of the diets of pregnant and lactating women on the intelligence of their offspring. *Metabolism, 5,* 555–562.

Jemal, A., Ward, E., Hao, Y., & Thun, M. (2005). Trends in the leading causes of death in the United States, 1970–2002. *Journal of the American Medical Association, 294*(10), 1255–1259.

John, T. T. J. (2000). Herd immunity and herd effect: New insights and definitions. *European Journal of Epidemiology, 16*(7), 601–606.

Laguna, J., & Carpenter, K. J. (1951). Raw versus processed corn in niacin-deficient diets. *Journal of Nutrition, 45*(1), 21–28.

Langmuir, A. D. (1963). The surveillance of communicable diseases of national importance. *New England Journal of Medicine, 268,* 182–192.

Last, J. M. (1988). What is "clinical epidemiology"? *Journal of Public Health Policy, 9,* 159–163.

Lindee, M. S. (1994). *Suffering made real: American science and the survivors at Hiroshima.* Chicago: University of Chicago Press.

Ma, W. W. (2007). Identification of H2N3 influenza A viruses from swine in the United States. *Proceedings of the National Academy of Sciences of the United States of America, 104*(52), 20949–20954.

Mokdad, A. H., Marks, J. S., Stroup, D. F., & Gerberding, J. L. (2004). Actual causes of death in the United States, 2000. *Journal of the American Medical Association, 291*(10), 1238–1245.

Mondy, C., Cardenas, D., & Avila, M. (2003). The role of an advanced practice public health nurse in bioterrorism preparedness. *Public Health Nursing, 20*(6), 422–431.

Monteiro, L. L. A. (1985). Florence Nightingale on public health nursing. *American Journal of Public Health, 75*(2), 181–186.

Morris, J. N. (2007). Uses of epidemiology. *International Journal of Epidemiology, 36*(6), 1165–1172.

Osterholm, M. M. T. (2005). Preparing for the next pandemic. *New England Journal of Medicine, 352*(18), 1839–1842.

Paul, Y. Y. (2004). Herd immunity and herd protection. *Vaccine, 22*(3–4), 301–302.

Plews, C., Billingham, K., & Rowe, A. (2000). Public health nursing: Barriers and opportunities. *Health & Social Care in the Community, 8*(2), 138–146.

Reverby, S. M. (1993). From Lillian Wald to Hillary Rodham Clinton: What will happen to public health nursing? *American Journal of Public Health, 83*(12), 1662.

Rothman, K. J. (1996). Lessons from John Graunt. *Lancet, 347*(8993), 37–39.

Shinya, K., & Kawaoka, Y. (2006). Influenza virus receptors in the human airway. *Uirusu Journal of Virology, 56*(1), 85–89.

Smith, H. V., & Spalding, J. M. (1959). Outbreak of paralysis in Morocco due to ortho-cresyl phosphate poisoning. *Lancet, 2*(7110), 1019–1021.

Smith, K., & Bazini-Barakat, N. (2003). A public health nursing practice model: Melding public health principles with the nursing process. *Public Health Nursing, 20*(1), 42–48.

Snow, J. (1991). On the mode of communication of cholera. 1855. [Sobre el modo detransmision del colera.] *Salud Publica De Mexico, 33*(2), 194–201.

Weiss, R. A. (2004). Social and environmental risk factors in the emergence of infectious diseases. *Nature Medicine, 10*(12), 70.

World Health Organization (WHO). (2010a). Fact sheet: The 10 leading causes of death by income group, 2004. Retrieved from http://www.who.int/mediacentre/factsheets/fs310_2008.pdf

World Health Organization (WHO). (2010b). Fact sheet: Smallpox. Retrieved from http://www.who.int/mediacentre/factsheets/smallpox/en

CHAPTER 2

Role of Epidemiology and Statistics in Advanced Nursing Practice

"Chance favors prepared minds."
—Louis Pasteur

Peter Wludyka

OBJECTIVES

- After completing this chapter the reader will understand that statistical methods and ideas as well as practical probability are essential to understanding epidemiology and its role in advanced nursing practice.
- The overall objective of the chapter is to familiarize the reader with the key elements of statistics (and statistical inference) including the role of level of measurement; methods for presenting, summarizing, and analyzing interval or categorical data; estimation; hypothesis testing; and modeling.
- The key epidemiological ideas of incidence and prevalence are defined, the distinction between rates and proportions is clearly made, and inferential methods associated with estimation of these parameters are presented.
- Statistical methods frequently used for examining the relationship between exposure and disease incidence, including survival analysis, the analysis of two by two tables, and regression modeling, are also discussed.

EASILY ACCESSIBLE RESOURCES IN EPIDEMIOLOGY AND STATISTICS

Many of the statistical ideas and methods in this chapter are discussed in more detail in van Bell, Fisher, Heagerty, and Lumley (2004). An excellent nonmathematical introduction to epidemiology can be found in Rothman (2002). For a more mathematical treatment of the statistical analysis of epidemiological data, Selvin (2004) is a solid resource. A comprehensive treatment of the analysis of means (ANOM) can be found in Nelson, Wludyka, and Copeland (2005). ANOM is a useful approach for analyzing stratified incidence (both proportions and rates) and prevalence data. Both SAS® and

PASW (formerly SPSS) were used to analyze data for examples in this chapter, and output (sometimes with the format modified) from these statistical packages appears throughout. OpenEpi, version 2 (Dean, Sullican, & Soe, 2009), which is available online, was also used and offers an easy way to statistically analyze epidemiological data. Cantor (1997) has an excellent discussion of survival analysis and explains how to use SAS to analyze survival data. Petrie and Sabin (2009) provide a very easy to read and understand general treatment of statistical methods useful in medical research, which also has an excellent glossary of statistical terms. There are several online glossaries of statistical and epidemiological terms, including Dorak (2010).

KEY IDEAS, DEFINITIONS, AND PRELIMINARIES

Epidemiology involves "the study of the distribution and determinants of disease frequency" (Rothman, 2002, p. 1970) and as such uses tools and intersects with many disciplines, including statistics, probability, demography, geography, and the biological sciences. Our interest in this chapter is statistics. The word "statistics" is used in two ways, illustrated by the following two sentences. "What is statistics?" "What are statistics?" The latter sense is the familiar one in which "statistics" are compilations or summarizations of data and includes the more technical use of the word "statistics" to describe characteristics (functions) of a sample. The former refers to the body of knowledge or discipline called "statistics." Both senses of the word are used in this chapter and the context determines which we use.

The "what is" aspect of statistics was first described to me by the late Professor Peter R. Nelson as "the art and science of dealing with variability." This captures the key idea: variability. When absent (which is almost never, and certainly never when one includes measurement error), there is no need for statistical methods. How much does a 5-pound bag of potatoes weigh? If one were studying 5-pound bags of potatoes, would statistical methods be appropriate? There are those who think of statistics as a science. Or even as an incarnation of the scientific method. But in practice art often seems to intervene. One of the most interesting (and distressing to some) aspects of statistics as a science is that two statistical analyses of the same phenomenon or process (even using the same data) can lead to different conclusions. Is this a result of ignorance? Mendacity? Honest disagreement?

The "what are" sense involves data, which is such a primitive idea that defining it might be impossible. Data can be thought of as "facts." These facts might be numbers or descriptors or almost anything. There are many sources for data, including government compilations (think Centers for Disease Control and Prevention, Census Bureau, etc.), private compilations such as those created by insurance companies and hospitals, or data arising from experiments and studies, including clinical trials. Typically, in the modern sense we think of these as data sets or databases (the latter having some formal structure relating the objects in it as well as methods for querying the database).

Data sets contain one or more variables. For example, a data set arising from a study of bedsores at a nursing facility might consist of cases (patients, typically being rows in a spreadsheet) along with facts about each patient such as the patient's gender, age, date at which the bedsore was discovered (recorded), comorbidities, severity of the bedsore (perhaps a score), the duration of the bedsore (date of "cure" minus date of discovery), numbers of sores, and so on. Each fact (often columns in a spreadsheet) is a variable. Interest in these variables arises primarily from the potential they have to vary; that is, different patients (or subjects or cases) may have different ages or may or may not have bedsores.

It is useful to classify variables with regard to their level of measurement: nominal, ordinal, interval, and ratio. Nominal data merely names (e.g., the variable gender is nominal). Ordinal data require that the data be capable of being ranked (e.g., severity of the bedsore might be scored on a scale of 1 to 4 in which 4 is the most severe and 1 the least). Note that $4 > 3 > 2 > 1$. Data of this type are sometimes referred to as being measured on a Likert scale. There is no need for ordinal data to be represented by numerals. The numerals in this example might correspond to 1 = "mild," 2 = "moderate," 3 = "severe," 4 = "extremely severe" so that in the data set the numerals are recorded (or in some cases the text itself is recorded). It is quite possible that the labels are reversed (4 = "mild"). In many circumstances severity scores such as these have clear definitions often based on checklists.

Interval data have the property that differences between values have a clear interpretation; for example, for the interval variable age, a patient 21 years of age is 9 years older than a patient 12 years of age. Ratio data have the property that ratios of values have a clear interpretation; for example, a patient with four bedsores has twice as many as a patient with two bedsores. The key property that identifies ratio data is the existence of a true (interpretable) zero. Zero bedsores means none is present (the patient does not presently have the disease of interest). Compare this with a temperature of zero degrees Fahrenheit. Observe that ratio data are interval, interval data are ordinal, and ordinal data are nominal; hence, one usually uses the highest level as the descriptor for a particular variable. Also note that interval data can always be converted into strictly ordinal data (e.g., small, medium, and large) by creating definitions.

In epidemiological studies all these types of variables may occur. Of special interest are counts (or count data). The number of bedsores on patient number 77 is an example of this; however, a more common epidemiological usage of counts might be the following: of 100 patients in the study, 26 were free of bedsores after 6 weeks of treatment. Or, using a slightly different type of counting, in the 100 patients in the study there were a total of 217 bedsores.

Why be concerned about level of measurement? The levels of measurement of the variables in a data set affect the method of data analysis. Most immediately, interval data can be analyzed using some of those things one learned in the fifth grade: adding, subtracting, and averaging. Or with nominal data one reverts to earlier grades in which one learned counting and perhaps later how to compute percentages (ratios).

So what is statistical data analysis? It almost always involves summarizing and organizing data. It frequently involves discovering and describing relationships between variables. In its more exotic forms it might involve creating models—something that may be going on unconsciously because a model is nothing more than a simplification of reality. A convenient definition of data analysis is drawing conclusions about some process or phenomenon using data. I prefer the more artistic characterization: determining and describing the story that a data set has to tell. This latter characterization allows different people (researchers) to tell different stories based on the same "set of facts" (data) collected about a process or phenomenon. Implied in the data analysis process are the notions of discovery and communication.

Data sets are of two general types: a census or a sample. The former is the totality of objects of interest (e.g., the USRDS database containing all dialysis patients in the United States for the year 2005). A sample is any subset of a population. Typically, there is little real interest in the sample itself. The interest lies in what the sample can tell us about the population. The activity of drawing conclusions about a population is called inference. If statistical methods are used, it is called statistical inference.

ROLE OF PROBABILITY IN EPIDEMIOLOGY

Probability is the study of the laws of chance. As a formal endeavor it arose in the study of gambling (games of chance) and as such it is naturally prospective. That is, it exists in reference to the future. This can be extended to ignorance (but that is often somewhat tenuous). In probability one deals with events. In the disease setting an event might be something like a patient with two bedsores. The probability of an event is a measure of the likelihood an event will occur. This measure is constrained to the interval [0, 1], in which a probability of 1 corresponds to absolute certainty and a probability of 0 is interpreted to mean that the event is impossible. This 0-1 characterization applies to all past or current events (but not necessarily to our knowledge about these events, which may be more problematic). That is, either they have occurred or they have not occurred. So does it make sense to say the probability that a 77-year-old nursing home patient has bedsores is 0.15? Either the patient does or does not have bedsores. The more practical approach is a frequentist characterization: In the population of nursing home patients we are interested in the fact that 15% of those 77-years-olds have bedsores. One can clothe this probabilistically by saying that a randomly selected patient from this population has a probability of 0.15 of having a bedsore; however, the frequentist characterization is more useful. In epidemiology probability is typically described as risk.

Probabilities can be assigned in three ways: subjectively, a priori, or empirically. The first of these might arise from panels of experts. The a priori assignment of probabilities arises frequently in simple games of chance, such as rolling dice. These methods involve some version of counting all outcomes, counting all "favorable" outcomes and forming a ratio to describe the probability. The exercise is purely deductive (mathematical). Epidemiological assignments of risk (probabilities) are almost always arrived at empirically; that is, through observation. For example, suppose one wishes to know the risk of bacteremia in dialysis patients in 2005. One can query the USRDS database to count the number of patients with bacteremia (I am making this much more simple than it actually is) and divide that by the number of patients in the database. This is a census, so the result is (apart from misclassification errors) a parameter (characteristic of a population). If one were to select a sample of patients from a clinic in which dialysis is performed, then a similar ratio could be formed; however, this number is an estimate. Estimates are subject to error. The error arises from the fact that a sample seldom is an exact replica of the population.

STATISTICAL INFERENCE AND THE LANGUAGE OF STATISTICS

Drawing conclusions from samples using statistical theory (methods) is called statistical inference. The subject is vast. Often, this discussion begins with the distinction between descriptive statistics and inferential statistics. For the most part this is a distinction without a difference because descriptives (this word is intended to include measures as well as graphical objects) quite naturally lead to attempts to draw conclusions. The advantage of formal inference is that the inferences can be associated with certain "probability" measures that tell one something about the likelihood that certain errors might occur. Strictly speaking, this probabilistic interpretation has meaning only before collecting the data.

Beginning with descriptives is useful. These are results from summarizing and organizing data. These can be summary measures or graphical objects. Recall that data analysis is discovering the story that a data set has to tell, so organizing and summarizing often make a good first step. No attempt will be made here to be complete. There are many standard statistics texts that are more complete (see, e.g., van Belle et al., 2004).

Summary Measures and Graphical Tools

A measure is a single number (or small set of numbers) used to describe a sample or population. With nominal data these are often percentages. It should be clear that using a single measure to describe a variable in a data set is futile if one's goal is completeness (recall that variability is the necessary condition for statistical methods to be useful). This reduction of a data set to a set of measures always involves (massive) loss of information. The benefit is conciseness and "understandability." The problem is addressed partly by using several measures that address aspects of the data. One approach is the LaSSO approach (useful for interval data): location, spread, shape, outliers. Addressing at least the first two of these is usually essential. Common measures of location are the mean and median. Common measures of spread are the standard deviation (SD; or its square, the variance), the range, and the average absolute deviation from the median (mean). The mean and SD have convenient mathematical properties, which is part of the reason they are so commonly used (as well as the fact that the normal model is completely described stochastically by these two parameters). Shape includes ideas such as skewness (the data have a long tail either left or right), bimodality (the data set consists of two piles or peaks), or more technical (and difficult to describe) notions such as kurtosis. Shape is usually best conveyed graphically using tools such as bar charts, histograms, and box plots. Outliers are "unusual" observations. Attempts at a formal definition are problematic. For univariate analyses graphs and plots (such as box plots) are useful for identifying potential outliers.

There are also summary measures useful for describing relationships among variables. The correlation coefficient (either Pearson or Spearman—along with others) measures the degree of linear association between two variables and is bounded on the interval negative 1 to positive 1 (where values near 0 indicate lack of correlation). The linear part of this is often suppressed or ignored by practitioners (and even more so by readers of research). That is, there is often a somewhat clear relationship between variables x and y but the correlation coefficient, r, is quite small in magnitude (near zero). Scatter plots often do a much better job of conveying relationships between interval variables, especially when curvature is present.

As an example consider a hypothetical nurse-based intervention study with diabetic patients. In the study the subjects in the treatment group were selected from an urban clinic and the control group was selected from another (but similar) city's clinic. At end of study HbA$_{1c}$ levels (an interval variable denoted HbA$_{1c3}$) were measured. **Figure 2-1** contains side-by-side box plots (sometimes called box and whiskers plots) of the HbA$_{1c}$ data by treatment group (a categorical/nominal variable). Box plots are useful for assessing the relationship between a categorical variable (in this case treatment group) and an interval variable (in this case HbA$_{1c}$). The vertical spread of the boxes measures variability. The solid horizontal line in each box is the median. The boxes capture the middle 50% of the observations, with the top of the box corresponding to the 75th percentile and the bottom of the box the 25th percentile. The vertical spread of a box is the interquartile range, which is a measure of variability of the middle 50% of the observations). Do HbA$_{1c}$ levels at end of study differ between the treatment and control groups? Because all the numbers used to construct these box plots are derived from samples, they are estimates so apparent differences could just be the result of random chance. This issue is treated later (in Inference, below). The treatment group has lower HbA$_{1c}$ levels based on the box plots; for example, about 75% of the treatment group has levels less than the median level for the control subjects. Both groups exhibit a great deal of variability (look at the distance from

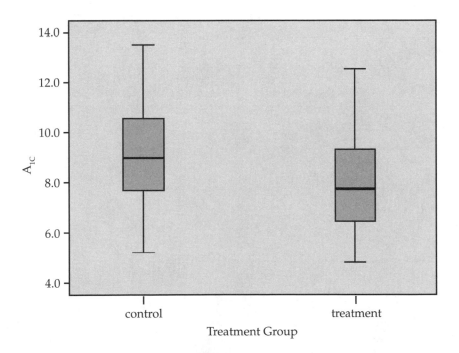

FIGURE 2-1   Box plot of variable HbA$_{1c}$ of both control and treatment groups.

whisker tip to whisker tip, which is the range when no outliers are present, as well as the vertical height of the boxes).

The same data can be summarized with statistical measures. Several are displayed in **Table 2-1**. This data set is a sample so the measures are statistics (estimates); hence, for some of them standard errors are displayed. The standard errors are measures (themselves estimates) of sample-to-sample variability of the estimates. From this one sees that the average HbA_{1c} level for the treatment group (7.967) is lower than the average for the control subjects (8.976). Which group has greater variability? The SDs are about the same (recall that the SD roughly measures the average distance of the observations from the mean); technically, the SD in Table 2-1 is the square root of the average squared distance from the mean multiplied by the square root of $[n/(n-1)]$. The factor $[n/(n-1)]$ is close to 1 for reasonably large n. Definitions of the

Table 2-1 Descriptives of HbA_{1c}		
Treatment Group	**Statistic**	**Std. Error**
Control		
Mean	8.976	0.2779
5% trimmed mean	8.950	
Median	8.900	
Variance	3.861	
Std. deviation	1.9650	
Minimum	5.3	
Maximum	13.5	
Range	8.2	
Interquartile range	2.8	
Skewness	0.122	0.337
Kurtosis	−0.350	0.662
Treatment		
Mean	7.967	0.2253
5% trimmed mean	7.907	
Median	7.900	
Variance	3.045	
Std. deviation	1.7450	
Minimum	5.0	
Maximum	12.4	
Range	7.4	
Interquartile range	2.6	
Skewness	0.460	0.309
Kurtosis	−0.010	0.608

measures in Table 2-1 can be found in any standard statistics text (e.g., van Belle et al., 2004).

One could convert the HbA_{1c} variable from interval to nominal by classifying patients as in control or not based on their HbA_{1c} level (e.g., less than 6.5 is in control). **Table 2-2** contains a cross-tabulation of HbA_{1c} by treatment group. Tables are often used to ferret out relationships between categorical variables. At end of study 12% of the control subjects are in control and 25% of the treatment group are in control.

The treatment groups are stratified by the presence or absence of hypertension (another categorical variable) in **Figure 2-2**. The dot above the whisker for treatment (without hypertension) is a potential outlier. What "story" does this figure have to tell?

When one wishes to examine the relationship between two interval variables, the scatter plot is a useful tool. In the nurse-based diabetes intervention study, one variable measured compliance (with good practices). **Figure 2-3** shows a scatter plot with HbA_{1c} on the vertical axis and of compliance on the horizontal axis. The data are stratified by treatment group. From the scatter plot one can see that as compliance increases, HbA_{1c} levels tend to decrease (for both treatment and control groups). This relationship can be measured with the correlation coefficient (r). For the treatment group $r = -0.44$, indicating that the two variables are inversely related (the negative sign for the correlation coefficient corresponds to the downward cast [negative slope] of the scatter plot as one goes from left to right).

Table 2-2 Cross-Tabulation of Treatment and Control Group of Variable HbA$_{1c}$				
		A$_{1c}$ In Control		
Treatment Group		**In Control**	**Not In Control**	**Total**
Control	Count	6	44	50
	% within treatment group	12.0%	88.0%	100.0%
Treatment	Count	15	45	60
	% within treatment group	25.0%	75.0%	100.0%
Total	Count	21	89	110
	% within treatment group	19.1%	80.9%	100.0%

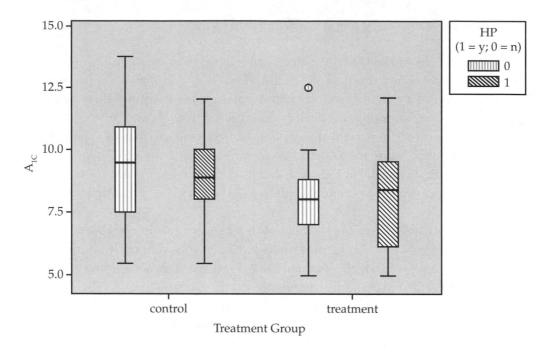

FIGURE 2-2   Box plot of variable HbA$_{1c}$ with and without hypertension.

Inference

Recall that inference is about using samples and statistical theory to draw conclusions about populations. Inference can be divided into three activities: estimation, hypothesis testing, and model fitting (building). These are not strictly distinct activities (although the first two are often presented in that way). The last of these involves the first and often the second.

Estimation and Population Modeling

The underlying idea is that for some populations (collection of individuals, a process or phenomenon) there are parameters that describe this population (or that some probability model describes the population). The parameters might be simple measures such as a percentage, the mean, the SD, the 25th percentile (or any other quantile or percentile), or other characteristics of the population. For example, the population of interest might be home-birth babies in a particular county in 2009. One might wish to estimate the percentage of home-birth babies that are premature, the average weight in grams of home-birth babies, the SD of the weights of home-birth

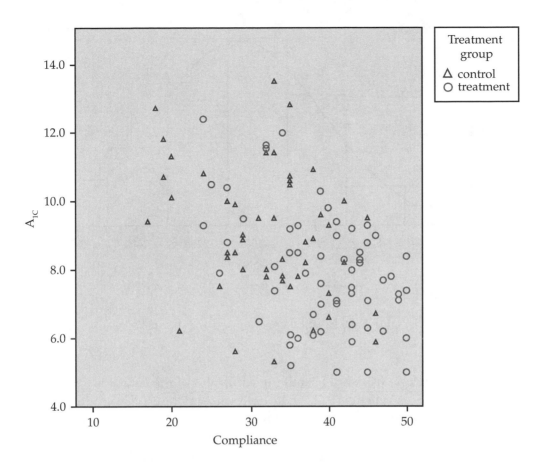

FIGURE 2-3   Scatter plot with HbA$_{1C}$ on *y*-axis and compliance on *x*-axis.

babies, or the 25th percentile of the weights. Each of these requires particular methods that are not discussed here. We distinguish between two types of estimates: point estimates and interval estimates.

Suppose that in County X data on 99 home births have been collected by a health department nurse. Typically, before engaging in formal inferences, gaining an understanding of the nature of the population of interest is wise. Suppose the weights of the babies are of interest. This is an interval/continuous measure so methods appropriate for that level of measure are used. **Figure 2-4** is a histogram of the data (which includes summary statistics). Based on the sample mean and SD, a normal curve has been superimposed on the histogram. Based on the histogram, it appears that the "normal model" is an appropriate statistical model for the birth

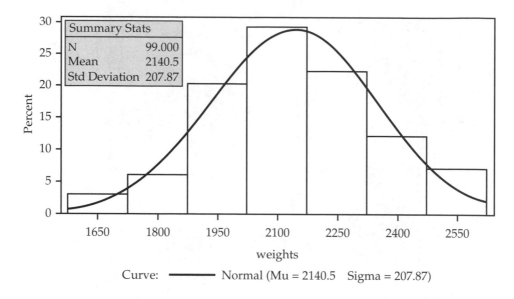

FIGURE 2-4   Histogram of baby weights superimposed with normal curve.

weight data. **Figure 2-5** shows a quantile-quantile plot of the data. This is a better tool for confirming normality (and can be used with any interval/continuous variable in fitting a particular distribution—probability model—provided the form of the model is completely specified). If the data conform to the distribution of interest, the plotted points fall along a straight line. This quantile-quantile plot offers no strong evidence against normality.

Researchers typically wish to estimate population parameters. Intervals of particular interest in this case are called confidence interval (CI) estimates. A point estimate is a single ("best number") guess. A CI is an interval with which there is associated a level of confidence. The level of confidence has a clear interpretation: If the "experiment" leading to construction of the CI is repeated many times, then the true population parameter will be trapped in the interval the percentage of times equal to the level of confidence. For example, in the home-birth study a 95% CI for mean weight is 2,099 to 2,182 g. This tells us nothing about whether the actual mean weight (pretend it is 2,150 g) is in the interval. It says only that if we use this method repeatedly, then 95% of the time the true mean will be captured in the interval; that is, if one constructed 100 intervals, then about 95 would contain 2,150. This is somewhat disappointing philosophically. Remedies have been suggested. In practice the CI approach leads to levels of belief in that there is stronger belief that the unknown

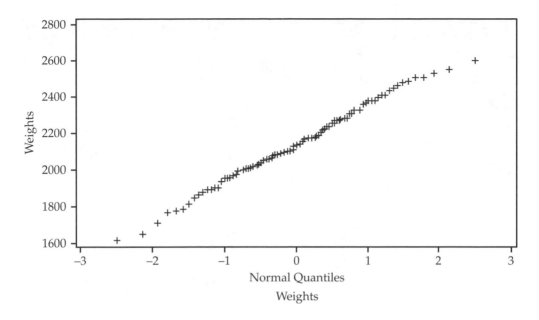

FIGURE 2-5 Quantile-quantile plot of baby weights.

parameter is in a 95% interval than a 90% interval. That is, the former interval is more likely to trap the parameter (which is achieved by widening the interval). Typically, interest focuses on the width of the interval, which is determined by the level of confidence (higher leads to wider), sample size (higher leads to narrower), and population variability (higher leads to wider). Hence, the typical interpretation of a 95% CI is a high level of belief that the parameter is in this interval. The researcher in the home-birth study is pretty sure that the average weight is in the interval 2,099 to 2,182 g.

A common misinterpretation of the CI is that 95% of babies weigh between 2,099 and 2,182 g. This is incorrect. To address this issue one needs a tolerance interval. A similar misuse would be to say that if a home birth is going to occur tomorrow, then there is a 95% chance the baby will weigh between 2,099 and 2,182 g. For this one needs a prediction interval. One could say that for the anticipated 200 home births next month the average weight of the babies will be between 2,099 and 2,182 with a high level of "confidence." Some other issues have crept in here and should be thought through. To continue this idea let's note that for epidemiological data any of the three types of intervals we have mentioned can be useful: CIs, prediction intervals, and tolerance intervals. **Table 2-3** contains interval estimates associated with birth weight data.

Table 2-3	Interval Estimates of Baby Birth Weights		
Confidence	**k**	**Prediction Limits**	
Approximate Prediction Interval Containing All of k Future Observations			
95.00%	1	1,726	2,555
95.00%	2	1,665	2,616
95.00%	10	1,540	2,740
Approximate Prediction Interval Containing the Mean of k Future Observations			
95.00%	1	1,726	2,555
95.00%	2	1,846	2,435
95.00%	10	2,004	2,277
Prediction Interval Containing the Standard Deviation of k Future Observations			
95.00%	2	6.531	473.192
95.00%	10	112.654	311.573
Confidence	**p**	**Tolerance Limits**	
Approximate Tolerance Interval Containing at Least Proportion p of the Population			
95.00%	0.9	1,751	2,530

All the interval estimates in Table 2-3 are based on the assumption that the data are a sample from the normal distribution and were produced using SAS. The interval at the bottom of Table 2-3 has the following interpretation: With 95% confidence 90% of the home-born babies in County X weigh between 1,751 and 2,530 g. One might compare this with the observed quantiles (percentiles) of the baby weight sample that appear in **Table 2-4** (note that these quantiles in Table 2-4 are properties of the sample but could be used as estimates of the corresponding population parameters). Ninety percent of the sample weights are between 1,776 (the 5th percentile) and 2,506 (the 95th percentile). Tolerance intervals incorporate uncertainty with respect to estimation of the mean and the SD as well as population variability. The key idea is that the interval "traps" a certain proportion of the population with a given level of confidence. Notice that an interval of this type contains information of an entirely different nature than a CI estimate (which is a guess about a parameter—a fixed but unknown number). It is possible (but unlikely) that none of the babies has

Table 2-4	Birth Weight Descriptives (Percentiles)
Quantile	**Estimate**
100% max	2,601
99%	2,601
95%	2,506
90%	2,433
75% Q3	2,278
50% median	2,134
25% Q1	2,006
10%	1,875
5%	1,776
1%	1,621
0% min	1,621

weights in the CI for the mean. Often, what are called the natural tolerance limits are used to estimate a proportion of the population; that is, a natural 95% tolerance interval is given by mean ± 2SD. Be aware that infinitely many intervals contain 95% of the population but only one is symmetrical about the mean (and this symmetry is unlikely to produce the narrowest interval unless the population is symmetric).

Prediction intervals are used to answer questions about the future (but are based on the assumption that the future is stochastically identical with the period over which the data were collected). For example, suppose one wants to guess the weight on the next home-born baby in County X. A 95% prediction interval is 1,726 to 2,555 g (top of Table 2-3, $k = 1$). A prediction interval incorporates uncertainty (potential error) from three sources: estimation of the mean, estimation of the SD, and the inherent variability in the population (as measured by its SD). Observe that a prediction interval for the average weight of the next 10 babies to be born is narrower than the estimate for a single birth (2,004–2,277 g, with $k = 10$ in Table 2-3).

Hypothesis Testing

Hypothesis testing has to do with assessing the "truthfulness" of statistical statements (hypotheses) using samples and statistical theory (methods). In its most commonly used and simplest form, it is a decision theoretic approach that leads to one of two mutually exclusive decisions regarding two mutually exclusive statements (the null hypothesis and the alternative hypothesis): One rejects the null hypothesis or one fails to reject the null hypothesis. The presumption is that there is a true state of nature (unknown to the researcher).

In testing a hypothesis one can commit two types of errors. A type I error is rejecting the null hypothesis when it is true. A type II error is failing to reject the null hypothesis when it is false. In repeated replications of an "experiment," these errors will occur with probability one (that is, with certainty). Why? Because the decision is based on a sample and sampling error will occur. The probability of a type I error is denoted alpha (α), called the level of significance of the test when alpha is expressed as a percentage. The probability of a type II error is a function of the value of the unknown parameter (in this example the true average birth weight). In most studies the level of significance is chosen before conducting the test (ideally before conducting the study). Typically, the mystical 5% level of significance is chosen because this has become something of an established scientific norm.

How do hypotheses arise? Typically, hypotheses arise from some sort of mind experiment. For example, a researcher wonders whether the average birth weight in this county is like the national average, which is 2,000 g. The null hypothesis is mean in County X = 2,000 g. The alternative can take many forms, but the typical two-sided alternative is mean in County X is not 2,000 g. Based on a sample, the researcher decides the hypothesis (this is equivalent to choosing between the null and alternative hypotheses). The basis for the decision is quite simple (but not one that is without critics): If the data are "inconsistent" with the null hypothesis, then one rejects the null hypothesis; otherwise, one fails to reject the null hypothesis. Now that statistical software packages are readily available, this decision is usually based on a p value, which is defined as the likelihood of observing a sample as different from the one hypothesized (in the null hypothesis) assuming that the null hypothesis is true. Along with this one must also make certain assumptions about the data to actually calculate a p value. One might ponder this for a moment to wonder why one supposes the null hypothesis is true to begin the formal analysis. For most parametric tests this is a very precise question. Let's continue the previous example in which a sample of 99 babies was selected. Having been to college, the researcher decides to perform a two-sided one-sample t-test. The test t is given by

$$t = \frac{(\text{sample mean}) - (\text{hypothesized mean})}{s/\sqrt{n}} = \frac{2{,}140.5 - 2{,}100}{207.87/\sqrt{99}} = 1.939$$

The p value = $2P (t > 1.939) = 0.0555$, in which the probability is based in the t distribution with 98 degrees of freedom (this test is described in detail in nearly all methods texts, e.g., van Belle et al., 2004). The t-test is appropriate because we verified the sample was "approximately normal" via the quantile-quantile plot. Now how is one to interpret this p value? Using the classical decision theoretic approach is straightforward: $p >$ alpha, then one fails to reject the null hypothesis (mean weight = 2,100 g). That is, there is not sufficient evidence to conclude that the null is false. Does the researcher believe that the average weight of home-born babies in Country X is 2,100 g? Recall that the point estimate was 2,140.5 g and the CI for the mean was 2,099 to 2,182 g. The issue can be dodged by saying that there is not sufficient evidence to conclude that County X is different from the national average for home-born baby birth weights.

Why is rejecting the null hypothesis 1 time in 20 of particular interest? That is, why is the 5% level of significance so embedded in scientific practice? One might wonder what the effect on science would have been had the generally accepted level of significance been 2.5%. Or 10%. There is no doubt that the choice of 5% has had serious ramifications.

Power

The power of a test is a measure of the likelihood of rejecting false hypotheses. This is of some importance because the null hypothesis is usually thought to be false. The power can be assessed prospectively (at the time the study is planned) or post hoc (after data collection and test selection). The former is primarily aimed at avoiding futility and in sample size selection. The latter is frequently used for explaining away nonsignificant findings. Preplanned power calculations typically require a set of assumptions (often including a statistical model for the phenomenon of interest) and should be regarded with some healthy suspicion. These power calculations are based on two critical choices: the null value of the parameter and a second value corresponding to the minimum clinically significant difference between the null value and this clinically significant value. In the home-born baby example, one might say something like I want to be 90% sure the null hypothesis will be rejected if the average weight in County X differs from the national average by 25 or more grams. After deciding on the test statistic and making assumptions about the distribution of weights, one can calculate power estimates to "determine" the appropriate sample size. Ideally, a considerable amount of sensitivity analysis ("what if" analysis) accompanies this sample size decision.

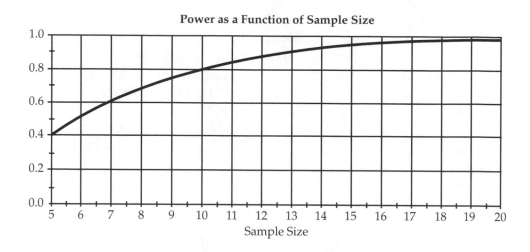

FIGURE 2-6   Power curve.

Graphs are an efficient method for doing what if analyses. The power curve in **Figure 2-6** is for a one-sample t-test for the mean with level of significance 5% and effect size $d = 1$. The effect size d is the magnitude of the difference between the null mean and the supposed mean measured in SDs. (See Cohen [1992] for a discussion of effect sizes.) For d (often applied to one-sample t-test, paired t-test, and two independent sample t-tests) an effect size of less than 0.2 is small, 0.8 is large, and 0.5 is medium. The effect size in Figure 2-6 corresponds, for example, to the null hypothesis in that the mean = 0 when the true mean is 1 and the population SD is 1. The power curve in Figure 2-6 has sample size on the horizontal axis and power on the vertical axis and applies to a specific test, effect size, and level of significance. The power increases as the sample size increases. If the effect size was smaller (e.g., 0.5), then the power would be lower (the curve would be below the one in Figure 2-6).

Power and Usefulness of Estimation

The key problem with classical hypothesis testing is that its primary use is in establishing what is not true when in fact scientific interest usually is in the truth. That is, for example, one wants to know something about the weights of home-born babies in County X. Suppose County X is in an affluent suburban area and researchers can reasonably guess that the birth weight distribution differs from the national one. In this case the null hypothesis is essentially a straw man. This is not atypical. Does a company engage in a clinical trial of a drug believing that it is no better than placebo? One solution to this problem is to report an effect size as well as a p value. Strictly speaking, effect sizes are unitless measures. For example, the effect size for this one-sample t-test is (mean − sample mean)/SD so that the effect size for the birth weight example is $d = (2140.5 − 2100)/207.87) = 0.192$, which is a small effect using Cohen's suggestions. This makes the effect size universally interpretable but at a price that is addressed in the next paragraph.

The advantage of a CI is that it is in the units associated with the analysis and makes a direct statement about the parameter of interest in terms that are easy to understand clinically; for example, with 95% confidence the mean weight of home-born babies in County X is between 2,099 to 2,182 g. The estimated difference from the national average is between 2,099 − 2,100 = −1 g and 2,182 − 2,100 = 82 g. The CI for this discrepancy is (−1, 82), which contains zero and hence indicates nonsignificance at the 5% level of significance. However, with 95% confidence home-birth babies in County X could be as much as 82 g on average higher (or as much as 1 g lighter) than the national average.

One approach to the significance issue is to carefully separate statistical significance from clinical significance. Strictly speaking, one establishes statistical significance first, which is tantamount to saying that the observed "difference" is not (or is unlikely) to be explained by random chance. It is important to realize that statistical significance is conditioned on the effect size as well as the sample size (and the predetermined level of significance). In a sense the sample size is only important in its effect on accuracy; it is not an attribute of the population. Having established statistical significance, one looks at the difference in terms of its clinical significance. In the above example, using the classical approach the question is answered once the p value is produced. A more nuanced approach might ask if a difference of as much as 82 g is important with respect to its health/disease consequences. By the way one might wonder whether the mean is that informative. One could look at the tolerance interval or estimated quantiles of the weight distribution to assess risks.

MEASURES OF DISEASE OCCURRENCE AND RISK

Measuring disease risk and occurrence is more complicated than might appear on the surface. The idea of risk seems easy to understand, and most people believe they understand it.

Incidence and Prevalence

Epidemiological measures of risk and disease occurrence require that a distinction be made between proportions and rates (even though these words are often used interchangeably, e.g., one speaks of immunization rates but is actually referring to the proportion [or percentage] immunized in a particular population). Time is implicitly or explicitly involved in these measures. Also, one should distinguish between snapshots (pictures of a population that are more or less instantaneous) and measures over time. The former can be described as prevalence measures and the latter as incidence measures.

Incidence Proportion

The notion of risk is widespread. The simplest measure of risk is a pure number (unitless) that might be thought of as a probability. If there are x new cases of disease during a 6-month period and N subjects are followed for those 6 months, then risk is defined as

$$\text{Risk} = \frac{x}{N} = \frac{\text{number of new cases of disease in time period}}{\text{number of subjects followed for time period}}$$

The risk defined above is also referred to as an incidence proportion or fraction. Although the time period may or may not be reported, it is critical to the proper understanding of the measure produced. Consider a nursing facility with 120 patients who at the beginning of the measurement period do not have bedsores. Over the next 6 months 30 of these patients develop bedsores. Then the risk or incidence proportion is $30/120 = 0.25$ (or 25%). The difficulty is that the actual phenomenon under study is seldom this simple and carefully defined. And one might wonder whether this adequately describes the bedsore "situation" at the nursing facility with respect to the risk of developing bedsores because the dynamics of the situation have been removed. What are some of these dynamics? The exposure time for the patients who complete the study is 6 months. For the 120 patients this is $6 \times 120 = 720$ person months. What if some of these 120 patients are discharged during the period of study? Then the total amount of exposure is less than 720 person months. In this case the risk is actually greater than the incidence proportion because not every patient was exposed for the full 6 months. One solution is to more carefully define incidence proportion:

$$\text{Incidence proportion} = \frac{x}{N} = \frac{\text{number of new cases of disease in time period}}{\text{number of subjects at beginning of time period}}$$

Notice that this does not completely solve the problem of how to measure risk. For that reason a more complicated measure is needed.

Incidence Rate

The incidence rate takes into account the total exposure of the subjects during the study period.

$$\text{Incidence rate} = \frac{x}{T} = \frac{\text{number of new cases of disease in time period}}{\text{person time at risk}}$$

Consider the bedsores example. Let's suppose that of the 120 patients beginning the study 110 patients were in the facility for the entire 6 months, 5 were discharged at the end of month 1 and another 5 at the end of month 4. Then the total exposure is $(110 \times 6) + (5 \times 1) + (5 \times 4) = 685$ person months. Hence, the incidence rate is 30/685 = 0.0438 per person month. For 6 months this becomes 0.26. Note that this is larger than the incidence proportion of 0.25 (per 6 months). Why? The incidence proportion understated the exposure. Typically, incidence rates are multiplied by a time factor so that the time unit is something familiar, such as person years (or in this case 100 to yield 4.38 cases per 100 person months).

There are two ways (methods) for counting cases when the disease of interest is potentially recurrent. One way is to count only first cases. The other is to count all the cases, allowing a single individual to have multiple episodes. Of course, this distinction does not apply when only one episode can occur, such as one ending in death. In the bedsores example a patient could have no bedsores at the beginning of the observation period, develop bedsores (say after 1 month), have the bedsores disappear (cured after an additional 6 weeks), and then have the bedsores recur at month 5 of the study. If the first episode approach is used, then the numerator is easily defined (the number of new first cases), but what about the denominator? The solution is to divide by the "time at risk of disease," which means that for those 30 cases of bedsores the clock stops ticking when they got bedsores (the first time). That is, their period of exposure ends.

Prevalence Proportion

Prevalence measures are attempts to describe a situation (phenomenon) at an instant in time. Prevalence addresses the question of how widespread the disease is in the population. For example, at the beginning of the previous surveillance there were 120 patients without bedsores. Then one might say at beginning of the study that the prevalence proportion or fraction was 0/120 = 0.0. Let's suppose that the facility at the beginning of the study had 140 patients (20 with bedsores and 120 without bedsores). Because in the previous section we were interested only in new cases, we used the denominator of 120 because these patients were disease free. That seems appropriate in the context of measuring risk in the sense that how likely is it that a disease-free patient will cease to be disease free during the period of study? However, if one is interested in a snapshot of the bedsores situation at the beginning of the study, then one can reasonably argue that the denominator should be 140 and the numerator 20. That is, the point prevalence at the beginning of the study (baseline) is 20/140 = 0.14 (14%).

Now, what about the prevalence at the end of the study? Well, one calculation might be (20 + 30)/140 = 0.36 (36%). This supposes that the 20 initial cases of bedsores and the 30 new cases that arose over the 6-month study period still have bedsores at the end of the 6 months (end of study). Notice that as a practical matter the nurse doing this study might take a much more direct approach (provided prevalence is the only measure of interest). At the beginning of the study the prevalence proportion is 20/140, which could be arrived at by simple enumeration. Then after 6 months the nurse counts the number of patients with bedsores, denoting this as y and forms the fraction $y/140$ (provided the head count at the facility is 140). Note that $y \leq (20 + 30)$—unless patients arrive at the facility with bedsores. The actual number of cases of bedsores could be reduced by some of the 50 cases of bedsores being cured.

Regardless of how the point prevalence fraction is calculated, it is unitless and is a snapshot of the disease situation at some moment in time. For that reason prevalence is a much easier measure (in a simple setting such as this nursing facility) to understand. When we calculated the incidence proportion, we implicitly took for granted that the head count at the facility and prevalence proportion depended in their calculation on key assumptions: There were 140 patients in the nursing facility at baseline and the same 140 patients were in the facility at end of study. Actual counting can be more complicated than that. Furthermore, implicit averaging is taking place when one uses units such as months when patients might be discharged (or die) at any time during the month.

Inferences for Incidence and Prevalence

Recall that inference is a process in which one uses data and statistical theory to draw conclusions about populations based on samples. Most of the theory is based on the notion that the data (sample) arose from some sort of random sample. The simple methods presented in this section are based on simple random sampling, which can loosely be defined as a sampling method in which each subject in the population is equally likely to be chosen (to be in the sample). Very seldom do epidemiological data meet this standard. One usually satisfies this assumption by arguing that the sample is representative of the population of interest. This often implies some limitation or restriction on what can be called the scope of inference. That is, what is the population to which the inferences apply? Questions of this type are sometimes outside the scope of statistics because they require subject matter knowledge to be properly answered.

Inferences About Incidence and Prevalence Proportions

Because the incidence proportion and the prevalence proportion are each proportions, inference in this case reduces to the study of proportions. If the underlying model for the data is assumed to be binomial (this is the typical assumption; see van Belle et al., 2004), then a $(1 - \alpha) \times 100\%$ (large sample) two-sided CI estimate for a proportion in which there are x "successes" out of N independent trials is

$$\frac{x}{N} \pm z \sqrt{\frac{\frac{x}{N}\left(1 - \frac{x}{N}\right)}{N}}$$

Alpha (α) relates the CI to level of significance, the idea being that for a 95% CI, $\alpha = 0.05$. Success is equated with observation of the disease (or not, because symmetry prevails). The point estimate is for the proportion in x/N, z is a quantile from the standard normal distribution (the z with $\alpha/2$ in the upper right hand tail of the distribution), and the quantity to the right of z in the equation is the (asymptotic) standard error of the estimate (which is a measure of the sample to sample variation in x/N). These days CI estimates are almost always generated using statistical software. SAS 9.1 was used to generate **Table 2-5**, which contains the incidence estimate for the bedsores example. One would say with 95% confidence the incidence of bedsores is between 0.1725 and 0.3275. Or more likely, the researcher might believe it is highly likely that between 17.25% and 32.75% of patients will develop bedsores over a 6-month period.

There are several important features of the CI estimate: The width of the interval is determined by N, the level of confidence, and x/N. Larger Ns are associated with narrower intervals, the higher the level of confidence the larger z is, and hence the wider the CI. The closer x/N is to 0.5, the wider the interval. Now what is the proper interpretation of this interval? Previously, we formally defined CI. For practical purposes that definition is not useful. The phrase "between 17.25% and 32.75% of

Table 2-5 Incidence (Proportion) Estimate of Bedsores Along With Confidence Intervals	
Proportion	0.2500
ASE (asymptotic standard error)	0.0395
95% Lower confidence limit	0.1725
95% Upper confidence limit	0.3275
Exact confidence limits	
95% Lower confidence limit	0.1755
95% Upper confidence limit	0.3373
Binomial proportion for disease status = bedsores	

patients" needs amplification. It is a fact that 25% of the disease-free patients in the nursing facility got bedsores during the observation period. What does the CI have to do with that? The answer is that the researcher was probably not interested (in a scientific sense) in this particular collection of 120 patients; rather, interest was in what these 120 patients tell us about some population of patients. Alternatively, the researcher might conduct a mind experiment that works something like this: Given another cohort of patients in the same facility, what can I expect to happen?

The second set of confidence limits is labeled "exact." These are also based on the binomial model but do not depend on the large sample properties of the binomial (asymptotic normality). There are also estimates that use a continuity correction factor as well as other methods designed to produce more accurate "coverage" probabilities (the likelihood before data collection that the parameter of interest is in the CI). Choices among these are partly a matter of taste. The key idea is that a CI is the preferred way to estimate incidence or prevalence proportions rather than a point estimate. A 90% CI (0.185, 0.315) for the incidence proportion is narrower.

Suppose that the researcher was motivated to conduct the bedsores study by an article in a nursing journal that stated the prevalence of bedsores for nursing facility patients was 22%. Based on the situation when the study began, the estimated prevalence was 20/140 = 0.14 (14%). Can the researcher conclude that the situation in her nursing facility is better that this national average? That is, can the discrepancy between the observed prevalence of 14% and the hypothesized prevalence of 22% be explained as being the result of random chance?

Table 2-6   Prevalence (Proportion) Estimates for Bedsores Along With Confidence Intervals

Proportion	0.1429
ASE (asymptotic standard error)	0.0296
95% Lower confidence limit	0.0849
95% Upper confidence limit	0.2008
Exact confidence limits	
95% Lower confidence limit	0.0895
95% Upper confidence limit	0.2120
Binomial proportion for disease status = bedsores.	

One approach is to examine the 95% CI for the prevalence (0.085, 0.200) to see whether the hypothesized value of 0.22 is in the CI (**Table 2-6**). Because it is not, one can conclude that the prevalence of bedsores at the nursing facility is different from the national average (with level of significance 5%; this is where the $(1 - \alpha) \times 100\%$ comes into play). Alternatively, one can perform a formal test of the hypothesis that prevalence equals 0.22 versus the alternative that prevalence is not equal to 0.22. The p value for this test is 0.0276 (**Table 2-7**), which is less than 0.05; hence, one rejects the null hypothesis and concludes that the prevalence at the nursing facility is not 0.22. Occasionally, one might wish to test the one-sided alternative that the prevalence is less than 0.22 (one should be cautious about doing this). For the one-sided alternative the p value is 0.0138 (which of course is also less than 0.05). These two approaches to testing a hypothesis about a proportion (the CI approach and the p value

Table 2-7   Output for the Statistical Test of the Hypothesis That Proportion = 0.22 Including p Value

Test of H0: Proportion = 0.22	
ASE (asymptotic standard error) under H0	0.0350
Z	−2.2034
One-sided Pr < Z	0.0138
Two-sided Pr > |Z|	0.0276

approach) occasionally lead to different conclusions because the former is based on the observed proportion and the latter on the hypothesized proportion.

Inferences About Incidence Rates

The most commonly used statistical model for incidence rates is the Poisson model (Rothman, 2002, p. 133 or for a more technical description see Selvin, 2002, p. 80). The Poisson model has a single parameter called the average rate and is used to model counts data. A large sample CI for the incidence rate (based on the normal approximation) is

$$\frac{x}{T} \pm z \sqrt{\frac{x}{T^2}}$$

Recall that the incidence rate for the bedsores example was 30/685 = 0.0438 per person month. Hence, a 95% CI for the incidence rate is

$$\frac{30}{685} \pm 1.96 \sqrt{\frac{30}{685^2}}$$

Hence, the lower confidence limit is 0.0438 − 1.96(0.0080) = 0.028 and the upper confidence limit is 0.059. That is, with 95% confidence the incidence rate is between 0.028 and 0.059 per person month. Using OpenEpi (Dean et al., 2009), one gets the results in **Table 2-8**, which show several of the many approaches to this problem. Note that the rates are in 100 person-months.

Table 2-8 Person-Time Rate and 95% Confidence Intervals: Per 100 Person-Time Units			
	Lower CL	**Rate**	**Upper CL**
Mid-*P* exact test	3.009	4.38	6.173
Fisher's exact test	2.955		6.252
Normal approximation	2.812		5.947
Byar approx. Poisson	2.954		6.252
Rothman/Greenland	3.062		6.264
Number of cases, 30; person-time, 685. Results from OpenEpi, Version 2, open source calculator—PersonTime1.			

Stratification

Often, it is useful to stratify epidemiological data. That can be planned or post hoc. If the post hoc analyses are done after data snooping (using data twice in an analysis such as examining the event rates in several districts and then comparing the district with the highest observed rate to the others in a formal statistical test is what is meant by "data snooping"), care should be taken to use the appropriate adjustments to the analysis. **Table 2-9** contains the bedsore data stratified by age. Both the incidence proportion and the incidence rate are shown for each of the three age groups.

Does the incidence proportion differ with respect to age group? The broader question is whether risk is related to age. There are several approaches to questions of this type. Two important factors are (1) the level of measurement one wishes to use for age (in Table 2-9 age is categorical) and (2) the measure of risk you wish to use. The case in which one treats age as interval/continuous is discussed below (see Regression Modeling; that section also includes logistic and Poisson regression modeling in which age is categorical). In this section the comparisons are done using the ANOM approach (for a comprehensive treatment see Nelson et al., 2005). This method has the advantage of producing a graphical solution to the problem (in the form of a decision chart).

Figure 2-7 contains the ANOM decision chart for the incidence proportion (produced using SAS). The null hypothesis is that the incidence proportions are the same for the three age groups. The center line has the overall incidence proportion (which is 0.25). The key idea is that if the three incidence proportions are "close" to one another, then they will be close to the center line. The observed incidence proportions for each group are plotted on the chart (top of the vertical lines). The dashed lines are the decision limits. If any one of the observed incidence proportions plots outside the decision limits, then one rejects the null hypothesis (at level of

Table 2-9	Data on Bedsores								
Age	New Cases	n	6 Months	1 Month	4 Months	T	Incidence Proportion	Incidence Rate	Incidence Rate per 100
<60	5	30	27	2	1	168	0.167	0.030	2.976
60-70	10	50	44	3	3	279	0.200	0.036	3.584
70+	15	40	39	0	1	238	0.375	0.063	6.303
Total/All	30	120	110	5	5	685	0.250	0.044	4.380

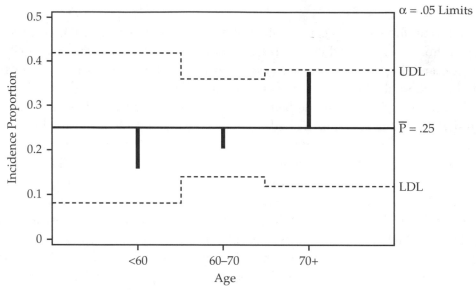

FIGURE 2-7   ANOM decision chart for incidence rate data.

significance = 5%). Because all three observed incidence proportions are within the decision limits, one cannot reject the null hypothesis. That is, there is not sufficient evidence to conclude that the incidence proportions are related to age.

There is some suspicion because the observed incidence proportions increase as one goes from left to right (perhaps this suggests an approach that takes this notion into account). If the level of significance increased (e.g., changed from 10% from 5%), the decision limits will move in toward the center line. The decision limits are different for each age group because the sample sizes are different. The vertical distance between the decision lines is inversely related to the sample sizes. The ANOM test for proportions is the analogue of the chi-squared test for the 3 by 2 table that can be constructed from the incidence proportion data. The underlying model is the normal approximation to the binomial.

ANOM analysis of the incidence rate data is based on the normal approximation to the Poisson model. The ANOM decision chart for the incidence rates (**Figure 2-8**) shows that the incidence rates differ among the age groups (at the 5% level of significance) because all three of the observed incidence rates plot outside the decision limits. The conclusions are that those younger than 60 and between 60 and 70 are at lower risk for bedsores than the overall average (the line labeled with $\overline{U}$ = 4.4); those older than 70 years are at greater risk than the overall average. That is, one

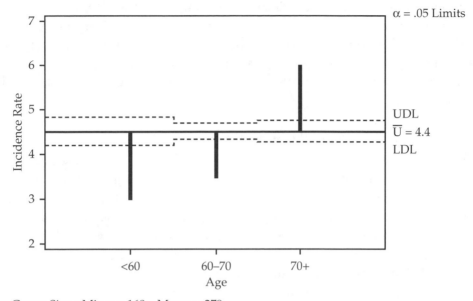

Group Sizes: Min n = 168   Max n = 279

FIGURE 2-8   ANOM decision chart for the incidence rates.

rejects the null hypothesis that three incidence rates are the same; in addition one can see the nature of the differences.

Survival Analysis

Survival analysis and modeling has its origins in mortality studies; however, the time to any well-defined event can be studied using survival analysis models. Let the random variable Y be the time at which an event occurs. For example, in the bedsores example of the 120 subjects free of bedsores at the beginning of the study, 30 got bedsores by the end of the study (after 6 months or 24 weeks). Given that a patient gets bedsores, let Y denote the time in weeks at which the bedsores are cured. That is, we are interested in how long it takes for bedsores to be cured. In the most general setting there is a function called the survival function, denoted $S(t)$, which is the probability that the time Y is greater than t; i.e.,

$$S(t) = P(Y > t)$$

In our example, $S(t)$ is the probability that the bedsores are still present after t weeks. In practice the survival function must be estimated from data. There are two general approaches: parametric estimation and nonparametric estimation. The former typically involves using models from the gamma family (e.g., exponential models), the Weibull, or others. In medical studies the nonparametric approach is the most commonly used (for a thorough discussion see Cantor, 1997). The most commonly used nonparametric estimate of the survival function is the Kaplan-Meier estimate.

Kaplan-Meier Estimation of the Survival Function

Several difficulties arise in estimating survival functions and survival distribution parameters. An example will help clarify these. Let's go back to the bedsores example. **Table 2-10** has data regarding the bedsores (of the 30 cases only a few are presented in Table 2-10 and the 30 are in no particular order) and contains something that in practice is not available—the actual duration of the disease in weeks. The patient identified as patient 1 had bedsores for 3 weeks. Patient 2 had bedsores for 25 weeks. But the study lasted for only 24 weeks, so this event was not actually observed during the course of the study. In fact, patient 2 did not acquire bedsores until week 10 of the study; hence, the maximum time that patient could be observed was 14 weeks.

So what do we know about that patient from observation? We know that the bedsores persisted for at least 14 weeks (see Table 2-10, Study Time). One approach to

Table 2-10	Data Tables Show Study Time					
Patient	Week of Diagnosis	Maximum Study Time	Disease	Diabetic	Study Time	Duration
1	9	15	0	1	3	3
2	10	14	1	1	14	25
3	13	11	1	1	11	23
4	8	16	0	1	9	9
.	.	.	.	.	.	.
27	7	17	0	1	5	5
28	8	16	0	1	14	14
29	15	9	1	1	9	9
30	14	10	1	1	10	10

estimating the average time to cure for bedsores is to only count the complete cases, but this will lead to underestimating the average duration of the disease. In the jargon of survival analysis this patient whose cure was not observed is censored. In the Disease column patient 2 has a "1" recorded, indicating that at the end of the study bedsores were still present. Patient 1 has a "0" in the Disease column because the bedsores were acquired at week 9 and the duration was 3 weeks, meaning that the bedsores disappeared before the study ended. Study Time contains the time during which a patient was observed to have bedsores. That and the Disease column are all that is required to produce a Kaplan-Meier estimate of the survival function. **Figure 2-9** shows the survival function (SAS 9.1). Like all survival functions, the function is nonincreasing. That is, it drifts downward over time.

How is one to read (use) this estimated survival function? The survival probability is on the vertical axis and the time to cure (Study Time) is on the horizontal. What is the probability that a bedsore will still be present after 10 weeks? Find 10 on the horizontal axis and go up until intersecting the curve from about 0.4. That is, about

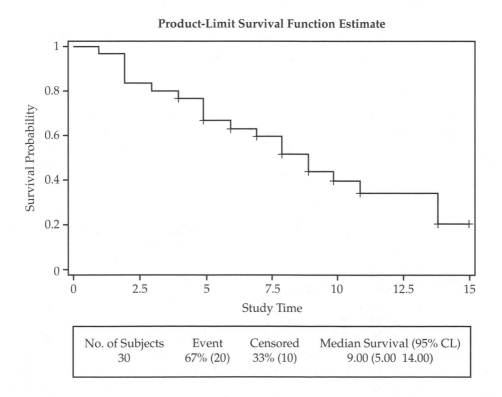

FIGURE 2-9 Survival function.

40% of the time a bedsore will take more than 10 weeks to be cured. What percent will be cured within 10 weeks? The relationship below tells us:

$$P(Y \leq t) = F(t) = 1 - P(Y > t) = 1 - S(t)$$

The probability that the bedsore is cured within 10 weeks is 1 minus the probability that it will take more than 10 weeks to cure. Hence, in about 60% of cases the cure will take place on or before week 10.

From Figure 2-9 one can see that of the 30 patients under study, 20 were cured and 10 were not (these censored times are indicated by a "+" in the graph). For example, there is a censored time at 4 weeks. The role of censoring in the construction of the curve is explained subsequently. The median survival time is 9.0; furthermore, with 95% confidence the median survival time is between 5 and 14 weeks. The median survival time is an estimate of the time by which 50% of cases of bedsores will be cured. More detail is available in **Table 2-11**, which has quartile estimates.

The estimated mean survival time (time to cure) is 8.62 weeks. The mean survival time was underestimated because the largest observation was censored and the estimation was restricted to the largest event time.

Details regarding the construction of Kaplan-Meier curves can be found in standard biostatistics texts (e.g., van Belle et al., 2004). For SAS details see Cantor (1997). The key idea is that the censored times do not alter the probability, but they reduce the number at risk at succeeding times. From the Kaplan-Meier (product limit) life table (**Table 2-12** is a partial listing), at time 1 week there was a cure. Because just before that there were 30 patients at risk (they had bedsores), the probability of a survival time greater than 1 week is 29/30 = 0.9667. There were four cures at week 2. The probability of surviving more than 2 weeks is (25/29) × 0.9667 = 0.8333 (note

Table 2-11	Quartile Estimates of Survival Time		
			95% CI
Percent	Point Estimate	Lower	Upper
75	14.0	10.0	
50	9.0	5.0	14.0
25	5.0	2.0	8.0

Table 2-12	Kaplan-Meier Life Table				
	Product-Limit Survival Estimates				
Study Time	**Survival**	**Failure**	**Survival Standard Error**	**Number Failed**	**Number Left**
0.0000	1.0000	0	0	0	30
1.0000	0.9667	0.0333	0.0328	1	29
2.0000	.	.	.	2	28
2.0000	.	.	.	3	27
2.0000	.	.	.	4	26
2.0000	0.8333	0.1667	0.0680	5	25
3.0000	0.8000	0.2000	0.0730	6	24
4.0000	0.7667	0.2333	0.0772	7	23
4.0000	.	.	.	7	22
5.0000	.	.	.	8	21
5.0000	.	.	.	9	20
5.0000	0.6621	0.3379	0.0871	10	19

that the survival probability is not updated until the row corresponding to the fourth cure for that time period and hence the preceding three rows are filled with periods to indicate that no calculations were made). When censored times occur (the first one is at 4 weeks), the denominator (those at risk) is reduced, but the probability is not affected.

Comparing Survival Functions and the Log-Rank Test

An interesting application of survival analysis is its value in comparing groups. This arises frequently when comparing treatments (e.g., interventions and drugs) or groups (these can be demographic or prognostic, e.g., disease severity for breast cancer). In the bedsores study the nurse also recorded comorbidities, one of which was diabetes (see the Diabetic column in Table 2-10 in which "1" corresponds to diabetic and "0" to not diabetic). The two survival functions are shown in **Figure 2-10**. From visual inspection one can see that the time to cure is longer for diabetic patients (the survival curve for diabetics is above the curve for nondiabetics). The median time to cure for diabetics is 14.0 weeks compared with 4.5 weeks for nondiabetic patients.

Is this apparent (observed) difference statistically significant? One commonly used test for homogeneity of survival curves is the log-rank test. In this example $p = 0.0001$ (chi-squared = 14.88 with 1 degree of freedom), so that the null hypothesis of homogeneous survival functions is rejected (e.g., $0.0001 < 0.05$). The formal hypothesis being tested is that the survival functions are the same for all time points t. It is worth noting that the Kaplan-Meier estimate of the survival function is unbiased (it equals the true survival function on average) and $S(t)$ is asymptotically normal so CIs can be constructed at any time t.

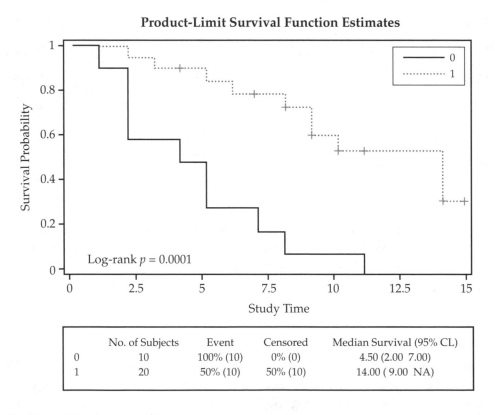

	No. of Subjects	Event	Censored	Median Survival (95% CL)
0	10	100% (10)	0% (0)	4.50 (2.00 7.00)
1	20	50% (10)	50% (10)	14.00 (9.00 NA)

FIGURE 2-10 Two survival functions.

Analysis of 2×2 Tables

Relationships between categorical variables can be explored by means of tables. Fundamental to this type of analysis are 2×2 tables, which are tables with two rows and two columns. The focus here is in measuring risk. **Table 2-13** contains hypothetical data collected about entering students at a university. Data were collected by a nursing team at student health services. We assume that the data were derived from a random survey of incoming students (even though the convenient numbers such as 100 cigarette smokers are suggestive of a different design; see Chapter 3 for a discussion of designs such as case-control studies). The exposure of interest is cigarette smoking and the response is marijuana smoking (both self-reported).

The population about which these inferences apply are not discussed, but the scope of inference depends on the manner in which the data were collected and other factors related to the comparability of these students with the entire entering class or of this university to others. The study of tables can be extended to tables with more than two rows and two columns as well as to sets of tables. Sets of tables frequently

Table 2-13   Frequency of Cigarette and Marijuana Use

Table of Cigarettes by Marijuana

Cigarettes Frequency Percent Row percent Col percent	Marijuana No	Yes	Total
No	175 58.33 87.5 74.47	25 8.33 12.5 38.46	200 66.67
Yes	60 20 60 25.53	40 13.33 40 61.54	100 33.33
Total	235 78.33	65 21.67	300 100

arise in multicenter studies in which one controls for center effect or through stratification (e.g., by gender or major). Cochran-Maentel-Haenszel methods are often used for sets of tables.

An immediate measure of the relationship between cigarette smoking and marijuana use can be made by testing whether the two categorical variables are statistically independent. The standard test is the chi-squared test (in this example chi square = 29.7; $p < 0.0001$). Based on the p value, the hypothesis of independence is rejected. This is equivalent to rejecting the hypothesis that the percentage of cigarette smokers that use marijuana is the same as the percentage of non–cigarette smokers that use marijuana. This conclusion, although interesting, is not as informative (useful) as risk estimates, which are discussed in the next section.

Risks, Relative Risks, and Odds Ratios

Is the risk of marijuana smoking the same for those who smoke cigarettes and those who do not? The (estimated) risk of marijuana smoking by those who do not smoke is 25/200 = 0.125 (12.5%) compared with 40/100 = 0.4 (40%) for cigarette smokers. Another measure of risk uses the notion of odds. In general, the odds of an event are the risk of the event divided by the probability the event does not occur; that is, odds = risk/(1 − risk). The odds of marijuana use in smokers is 0.4/0.6 = 0.67. Note that the odds are less than 1.0, which means there is less than a 50% chance the event (marijuana use) occurs. For those not smoking cigarettes the odds (in favor of) marijuana use are 0.125/0.875 = 0.143.

Two commonly used measures useful for comparing risks are relative risk (RR) and the odds ratio (OR). The former is much more intuitive but can be meaningfully calculated only under certain data collection circumstances (which is addressed in Chapter 3). The RR = 0.4/0.125 = 3.2. That is, the risk of marijuana use among smokers is 3.2 times greater than that of nonsmokers. A 95% CI for the RR is (2.06, 4.96); that is, the risk is between 2.06 times greater and 4.96 times greater for cigarette smokers. Because this CI does not contain 1, the RR is statistically significant at 5% level of significance. The OR = 0.67/0.143 = 4.667 (95% CI: 2.61, 8.33); that is, the odds of marijuana use among cigarette smokers are between 2.61 and 8.33 times greater with 95% confidence. Again, this CI does not contain 1, which means the result is statistically significant at the 5% level of significance.

It is worth pointing out here that the measures of relative risk (RR and OR) are best understood in the context of absolute risk. If the exposed are 30 times more likely to be diseased than the unexposed but the absolute disease risk is 1 per million (per year) for the unexposed, then how daunting is the exposure? This shortcoming of RR and OR as comparative measures is addressed in the next section by presenting additional measures.

Effect Measures Including Attributable Risk and Etiological Fraction

Does cigarette smoking cause marijuana smoking? This question makes a different impression than asking whether asbestos exposure causes cancer. Nevertheless, the first question raises the issue of causal effects. We have just finished comparing the risks of marijuana smoking for smokers and nonsmokers (compared the exposed with the nonexposed). Can we be certain that the differences in risk are attributable to exposure? "The ideal comparison would be of people with themselves in both an exposed and unexposed state" (Rothman, 2002, p. 45). This would be the counterfactual ideal. Instead, we settle with comparing the exposed and unexposed, believing that the two groups are identical apart from exposure (in some circumstances this can be investigated using statistical or other methods).

Define the risk difference as the difference between the risk for those with exposure and the risk for those without exposure (there is an analogous measure for rates). This requires that from data at hand one can estimate disease risk given exposure (more about this in Chapter 3 in which study design is discussed). Some epidemiologists call this quantity attributable risk. When discussing effects, there is not complete consistency among epidemiologists with regard to definitions. For the most part we either use or modify the terminology in Rothman (2002). The key idea is that attributable risk (risk difference) is the portion of the incidence of a disease in the exposed that is associated with (due to) the exposure. "It is the incidence of a disease *in the exposed* that would be eliminated if exposure were eliminated" (Kirch, 2008, p. 54). Attributable risk is sometimes referred to as excess risk. The attributable risk can be used to define the relative effect:

$$\text{Relative effect} = \frac{\text{RD}}{\text{risk in unexposed}} = \frac{\text{AR}}{\text{risk in unexposed}} = \text{RR} - 1$$

The right-hand part of the equation is the result of elementary algebra. In the cigarette exposure example the risk difference is $0.40 - 0.125 = 0.275$ and the relative effect is $0.275/0.125 = 2.2$, which is $\text{RR} - 1 = 3.2 - 1 = 2.2$. The rationale for this is that when there is no exposure effect the relative risk is 1; hence, subtracting the 1 makes it an incremental measure. Note that the above risk difference is a point estimate (that is, 0.275 is based on a sample); hence, one could construct a 95% CI estimate, which is 0.169 to 0.381 (or 16.9 per 100 to 38.1 per 100). This indicates considerable uncertainty regarding the true attributable risk based on this relatively small sample.

In addition to measuring the relative effect by dividing the risk difference by the risk in the nonexposed, one can calculate what is called the attributable risk fraction by dividing by the risk in the exposed. That is,

$$\text{Attributable fraction} = \frac{RD}{\text{risk in unexposed}} = \frac{AR}{\text{risk in exposed}} = \frac{RR - 1}{RR}$$

Again the right-hand expression is the result of elementary algebra. This fraction can be expressed as a percentage. In the cigarette exposure example the attributable fraction is 0.275/0.40 = 0.687, or 68.7%. Pushing this to its logical limits (achieved partly by assuming that all bias has been removed from differences between the exposed and unexposed groups), one can say that were cigarette smoking to end, the risk of marijuana smoking would be reduced from 40 per 100 to 12.5 per hundred in the exposed group, which is a 68.7% reduction. Be aware that there are a number of ways to express percentages. In our example the RR was 3.2 (the relative effect was 2.2), which corresponds to a 220% increase in risk (from 12.5 cases per 100 to 40 cases per 100, which is [(40 − 12.5)/12.5] × 100% = 220%).

The population attributable risk is the portion of the incidence of a disease in the population (exposed plus unexposed) that is a result of exposure. It is the incidence of a disease in the population that would be eliminated if exposure were eliminated. Hence, population attributable risk equals the disease incidence in the population minus the disease incidence in the unexposed. Note that the comparison is being made to the existing pattern of exposure. For the cigarette example the incidence of marijuana smoking in the population is 65/300 = 0.217 (21.7%). Hence, population attributable risk = 0.217 − 0.125 = 0.092. That is, were cigarette smoking to end, marijuana smoking would be reduced by 9.2 per 100 students. The population attributable risk fraction is found by dividing population attributable risk by the population incidence, which in this example is 0.092/0.217 = 0.423. This can be expressed as a percentage; that is, cessation of cigarette smoking would lead to a 42.3% reduction in the incidence of marijuana smoking in the student population (from 21.7 per 100 to 12.5 per 100). The comparison (denominator) is to the existing exposure–disease relationship.

Let's return to the question: Does cigarette smoking cause marijuana smoking in university students or some appropriate population? Until now we have seen that it appears to play a role. One might ask whether it preceded marijuana use. One might even have some theory or even biological evidence to back up such an assertion. Instead, we rely on a purely epidemiological approach by defining the etiological fraction (EF) as the proportion of the cases in which the exposure played a causal role in its development. That is,

$$EF = \frac{N_{ED} - N_{UD}}{N_{ED}}$$

In the above equation N_{ED} is the number of exposed persons in the population that are diseased and N_{UD} is the number of unexposed persons in the population that are diseased. If one were estimating EF based on the data in Table 2-13, then

$$EF = \frac{N_{ED} - N_{UD}}{N_{ED}} = \frac{40 - 25}{40} = 0.375$$

In the preceding equation, EF is an estimate and the Ns are observed counts.

Regression Modeling

Regression modeling has to do with building models to describe a phenomenon. In this chapter we consider only models for which there is a single response variable (sometimes called the dependent variable); models of this type are called univariate (whereas models with more than one response variable are multivariate). Typically, the modeler "fits" a function that explains the response. This function is typically a mathematical expression involving one or more explanatory (predictor) variables. One way to look at this is to think of the response as the left-hand side of an equation and the predictors as being on the right-hand side. In the case in which there is a single explanatory variable, the model is called "simple," and when there is more than one explanatory variable, the model is referred to as a multiple regression model. The function can take many forms, but the linear model is the most commonly used, where "linear" allows for various transformations of the explanatory variables to appear (such as quadratics or square roots).

Linear regression has been extensively studied. What distinguishes statistical models from mathematical models is the inclusion of stochastic properties in the model relationship. The nature of the stochastic component in the model influences how the model is fit, where fitting usually refers to estimating the parameters in the model. Often, these parameters include model coefficients in the function form.

The level of measurement of the response variable is typically used to describe the form of regression model one is using. In the case in which y is an interval continuous variable (or approximately so), standard regression modeling is used. For example, the response might be systolic blood pressure (SBP) in obese patients. In the case in which y is dichotomous (or ordinal), one can adopt logistic regression methods. For example, the response might be A1c in control versus A1c not in control. When dealing with counts data, one can use Poisson regression (although there are other choices), which can be described as various generalized linear models. For example, the response might be emergency department visits during the last 6 months by asthmatic children.

Linear Models With an Interval Continuous Response

A linear regression model has the form

$$y = \beta_0 + \beta_1 x_1 + \beta_2 x_2 + \cdots + \beta_k x_k + \epsilon$$

The response is y, the explanatory variables are x (of which there are k), the betas are the coefficients, and epsilon is the random error term. The random error term is intended to capture the effects of variables not in the model—these often include idiosyncratic characteristics of patients as well as variables either not considered by the investigator or not available to the investigator. The nature of the random error term affects inference and model fitting (this refers to estimating the betas as well as estimating parameters associated with the random error such as its variance). The mechanics and theory of fitting regression models is not our concern here. Computer packages are now used to fit models regardless of the method used. Once the model has been fit, the betas are replaced with numerical estimates and one may "predict" y by "plugging in" values for x. The betas are slope parameters and their estimates determine the linear change in y associated with changes in an x. For example, a fitted model might be

$$y = 140 + 3x_1 - 8x_2$$

Such an equation is often referred to as a regression equation. Suppose this model is used to predict SBP in obese individuals. The first predictor is the amount by which body mass index (BMI) exceeds 30 and the second predictor is gender (male = 0 and female = 1). The latter is called a dummy or indicator variable. Then the predicted SBP for a male with a BMI of 30 is 140. For each one unit increase in BMI, the expected SBP increases by three units. On average SBP is eight units lower for females. In this model the effect of BMI is independent of gender. In a model in which these factors interact, the slope coefficient for BMI would be different for males and females. Geometrically, this regression equation can be represented as two parallel lines (one for males and one for females). If there was an interaction, the lines would not be parallel.

One can construct CIs for the slope coefficients. If a CI does not contain 0, then the corresponding predictor is significant. In the final model typically only significant variables are included. The overall fit of the model can be assessed in several ways. The typical method for reporting effect size in regression is R^2. Higher values (as one approaches from below 1, the maximum value for R^2) indicate a greater effect size. Given a fitted model, inferences about a particular coefficient depend on the other variables in the model. A regression model can have several uses, including prediction, establishment of association (e.g., for the population under study gender and BMI are related to SBP), and assertions about the exact nature of relationship (for each unit increase in BMI one can expect a three-unit increase in SBP).

With respect to prediction there are two general types: One can estimate the average value for y given values for the predictors, or one can predict the value of y given values for the predictors. The point estimates are the same in either case, but the interval estimates differ. Prediction intervals (the second case) are wider than CIs for the average value of y. Consider the SBP model. Given a female with a BMI of 36, the predicted SBP is $140 + 3(6) - 8(1) = 150$. If a patient enters a clinic and one wishes to guess this patient's SBP, then one needs a prediction interval (note that this is not an interval for the actual SBP reading but the patient's true SBP). If one wishes to guess the average SBP in a large group of female persons with BMIs of 136, then one should use a CI.

Logistic Regression

Only dichotomous logistic regression is discussed. The basic idea is that the response can take on only two values, such as lived/died or blood sugar under 110 versus not under 110. Usually, interest is in estimating probabilities and odds ratios as well as identifying variables associated with occurrence of the event of interest. A dichotomous outcome can be coded (e.g., 0 and 1), but fitting a standard regression model to the data with the hope of using the regression equation to predict probabilities of particular outcomes in unlikely to be satisfactory because predicted values outside the interval [0, 1] may occur. There are also other problems associated with this approach.

The previous example concerning the relationship between cigarette smoking and marijuana use was based on a 2×2 table. Data of that type (and any 2×k table) can be analyzed using logistic regression; however, the main benefits of logistic modeling are that one can conveniently include more than one predictor and in addition one can use interval/continuous predictors without explicitly converting them to categorical variables.

The idea behind dichotomous logistic regression is to model the log odds of the event of interest. Let p be the probability of the event of interest (e.g., patient has a stroke). Hence, one fits a model of the form

$$\text{log odds(event)} = \log\left(\frac{p}{1-p}\right) = \beta_0 + \beta_1 x_1 + \beta_2 x_2 + \cdots + b_k x_k$$

Having fit the model, one can recover estimates for p by exponentiating the result (raising the log odds to the power e), which produces an estimate of the odds of the event. Then $p = 1/(1 + \text{odds})$. Fortunately, computer packages can perform these computations.

Suppose the data for the study relating cigarette smoking and marijuana use can be stratified by gender (**Table 2-14**). Fitting a main effects logistic regression model with gender and cigarette smoking as predictors (these are main effects) showed that gender was not significant; however, fitting a model with the interaction between gender and cigarette smoking showed that the interaction was significant. **Table 2-15** contains parameter estimates for the logistic model. Cigarettes ($p < 0.0001$) and the cigarettes gender (cigarettes × gender) interaction ($p < 0.0001$) are significant. Gender alone was not ($p = 0.2379$) but was left in the model because the interaction was in-

Table 2-14	Frequency of Cigarette and Marijuana Use Based on Gender		
Cigarettes	**Marijuana**	**Gender**	**Count**
Yes	Yes	M	10
Yes	Yes	F	30
Yes	No	M	30
Yes	No	F	30
No	Yes	F	12
No	Yes	M	13
No	No	M	75
No	No	F	100

Table 2-15 Logistic Regression: Analysis of Maximum Likelihood Estimates

Parameter		df	Estimate	Standard Error	Wald Chi-Square	$p > \chi^2$
Intercept		1	−1.2428	0.1548	64.4298	<0.0001
Cigarettes	No	1	−0.6935	0.1548	20.0627	<0.0001
Gender	F	1	0.1827	0.1548	1.3929	0.2379
Cigarettes × gender	No × F	1	−0.3666	0.1548	5.6049	0.0179

cluded (this is a matter of taste). **Figure 2-11** shows the predicted probabilities (risks of marijuana use on the vertical axis) from which one can see the nature of the interaction. Cigarette smoking in females is associated with a much higher marijuana use risk.

With logistic modeling one can use any mixture of interval and categorical predictors. Consider a variant of the bedsore analysis based on data from another nursing facility in which through a retrospective chart review data were collected on the incidence of bedsores during a 1-year period. Included in the data collected were age of the patient at diagnosis and whether the patient was diabetic. Data on 50 patients were collected (19 with bedsores) of which 22 were diabetic (**Table 2-16**). To investi-

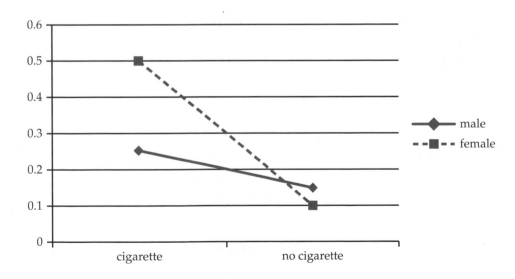

FIGURE 2-11 Predicted probabilities of marijuana and cigarette use.

Table 2-16   Frequency of Bedsores Based on Diabetes

Diagnosis/Statistic	Bedsores		Total
	Present	Not Present	
Diabetic			
Frequency	16	6	22
Percent	32	12	44
Row percent	72.73	27.27	
Column percent	84.21	19.35	
Not diabetic			
Frequency	3	25	28
Percent	6	50	56
Row percent	10.71	89.29	
Column percent	15.79	80.65	
Total	19	31	50
Percent of total	38	62	100

gate the relationship between bedsores and age as well as a diagnosis of diabetes, a logistic regression model was fitted. **Table 2-17** shows the coefficient estimates, from which one can see that both age ($p = 0.0056$) and diabetes ($p = 0.0007$) are significant. **Table 2-18** contains estimated ORs as well as CIs for them. Neither CI contains 1 (which would indicate no relationship), and the intervals are positive. The odds of bedsores are 263 times greater for diabetics (while accounting for age). Compare this with the OR of $22.2 = (16 \times 25)/(3 \times 6)$ from Table 2-16. The total picture is most easily portrayed in **Figure 2-12**, which contains the graphs of the estimated probability of bedsores for the two disease groups.

Table 2-17   Coefficient Estimates: Analysis of Maximum Likelihood Estimates

Parameter	Diabetes Present	df	Estimate	Standard Error	Wald Chi-Square	$p > \chi^2$
Intercept		1	−17.5	6.2318	7.9341	0.0049
Age		1	0.273	0.0986	7.666	0.0056
Diabetic diagnosis	Diabetic	1	2.768	0.812	11.6198	0.0007

Table 2-18 Odds Ratio Estimates			
Effect	**Point Estimate**	**95% Wald Confidence Limits**	
Age	1.314	1.083	1.594
Diabetic vs. not diabetic	253.68	10.517	>999.9

SUMMARY OF EPIDEMIOLOGICAL MEASURES OF DISEASE RISK

Table 2-19 is a general 2×2 table that can be used to estimate epidemiological parameters. The body of the table contains observed counts (e.g., n_{ED} is the number of exposed persons for whom the event [disease] occurred and n_{Ed} is the number of exposed persons for whom the event did not occur). The edges contain sums, all of which are sample values (e.g., N_E is the number of person in the sample that suffered exposure). **Table 2-20** shows via formulas the estimators (and in effect the definitions of the risk measures being described). Underlying this is some population from which this sample was collected. The implicit assumption is that the design (see Chapter 3) was such that the parameters in the table are estimable. To avoid unnecessary complications, symbols for the parameters are not given.

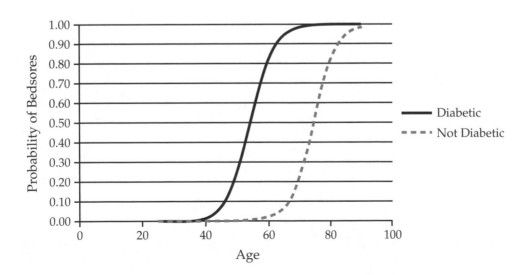

FIGURE 2-12   Estimated probability of bedsores for two disease groups.

Table 2-19   Exposed and Nonexposed Calculations

	Event (D)	No Event (d)	
Exposed	n_{ED}	n_{Ed}	$N_E = n_{ED} + n_{Ed}$
Unexposed	n_{UD}	n_{Ud}	$N_U = n_{UD} + n_{Ud}$
	$N_D = n_{ED} + n_{UD}$	$N_d = n_{Ed} + n_{UD}$	N

Table 2-20   Formulas

Parameter	Parameter Description	Estimator (formula)
r_E	Incidence (risk) of disease in exposed	n_{ED}/N_E
r_U	Incidence (risk) of disease in unexposed	n_{UD}/N_U
RR	Relative risk	r_E/r_U
OR	Odds ratio	$$\frac{r_E}{1-r_E} \Big/ \frac{r_U}{1-r_U}$$
AR	Attributable risk	$r_E - r_U$
ARF	Attributable risk fraction	$(r_E - r_U)/r_E$
PPE	Proportion of population exposed	N_E/N
r_P	Incidence (risk) of disease in population	N_D/N
PAR	Population attributable risk	$r_P - r_U$
PAF	Population attributable risk fraction	$(r_P - r_U)/r_P$
EF	Etiological fraction	$(n_{ED} - n_{UD})/n_{ED}$

Vital Statistics

Statistics of birth, death, marriage, and divorce rates in a community can be calculated by using the following formulas.

Crude birth rate is defined as number of live births per 1,000 population.

$$\text{Crude birth rate} = \frac{\text{number of births}}{\text{estimated midyear population}} \times 1,000$$

Crude death rate is defined as number of deaths per 1,000 population.

$$\text{Crude death rate} = \frac{\text{number of deaths}}{\text{estimated midyear population}} \times 1,000$$

Crude divorce rate is defined as number of divorces per 1,000 population.

$$\text{Crude divorce rate} = \frac{\text{number of divorces}}{\text{estimated midyear population}} \times 1,000$$

Crude marriage rate is defined as number of marriages per 1,000 population.

$$\text{Crude marriage rate} = \frac{\text{number of marriages}}{\text{estimated midyear population}} \times 1,000$$

Fetal death rate is defined as number of fetal deaths (20 weeks or more gestation) per 1,000 live births plus fetal deaths.

$$\text{Fetal death rate} = \frac{\text{number of fetal deaths (20 + Weeks Gestation)}}{\text{number of live births} + \text{number of fetal deaths}} \times 1,000$$

Fertility rate is defined as the total number of births in a year per 1,000 female population aged between 15 and 44 years

$$\text{Fertility rate} = \frac{\text{number of live births}}{\text{estimated midyear female population aged between 15–44 yrs}} \times 1,000$$

Infant mortality rate is defined as deaths to individuals less than one year old per 1,000 live births.

$$\text{Infant mortality rate} = \frac{\text{number of infants deaths}}{\text{number of live births}} \times 1,000$$

Maternal mortality rate is defined as the number of deaths as a result of complications of pregnancy, childbirth, abortion, or the puerperium per 10,000 live births.

$$\text{Maternal mortality rate} = \frac{\text{number of maternal deaths}}{\text{number of live births}} \times 10,000$$

Neonatal mortality rate is defined as deaths to individuals less than 28 days old per 1,000 live births

$$\text{Neonatal mortality rate} = \frac{\text{number of deaths} < 28 \text{ days}}{\text{number of live births}} \times 1,000$$

Perinatal mortality rate is defined as fetal deaths (20 weeks or more gestation) plus neonatal deaths (occurring in the first 27 days of life) per 1,000 live births plus fetal deaths.

$$\text{Perinatal mortality rate} = \frac{\text{number of fetal deaths} + \text{number of neonatal deaths}}{\text{number of fetal deaths} + \text{number of live births}} \times 1,000$$

Graphical Representation of Data

The data can be organized in the form of two-dimensional graphs. These visuals feed information faster and conserve readers' time and energy. To create these data graphs one can use Microsoft excel, PASW (SPSS), SAS, and many other statistical packages available in the market.

The following are examples:

- The following are comparative histograms with superimposed normal curves. The histogram was generated using SAS, version 9.1 The vertical axis in each case represents the relative frequency (percent) for age at diagnosis. The data have been stratified by race (AA = African American; Not AA = not African American). Summary statistics are in the upper left-hand corner. Note that the age at diagnosis is lower for African Americans; however, the variability is about the same.

Comparative Analysis of Age at Diagnosis With Superimposed Normal Curve

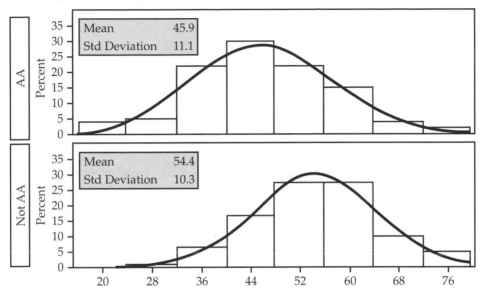

Age at Diagnosis of Type II Diabetes

- The following is a bar chart created from gender (1 = male; 2 = female) percentage values involved in a study.

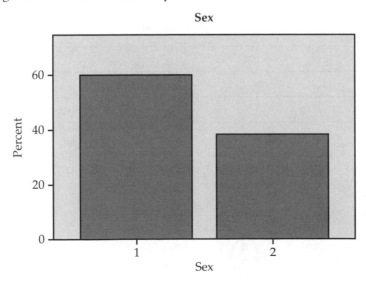

- These are cases at an urban clinic for a one month period. The table has cases and the pie chart has percentages.

Stage	Cases
Stage 0	22
Stage I	14
Stage II	12
Stage III	8
Stage IV	6

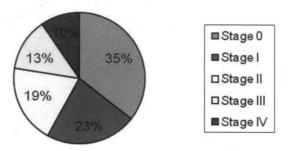

- The following line graph was created based on 10-year incidence rates of campylobacteriosis.

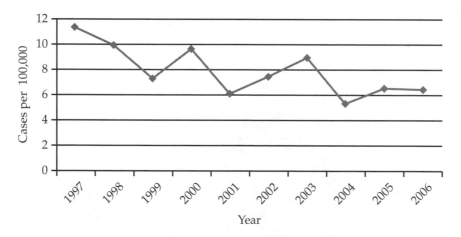

- The following is an example of a geographical information system software output file. Health data based on zip codes, counties, and states can be shown in maps.

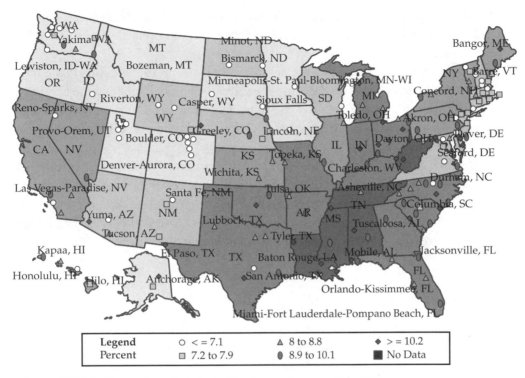

Legend	○	< = 7.1	▲	8 to 8.8	◆	> = 10.2
Percent	□	7.2 to 7.9	●	8.9 to 10.1	■	No Data

Source: CDC, http://www.cdc.gov/brfss/index.htm; Accessed on June 10th, 2010.

- P-P plots, Q-Q plots, and scatter plots already shown in the chapter are graphical tools for analyzing and presenting data.

KEY POINTS

- Epidemiology is concerned with disease. A common focus is on the relationship between exposure and disease where exposure can be taken to have quite a broad meaning.
- Almost all epidemiological data, especially data arising in clinical epidemiology, are samples.
- Samples can be described using graphical as well as summary measures. The level of measurement of data influences methods of presentation and analysis.
- Inference, drawing conclusions about populations based on samples and statistical theory, consists of estimation, hypothesis testing, and modeling. Estimation is fundamental, and interval estimates are almost always more useful than tests.

- All inference is subject to error associated with sampling. Regarding a particular decision concerning a statistical test, one never knows whether an error has occurred.
- Key epidemiological measures of disease risk are prevalence, incidence fraction, and incidence rate. Rates are measured in units of person-time exposure. Although rates are frequently thought of as more accurate measures of risk, they are more difficult to interpret and effectively communicate than risk measured by a proportion.
- Relationships between exposure and disease can be statistically analyzed (modeled) using an assortment of tools including (but certainly not limited to) CIs, prediction intervals, tolerance intervals, parametric tests (such as t-tests, chi-squared tests, ANOM, and analysis of variance), survival curves, 2×2 tables, and regression modeling (including logistic regression).

CRITICAL QUESTIONS

1. Why and in what manner are CI estimates superior to point estimates?
2. Suppose that a 95% CI for the odds ratio for a disease event given exposure compared with nonexposure is (0.95, 3.53). What does this tell you about the risk associated with exposure? What does this tell you about a formal statistical test of the hypothesis that the OR is 1.0 (at what level of significance?). Suppose a 90% CI is (1.05, 3.17).
3. Suppose a researcher is interested in SBP in a population of individuals in high stress jobs and takes SBP readings from 100 subjects selected from the population. What would be more useful: a 95% CI estimate for the mean SBP or a 95% tolerance interval estimate for 90% of the population? In the first case, what would the lower end point of the interval tell you? In the second case, what would the lower end point of the interval tell you?
4. In what circumstance is logistic regression modeling most useful in assessing the relationship between exposure and disease? Consider the level of measurement of the predictors and the number of predictors in your answer.
5. What are the consequences of ignoring (or being unaware of) interaction between exposure and some demographic characteristic (or between two exposures) in modeling the relationship between exposure and disease (or behavior)? Examine this question by constructing an example on which you can perform mind experiments associated with different scenarios such as synergistic interaction, antagonistic interaction, and no interaction.

6. In judging risky behavior, which is more informative: relative risk or attributable risk? Think of this in terms of making a decision yourself or advising someone considering engaging in risky behavior.

REFERENCES

Cantor, A. (1997). *Extending SAS® survival analysis techniques for medical research*. Cary, NC: SAS Institute.

Cohen, J. (1992). A power primer. *Psychological Bulletin, 112*, 155–159.

Dean, A. G., Sullican, K. M., & Soe, M. M. (updates 2009/2005). *OpenEpi: Open source epidemiologic statistics for public health*. Retrieved from http://www.OpenEpi.com

Dorak, M. T. (updated April 2010). *Common concepts in statistics*. Retrieved from http://www.Dorak.info/mtd/glosstat.html

Kirch, W. (Ed.). (2008). *Encyclopedia of public health*. Danvers, MA: Springer.

Nelson, P. R., Wludyka, P. S., & Copeland, A. F. (2005). *The analysis of means: A graphical method for comparing means, rates, and proportions*. SIAM, Philadelphia, ASA, Alexandria, VA: ASA-SIAM Series on Statistics and Applied Probability.

Petrie, A., & Sabin, C. (2009). *Medical statistics at a glance*. Chichester, UK: John Wiley & Sons.

Rothman, K. J. (2002). *Epidemiology: An introduction*. New York: Oxford University Press.

Selvin, S. (2004). *Statistical analysis of epidemiological data*. New York: Oxford University Press.

van Belle, G., Fisher, L. D., Heagerty, P. J., & Lumley, T. (2004). *Biostatistics: A methodology for the health sciences*. Hoboken, NJ: John Wiley & Sons.

CHAPTER 3

Study Designs and Their Outcomes

"Natural selection is a mechanism for generating an exceedingly high degree of improbability."
—Sir Ronald Aylmer Fisher

Peter Wludyka

OBJECTIVES

- Define research design, research study, and research protocol.
- Identify the major features of a research study.
- Identify the four types of designs discussed in this chapter.
- Describe nonexperimental designs, including cohort, case-control, and cross-sectional studies.
- Describe the types of epidemiological parameters that can be estimated with exposed cohort, case-control, and cross-sectional studies along with the role, appropriateness, and interpretation of relative risk and odds ratios in the context of design choice.
- Define true experimental design and describe its role in assessing cause-and-effect relationships along with definitions of and discussion of the role of internal and external validity in evaluating designs.
- Describe commonly used experimental designs, including randomized controlled trials (RCTs), after-only (post-test only) designs, the Solomon four-group design, crossover designs, and factorial designs.
- Define quasi-experimental design and compare it with true experimental design with respect to validity and assessing causal relationships.
- Describe commonly used quasi-experimental designs, including nonequivalent control group design, after-only nonequivalent control group design, and single-group designs.
- Describe repeated measures designs and how they might naturally be used.

INTRODUCTION

Most of science can be described as efforts to describe some process or phenomenon or as efforts to discover relationships among entities in the physical world. Particular goal-oriented scientific activities are often called studies. This chapter is concerned with study design, which is used interchangeably with research design or, when appropriate, experimental design. The design arises from (or is structured to fit) the objectives of the study, which is a set of activities undertaken to answer some research question. The idea is rather primitive and hard to define precisely but is typically an attempt to gain understanding about some process or phenomenon. "Research design provides the glue that holds the research project together. A design is used to structure the research, to show how all of the major parts of the research project—the samples or groups, measures, treatments or programs, and methods of assignment—work together to try to address the central research questions" (Trochim, 2006).

There are many different types of studies with many different purposes. The studies we are interested in concern disease (used very broadly) and its relationship to exposure (again used very broadly). Most studies we are interested in have the following properties:

- A study is conducted to answer some research question.
- The studies we are interested in involve observation (recording, measuring, and such).
- Often, a rather general statement of the research question is turned into a precise statement.
- The research question usually involves the "measurement" of one or more outcomes/responses. Generically, one may denote this as y, which can stand for a single outcome measurement (one variable) or several (more than one variable).
- Typically, other variables are "measured" either at the same time or before measurements of y. Let's use x to stand for these. Note that x might be something as simple as a dichotomous variable that identifies treatment subjects and control subjects.
- Usually, the researcher is interested in the relationship between x and y.

Studies can be described by their features such as randomization, type and degree of control, blinding, timing, whether manipulation or an intervention takes place, as well as the nature of the associated statistical analysis plan.

The study protocol is a detailed description of what will be done and how it will be accomplished. A statistical (data) analysis plan usually accompanies a protocol. For a particular study the protocol and the embedded data analysis plan may be quite detailed. In this chapter, and consistent with usual practice, a design is a more abstract notion and the phrase "study design" is typically used to describe a study with respect to its major aspects in a manner that is often independent of a specific study. That is, design is often a shorthand description of a study that is generic in that many very different studies with very different purposes can be described as having the same design. This approach allows certain commonly used designs to have names and also allows for discussion of strengths and weaknesses of particular designs (or aspects of designs) often with respect to validity (a subject with many forms and aspects discussed later is this chapter).

The design taxonomy in this chapter divides designs into nonexperimental, experimental, quasi-experimental designs, and time series (repeated-measures) designs. A rather detailed list and description of experimental and quasi-experimental designs appears in Garson (2010). A discussion of nonexperimental designs appears in Rothman (2002).

NONEXPERIMENTAL DESIGNS

Nonexperimental designs are missing some or all of the features associated with experimental designs, namely

- Manipulation or an intervention
- Randomization
- Control

More will be said about this later in this chapter. Nonexperimental designs can lead to useful information, and certain conclusions can be drawn from data arising from these designs. Causality is difficult to demonstrate with these designs; that is, typically one has to settle for statements regarding association. Importantly, there are circumstances in which experimental designs are not appropriate (typically for ethical reasons) or impossible. Long-term studies that span several years or decades are difficult to arrange as experimental studies.

Cohort

In epidemiology a cohort is any group of individuals sharing a common characteristic and observed over time. There is no randomization and no intervention (manipulation) has occurred. Measuring disease within one or more cohorts is the goal of cohort analysis. Characteristic(s) defining the cohort may be ethnic, exposure, geographical, or almost anything that creates a grouping of value in studying disease distribution and occurrence. This is seldom as easy as it appears, especially for large cohorts. Typical complications (questions to be addressed) are as follows:

- Who should be followed?
- What counts as a disease occurrence?
- How are incidence (rates and risks) and prevalence measured?
- What constitutes exposure?

The diagram in **Figure 3-1** displays the structure of a cohort design. In this general case the defined population is independent of exposure. That is, selection took place before any of its members became exposed or before their exposures were identified. In a study of this type many exposures can be studied simultaneously. In addition, for many of the subjects in the study precedence relationships can be established (e.g., did exposure to tobacco occur before the occurrence of chronic obstructive pulmonary disease?).

A cohort study can be retrospective (e.g., the study covers 20 years: the researchers begin in 2010, but the subjects in the study are studied beginning in 1990). This type of study might consist of chart data, public records, or whatever sources of data are available. A cohort study may be concurrent (prospective); for example, it may commence in 2010 and consist of newborn babies in a rural hospital with the plan of studying the subjects until they are 12 years old. If this cohort consists of babies born only in 2010, then it is a closed cohort. If the researchers plan to continue to "enroll" babies over the course of the study, then the cohort is open. Several famous cohort studies were geographically defined (e.g., the still ongoing Framingham Heart Study [Shindler, 2010]). Cohort studies can be retrospective, concurrent, or a combination of these. In cohort studies there is often interest in what can be called the "cohort effect." In this context one might be thinking of a complete cohort study as consisting of cohorts as defined typically by the period during which subjects were born, such as decades.

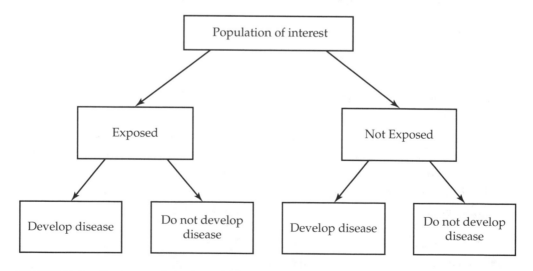

FIGURE 3-1   Structure of a cohort design.

Exposed Cohort

An exposed cohort is one in which exposure is the basis for selection (**Figure 3-2**). For example, exposure might be "parent smokes" and the disease of interest might be "child develops asthma." In this type design one might simultaneously study several diseases (or other attributes of the children of smokers). Furthermore, data may be collected on demographics, actual smoking behavior (e.g., "always smoke outside the house"), or other variables of interest. In a cohort study of this type, the subjects in the study are observed over time. Deciding how and at what particular times observation is made are critical issues. Loss to follow-up can also be a critical issue.

Data of any level of measurement (see Chapter 2) can be recorded and analyzed. In epidemiological studies counts are frequently of interest. **Table 3-1** shows how counts data from an exposed cohort study can be arranged in a 2×2 table in which the rows are exposure versus no exposure and the columns are disease versus no disease (in place of disease one could have any well-defined event, such as for example "death prior to age 50"). Note that a, b, c, and d represent counts in which a is the number of those who were exposed and in whom the disease appeared. In a table of this type $n = a + b + c + d =$ the total number of subjects. The key is that in an exposed cohort study the researcher determines the number exposed ($a + b$) and the number with no exposure ($c + d$). For example, suppose that 30 subjects with exposure were selected and 170 with no exposure were selected. What can be estimated from the 2×2 embedded in Table 3-1 that is identified as sample 1 (in which $n = 200$)? One can clearly estimate proportions from the data present (that is, incidence or prevalence proportions). If one wanted to estimate rates, then a different measure of exposure would be needed. For now let's focus on proportions.

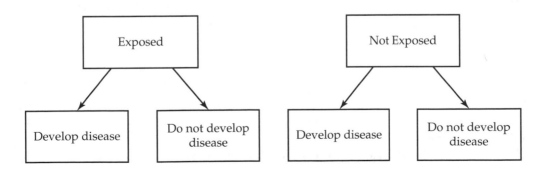

FIGURE 3-2   Exposed and nonexposed groups.

Table 3-1   Calculations

		Observed Counts and Proportions			
		Disease	No Disease	sum	prop
Exposure		a	b	$(a + b)$	$a/(a + b)$
No exposure		c	d	$(c + d)$	$c/(c + d)$
	sum	$a + c$	$b + d$	n	
	prop	$a/(a + c)$	$b/(b + d)$		

		Sample Size 1			
		Disease	No Disease	row sum	
Exposure		20	10	30	**0.67**
No exposure		80	90	170	**0.47**
	sum	100	100	200	
	prop	0.2	0.1		

		Sample Size 2			
		Disease	No Disease	row sum	
Exposure		20	10	30	**0.67**
No exposure		160	180	340	**0.47**
	sum	180	190	370	
	prop	0.11	0.04		

Without loss of generality in the example, the proportions are referred to as prevalence. Consider the following hypothetical study. A nurse researcher selects 30 children about whom it is known that a parent smokes and 170 who do not have a parent who smokes. The children are selected from a pediatric clinic in an urban hospital. Over the course of 1 year episodes of colds or respiratory infection are recorded for the children, and each child is classified as having had an episode defined in this manner (disease) or not (no disease). Data from the study are shown in Table 3-1 (under sample size 1). The researcher can estimate the prevalence of disease given exposure, which is $a/(a + b) = 20/30 = 0.67$, as well as the prevalence given no exposure (0.47). Hence, the relative risk can be estimated, which is $0.67/0.47 = 1.42$ (see more about this subsequently). But the researcher cannot estimate the prevalence of exposure given disease, $a/(a + c)$, because just increasing the number of subjects in the no exposure group (which is 170 in sample size 1 and 340 in sample size 2) can alter the estimate from $20/100 = 0.2$ to $20/180 = 0.11$. Note that the estimate for disease given exposure is invariant (because the difference between sample 1 and sample 2 is that in sample 2 the number with no exposure has been doubled, keeping the risk of disease fixed). Typically, this would be summed up by saying that, based on data from an exposed cohort study, prevalence can be estimated. That means that parameters derived from risk estimates can be estimated, including attributable risk (see Table 2-19 and the section **Analysis of 2×2 Tables** in Chapter 2, which includes a definition and discussion of attributable risk in subsection Effect Measures Including Attributable Risk and Etiological Fraction) as well as population attributable risk. As a caution, one should not interpret Table 3-1 to mean that, with the proportionate increase in exposure or nonexposure, sample values would be identical. The exercise is strictly theoretical.

Case-Control

In a case-control study the researcher selects cases and a corresponding set of subjects as control subjects (for a thorough discussion see Schlesselman, 1982). The manner in which the control subjects are selected is important with respect to interpretation and method of analysis. There is no generally agreed-on method for selecting control subjects, and the purposes of the study impact the choice mechanism. Broadly, there is group matching and forms of case matching (with one or more control subjects matched to each case). **Figure 3-3** displays the choice mechanism. The key point is that cases are selected and then exposure is determined; this is performed similarly for control subjects.

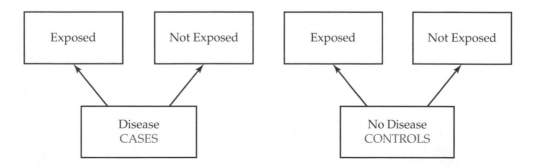

FIGURE 3-3 Case-control study design.

Table 3-2 shows the arrangement of a case-control study into a 2×2 table. The definitions are identical to those that apply to Table 3-1. The key idea is that the column sums are fixed (i.e., chosen by the researcher) because the researcher chooses the number of cases and the number of control subjects. The difference between sample 1 and sample 2 is that sample 2 has five times as many control subjects (but the underlying distribution of the control subjects between those exposed and those with no exposure is the same for both samples).

Fixing the column totals implies that one can estimate the prevalence of exposure given disease, which is $a/(a + c)$. Similarly, one can estimate the prevalence of exposure given no disease. The flip side is that one cannot estimate prevalence of disease given exposure, which is $a/(a + b)$, because just increasing the number of subjects in the no disease group can alter the estimate from 0.67 in sample 1 to 0.29 in sample 2. Hence, one cannot directly estimate relative risk. That means parameters derived from risk

Table 3-2	**Formulas and Calculations**				
		Case-Control Design: a + c fixed; b + d fixed			
		Disease	**No Disease**	**row sum**	**prop**
Exposure		a	b	$(a + b)$	$a/(a + b)$
No exposure		c	d	$(c + d)$	$c/(c + d)$
	sum	$a + c$	$b + d$	n	
	prop	$a/(a + c)$	$b/(b + d)$		
		Sample Size 1			
		Disease	**No Disease**	**row sum**	
Exposure		20	10	30	**0.67**
No exposure		80	90	170	**0.47**
	sum	100	100	200	
	prop	0.2	0.1		
		Sample Size 2			
		Disease	**No Disease**	**row sum**	
Exposure		20	50	70	**0.29**
No exposure		80	450	530	**0.15**
	sum	100	500	600	
	prop	0.2	0.1		

estimates, including attributable risk, cannot be estimated, directly from case-control data; that is, data/estimates from other sources must be found. An alternative measure is the odds ratio. This can be estimated with case-control data and will be discussed subsequently in the Odds Ratios section.

Cross-Sectional

A cross-sectional study is a snapshot based on a sample of size n—that is, the numbers of diseased or exposed subjects is determined by chance within the context of characteristics of the population. The schematic in **Figure 3-4** displays how it works. The key idea is data on exposure and disease are gathered simultaneously. Hence, all that can be concluded from such data is association. However, because neither the row sums (exposures) nor column sums (disease counts) are fixed (predetermined by the researcher) one can estimate both the prevalence of disease given exposure and the prevalence of exposure given disease (**Table 3-3**). The difference between sample 1 and sample 2 is n has been doubled. The cell counts are increased proportionately. The fact that risk of disease given exposure can be estimated means that parameters derived from risk estimates can be estimated, including attributable risk as well as population attributable risk.

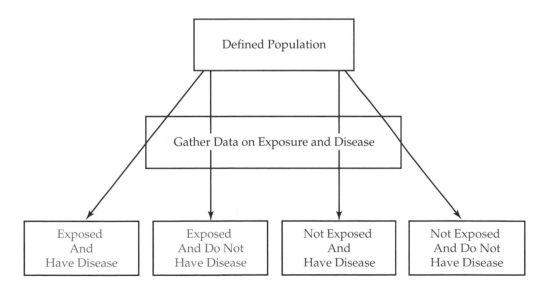

FIGURE 3-4   Cross-sectional study.

Table 3-3	Cross-Sectional Study				
Cross-Sectional Study: $n = a + b + c + d$ **is fixed**					
		Disease	**No Disease**	**row sum**	**prop**
Exposure		a	b	$(a + b)$	$a/(a + b)$
No exposure		c	d	$(c + d)$	$c/(c + d)$
	sum	$a + c$	$b + d$	n	
	prop	$a/(a + c)$	$b/(b + d)$		
Sample Size 1					
		Disease	**No Disease**	**row sum**	
Exposure		20	10	30	0.67
No exposure		80	90	170	0.47
	sum	100	100	200	
	prop	0.2	0.1		
Sample Size 2					
		Disease	**No Disease**	**row sum**	
Exposure		40	20	60	0.67
No exposure		160	180	340	0.47
	sum	200	200	400	
	prop	0.2	0.1		

Odds Ratios

Whether the data arise from an exposed cohort study, a case-control study, or a cross-sectional study, the association between exposure and disease can be measured using an odds ratio, and in each case the calculations are the same. Consider first the exposed cohort (Table 3-1). The risk of disease given exposure is equal to $a/(a + b)$. The odds are defined as risk/(1 − risk). Hence, the odds that an exposed person develops disease are

$$\frac{a / (a + b)}{b / (a + b)} = a / b$$

The odds that a nonexposed person develops disease are

$$\frac{c/(c+d)}{d/(c+d)} = c/d$$

Hence, the odds ratio (odds of disease in exposed divided by odds of disease in nonexposed) is

$$\frac{a/(a+b)}{b/(a+b)} \sqrt{\frac{c/(c+d)}{d/(c+d)}} = \frac{a/(a+b)}{b/(a+b)} \times \frac{d/(c+d)}{c/(c+d)} = \frac{a}{b} \times \frac{d}{c} = \frac{ad}{bc}$$

Using the counts in Table 3-1 for sample size 1 yields the following:

1. Odds of disease given exposure = a/b = 20/10 = 2.0
2. Odds of disease in the nonexposed = c/d = 80/90 = 0.89
3. Odds ratio = 2.0/0.89 = 2.25 or more directly ad/cb = (20 × 90)/(80 × 10) = 2.25

Using the smoking example, the following is found:

1. For children with a parent who smokes, the odds of developing colds or respiratory infection are two times the odds of not developing colds or respiratory infection. The fact that the odds are greater than 1 means that the event (colds or respiratory infection) is more likely than the nonevent (no colds or respiratory infections).
2. For children with a parent who does not smoke, the odds of developing colds or respiratory infection are 0.89 times the odds of not developing colds or respiratory infection. The fact that the odds are less than 1 means that the event (colds or respiratory infection) is less likely than the nonevent (no colds or respiratory infections).
3. For children with a smoking parent, the odds of the event (colds or respiratory infection) are 2.25 times greater than the odds for children whose parent does not smoke. The odds ratio is greater than 1.0, which means that the event is more likely in the children with a smoking parent.

Several points should be made. First, the choice of making colds or respiratory infections the event of interest was arbitrary; that is, the analysis could have proceeded with the event of interest being no colds or respiratory infections. In that case the odds are b/a and the other calculations are arrived at similarly. Typically, one focuses on disease. Second, the counts we used are estimates and hence subject to sampling error. It is possible to construct confidence interval estimates for any of the quantities as needed. Third, the odds ratio (as well as the odds) is much harder for most practitioners to understand than relative risks (and risk). For example, the risk of disease in the exposed group is 0.67 compared with 0.47 in the nonexposed; furthermore, the relative risk is 0.67/0.47 = 1.42. The latter, which leads to the statement that colds or respiratory infections are 1.42 times more likely when a parent smokes, has an immediate interpretation: In a population similar to the one from which the sample was drawn, the risk of the event is 1.42 times greater. The odds ratio (2.25) has no such immediate interpretation.

Chart Reviews and Case Review Studies

A chart review is a careful compilation of information from a collection of cases, typically cases concerning a single disease, procedure, or other defining characteristic. A case review is just an analysis of a single case. This type of study can be useful in identifying potential relationships (e.g., in a review of 30 prenatal intensive care unit cases of H_1N_1 flu infection, length-of-stay data might be analyzed to determine its relationship to time to treatment). These studies are retrospective in nature and may offer insights into associations and certainly might offer clues regarding fruitful areas for additional research. One shortcoming of chart reviews is that chart data are often incomplete and, compared with a carefully designed prospective study, information on key variables may be missing. Compare this with a case-control study and you will see that the only comparisons one can make are internal to the collection of cases.

EXPERIMENTAL DESIGNS

Features of True Experimental Designs

True experimental designs have each of the following features: (1) manipulation or an intervention, (2) randomization, and (3) experimental control. There is also some measure or collection of outcome measures that are connected with the purposes of the study. These are defined in the study protocol and should be logically connected to the research question that motivates the study. In what follows the studies are for the most part pictured (described) as consisting of two treatment groups. This is merely for convenience (simplicity) because there is no limit to the number of treatment groups in an experimental study. Labeling the groups as "treatment group" and "control group" is also for convenience. To have randomization between groups one must have at least two groups, and typically one is the control group (a comparison group that comprises the standard treatment); however, this may not be the case in a particular study.

The language of study design arises from several sources, two important ones being industrial/agricultural experimentation (scientific areas in which true experimental studies routinely take place) and psychology/education. The latter probably accounts for use of terms such as "pretest/posttest" designs, which are used even when the outcome measures are not strictly speaking something that could be described as a test. The former are the source for terms such as "split plot" designs, which suggest agricultural experimentation.

Previously, we discussed nonexperimental designs. These were observational in nature. Nonpejoratively they can be described as passive—the approach is basically let's see what happens. Many useful scientific conclusions are arrived at in this manner (think astronomy).

Manipulation or Intervention

In experimental studies something is done that is intended to affect subjects in the study. It might be the administration of a drug or a change in protocol by the pharmacy or almost anything thought to affect an outcome. This intervention divides the subjects in the study into groups (defined by the intervention). A simple division is one in which one group receives a treatment (treatment group) and another group receives no treatment (control group).

Randomization

Randomization refers to the introduction of chance into the selection or assignment of subjects to treatments. Randomization can occur at two levels: one described as random selection and the other described as random assignment. *Random selection* refers to how one draws the sample of people (subjects) for the study from a population. In most nursing and medical studies, this is desirable but not achievable; however, some studies do have random selection. The form of random selection can be simple (characterized loosely as "each subject in the population has an equal chance of selection") or more complicated (such as using stratification and clustering). These more complex methods of selection are often used in surveys. *Random assignment* refers to how one assigns the subjects in the sample that is drawn to different groups or treatments in the study. Random assignment is sufficient for a study to be referred to as experimental. Patients who enter a clinic and are diagnosed with disease A are randomly assigned to "old treatment" and "new treatment." This is not a random sample of patients from which assignment is made.

This is typically referred to as a convenience sample. However, the random assignment has made it possible to argue that different outcomes are attributable to the treatment and hence the design is an experimental one.

The purpose behind randomization is to remove the effects of systematic variation in the subjects (e.g., the sickest are assigned to treatment) that might confound (confounding factors are factors other than the intervention that might be used to explain the observed outcomes) the results. Underlying randomization theory is the notion of potential differential effects; that is, attributes of the subjects (known or unknown to the researcher) might mediate the impact of the intervention. The idea behind randomization is that these differential effects are "averaged out"; that is, all those characteristics of the subjects that impact on the outcome (measure) are distributed evening among the treatment groups. This ideal is often not achieved and in small samples is possibly unachievable. Also, the researcher must contend with "bad luck." If you are living on luck (randomization), then one result is bad luck. In practice this means that the groups (those defined by the intervention) are not similar with respect to the subjects assigned to the groups. Note that the implied "comparison" can be made explicitly only with known aspects of the treatment groups, but faith in the randomization leads the researcher to believe that those factors unknown to the researcher (or factors with respect to which no data have been collected) have been averaged out.

Experimental Control

Control (experimental control) is concerned with consistent administration of the intervention. In simplest terms, a well-controlled experiment is one in which the treatment groups are managed identically with respect to both the administration of the intervention and any aspects of the study (factors) that might influence the outcome, both known and unknown to the researcher. Key among these is "attention control"; that is, ensuring that those in different treatment groups receive the same level of attention (including surveillance). This is frequently achieved in clinical settings by adhering to a well-designed protocol. Inclusion of blinding is a form of control. Blinding the subjects means that the subjects do not know what form of treatment they are receiving. Those administering the study may also be blinded (as well as those performing statistical analyses). Blinding is often easy to achieve in drug studies, but in other studies it is impossible (e.g., surgery versus radiation in prostate cancer).

Notes on the Narrow Definition of Experimental Study

It is worth noting that the definition of an experimental design we are using is quite narrow and excludes certain things that one might think of as experiments. Suppose one randomly selects depressed subjects infected with human immunodeficiency virus from an urban clinic database to study their response to a nurse-based program of laughter therapy. At the end of the study, subjects are administered an instrument that measures depression. One might learn useful information from this study, but there has been no random assignment because there is only one treatment group. This design could be characterized as a one-group-only posttest design, where posttest is shorthand for the idea that measurements are made only after the intervention. This study could be designed to allow for preintervention measurement of depression. This leads to another form of division in which subjects are measured initially (baseline), then the intervention occurs, and then subsequent to the intervention the subjects are measured again (these types of studies in the simplest form are referred to as pre–post studies; when more than one postintervention observation is made, these may be called repeated-measures studies or perhaps longitudinal studies). A one-group pre–post design is sometimes called preexperimental (and would not conform to our definition of experimental).

Laboratory or certain industrial experiments are frequently designed as one-group posttest studies when the phenomenon is well understood. For example, the breaking strength of metal wire of a certain composition might be known (actually the distribution of breaking strengths) and the researchers wish to study the effect of a change in composition (e.g., tungsten is added). Ten pieces of wire with the new composition are tested, and the breaking strength is measured with the intention of comparing these measurements with a known outcome (e.g., average braking strength). Those performing this study would consider the study to be experimental. Research on human subjects is usually more complicated than this. Furthermore, the effects of a human subject's intervention in general tend to be more varied in the response often because of idiosyncratic attributes of the subjects (that are unknown or not understood by the researcher).

Purposes Behind the Use of Experimental Designs

Why are studies undertaken? Fundamentally, the researcher wishes to gain and communicate knowledge about some process or phenomenon. In epidemiological studies (which include clinical research and related activities) the subject is disease. With nonexperimental designs one can establish association, but it is difficult to develop compelling arguments regarding causality, although occasionally this has been done with some success. In experimental studies one can come closer to establishing cause and effect.

Cause and effect in human subject studies is not only hard to establish; in most cases it has to be carefully circumscribed because the effects of an intervention are typically differential—that is, the intervention does not affect all subjects to the same degree or at all. For example, under controlled circumstances a Newtonian apple always falls toward earth when it falls from a tree. Every apple falls. Even in cases of perfect experimental control in a cancer study, perhaps in 50% of subjects tumor size is reduced. Not only did only some of the subjects respond to the treatment, but some responded without the treatment (because of placebo or other unknown causes). Often in intervention studies the response rate is described in terms such as these. This is not classical causality (if x then y; if not x then not y). Human subjects are extremely idiosyncratic. In addition, other causes can operate to complicate the explanation. Hence, cause and effect in studies on human subjects is more problematic. Finally, does one ever observe cause and effect in studies on human subjects? One can argue that only correlation (association) is ever observed (where correlation is defined more broadly than a linear relationship).

Internal Validity

In assessing internal validity, one answers the question of whether the study measures what it set out to measure. Often, and more importantly, did x really change y? This issue is not relevant to most observational studies (e.g., cohort or case-control studies), although such studies have been used to argue causality (and in this circumstance the issue of internal validity arises). For intervention studies internal validity is crucial, so true experimental and quasi-experimental designs can be evaluated with respect to the degree of interval validity particular designs possess. Put simply, internal validity addresses the question of whether observed changes in outcomes can be attributed to the intervention (manipulation) and not to possible other causes. In the real world this ideal can never be completely achieved. In that sense one can think of degrees of internal validity.

Internal validity applies to a specific study. That is, when one has internal validity, then one can claim that "what was done" did affect the outcome. One can examine the construct validity of a study, which refers to the connection of your study to its theoretical constructs. For example, in a study of regular nurse visits to elderly shut-ins, the visits improved scores on a quality of life survey (compared with the control subjects, who received no visit). Properly designed, this study had high internal validity. Suppose in another study there were three arms: no visit, nurse visit, and meals-on-wheels delivers a hot lunch. In this study there is no difference between the quality of life scores for the nurse visits and the meals visits. In the first study the outcome is attributed to the nurse visit, and it is true the visit led to higher quality of life scores (hence internal validity was high), but human contact seems to be the true explanation of the effect (as established in the second study). Or was it the hot lunch?

Below are some commonly identified threats to internal validity. When examining a particular study, one can examine each of these with respect to its perceived impact on internal validity.

- *History:* Did some other current event effect the change in the dependent variable? Typically, the event occurs between a first and second measurement (between pre and post).
- *Maturation:* Were changes in the dependent variable the result of normal developmental processes? This would include any change associated with the passage of time independently of treatment.
- *Statistical regression:* Possible if groups are selected on extreme scores or other extreme characteristics. This is classically referred to as "regression to the mean."
- *Selection:* Were the subjects self-selected into experimental and control groups, which could affect the dependent variable? The usual remedy is random assignment, but this is not always effective.
- *Experimental mortality:* Dropouts and loss to follow-up. How were missing data treated in the statistical analysis?
- *Testing:* Did the pretest affect the scores on the posttest?
- *Instrumentation:* Did the measurement method change during the research?
- *Design contamination:* Did the control group find out about or interact with the experimental treatment? This includes contamination via personnel administering the "intervention," such as nurses who are involved in different arms of the study communicating.
- *Selection–maturation interaction:* The selection of comparison groups and maturation interacting that may lead to confounding outcomes and erroneous interpretation that the treatment caused the effect.

External Validity

External validity refers to generalizability. That is, to what populations do the conclusions of a study pertain? This is not relevant in the absence of internal validity. Construct validity also relates to generalizability in as far as this measures the degree to which the theoretical constructs being measured in the study are valid. Ideally, a study should have high interval validity and high external validity. Actually defining the population to which the conclusions of a study apply is nontrivial and often likely to be overstated.

A threat to external validity is an explanation of how you might be wrong in making a generalization regarding the findings from some study. Generalizations typically involve extending the study to different people, places, or times. These errors of generalization can occur at the researcher level (that is, those who performed the study can make invalid claims) or by users of the study (you, if you are engaged in advanced nursing practice and apply findings in a way that is inconsistent with the study's generalizability). Perceived or potential threats to external validity can be the inspiration for additional research in which the original study is replicated with new people, places, or times. Below are listed some commonly identified threats to external validity:

- Unique program features.
- Effects of selection: The pool from which random assignment was made is often a large convenience sample, not random selection from some well-defined population. This makes generalizability problematic.
- Effects of setting/situation: All situational specifics (e.g., treatment conditions, time, location, lighting, noise, treatment administration, investigator, timing, scope and extent of measurement, etc.) of a study potentially limit generalizability.
- Effects of history: If historical circumstances were different at the time the study was conducted, findings no longer apply.
- Effects of testing: In general, testing will not occur and certainly not pretesting. For example, implementation of a program (intervention) to improve quality of life probably will not include testing.
- Reactive effects of experimental arrangements: Subjects know they are in study. Another aspect of this revolves around the question of whether those that participate in studies are different from those who do not or did not have an opportunity to participate.
- The Pygmalion effect, or Rosenthal effect: The phenomenon in which the greater the expectation placed on people, often children or students and employees, the better they perform. This is related to the reactive effects of experimental arrangement points.

Important Examples of Experimental Designs

The literature of experimental design is vast and typically is presented in the context of statistical analysis. The designs selected for discussion in this chapter are typical of those that arise in health-related studies that would be encountered by those engaged in advanced nursing practice.

Randomized Controlled Trial

In the jargon of experimental design (as a subject area of statistics), a completely randomized design is one in which experimental units are randomly assigned to treatments. In most clinical and epidemiological studies the experimental units are human subjects, and studies (designs) of this type are typically referred to as randomized controlled trials (RCTs). For a single study these are often considered the best designs (that is, internal validity is high) or the gold standard. The other designs considered in this chapter are variants of this fundamental design. The basic outline appears in **Figure 3-5**.

This description is quite general and covers many possible variations with respect to details. Some key points are as follows:

- The sampling may take many forms, including convenience sampling. This can greatly affect external validity.
- This is a pre–post design if measurements of the response variable(s) are made at baseline (e.g., quality of life instrument is administered) and postintervention.
- Data collected may be nominal, ordinal, or interval, which affects the data analysis and the type of conclusions drawn.

Consider the following simple example, which begins with the research question: Does adding a video to predischarge education by nurses increase patients' (who have had colostomy surgery) knowledge about infection risks? In outline, the study design is as follows: (1) 1 day before discharge (and after the standard nurse conducted education) all patients are given a 10-question "test" designed to measure their knowledge of risks and good practices. (2) Those in the intervention group (randomly selected) are shown a video before discharge. All patients are given the same test at discharge.

In this example the key features of the RCT are easily identified. There is an intervention, which is the video. The treatment groups are created by randomization and consist of those who received the "standard education" and those who received the standard education plus the video. There is at least one clearly defined outcome variable that in this study is derived from the test administered pre (subsequent to the standard nurse conducted education) and post (that is, subsequent to the video). The test might be scored (e.g., percent correct answers), or individual questions on the test may be considered as outcomes. Observe that this study cannot be blinded with respect to subjects because as those receiving the intervention will certainly know they saw the video. The study protocol should clearly describe how the intervention is to be administered (e.g., is there a question-and-answer period after the video) as part of experimental control.

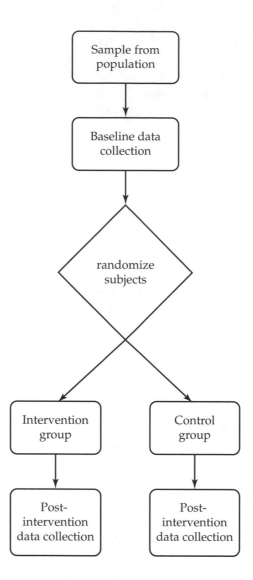

FIGURE 3-5   Randomized controlled trial outline.

After-Only (Posttest Only) Design

In an after-only design the subjects are randomized into treatment groups without preintervention measurement of response (outcome) measures (**Figure 3-6**). This does not mean certain data cannot be collected before randomization (these may be covariates such as age, gender, education); however, no measure of the response (outcome variable) is made preintervention. In some studies only postmeasurements may

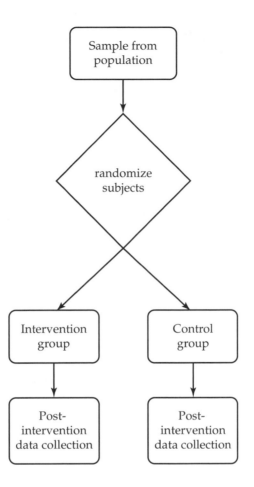

FIGURE 3-6 Post-test design.

be taken; for example, a study of post surgical hospital readmits for groups randomized between two predischarge instruction methods for wound care. The after-only design results in data from two independent groups (a consequence of random assignment). Variability within the groups could be quite large, which means that successfully detecting differences between the groups may require large samples. In studies involving quality of life, the acquisition of knowledge, and assay or other physiological measurements, collecting preintervention measurements can increase the power associated with statistical analyses because inherent human subject variability can be reduced taking preintervention measures into account when performing analyses. However, randomization alone is a sufficient basis for declaring differences between treatment groups are associated with treatment (intervention).

Solomon Four-Group Design

The Solomon four-group design is appropriate when the researcher suspects that preintervention measurement has an effect on the response. That is, this design considers the possibility that baseline measurement affects postmeasurements; for example, taking pretest influences posttest (typically either through learning or increased awareness). The four groups are as follows (**Figure 3-7**):

- A: Baseline data collected and subjects receive intervention (treatment)
- B: Baseline data collected and subjects are in the control group (standard treatment)
- C: No baseline data collected and subjects receive intervention (treatment)
- D: No baseline data collected and subjects are in the control group (standard treatment)

This design can be modified so that certain baseline data are collected from all four groups and other baseline data are not. That is, outcome measures data are omitted in "no baseline data" but certain other (covariate) data (e.g., age, gender, race and such) might be collected.

What is the idea behind this design? Suppose a study is intended to measure the effects of a nurse-based intervention for transitioning adolescent diabetics into adulthood. Observations are to be taken at baseline and end of study 12 months later. One measure in the study is adherence to good practices as measured by a survey instrument. Does just taking the survey (which serves to remind the subjects of certain good practices) affect behavior? One way to answer that question (and simultaneously guard against this effect) is the four-group design. By comparing groups A and C with respect to end-of-study responses with the survey, one can assess the impact of taking the survey preintervention. What is learned from comparing groups A and D at end of study? The cost of this design is greater than a classical RCT because there are four groups. One additional issue is the lack of a generally agreed-on method of statistical analysis for this design. That is, how does one model it? In itself this is not that serious a drawback because using several approaches to the resulting data can lead to answers to key research questions. There are several approaches to analyzing RCT data, but that has not reduced interest in using this design.

Crossover

In the most elementary version of a crossover design, all subjects in the study receive all treatments. This design closely corresponds to the counterfactual ideal in epidemiological studies in which, instead of comparing disease outcomes for those who are

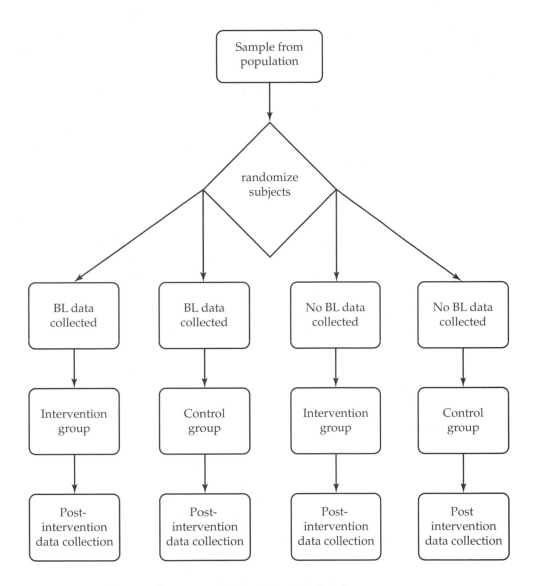

FIGURE 3-7 Solomon four-group design. *Note:* BL, baseline.

exposed and those who are not exposed, the same individual experiences both exposure and nonexposure. Crossover designs are often used in clinical trials. The study is divided into periods, and patients receive different treatments in these periods. There can be several periods, but in the simplest case there are two. Compare this with the previous parallel designs in which the (two) treatment groups simultaneously receive treatment (this is an abstraction because in practice patients are typically enrolled over time). In the crossover design there is not a separate comparison group. Each subject acts as his or her own control.

Because each subject acts as his or her own control, there is no possibility of covariate imbalance. However, in more complicated versions this can arise (i.e., not all subjects receive all treatments). Randomization enters the picture with respect to the order in which the treatments are administered. Types of randomization can arise in other circumstances. The rule of thumb is when in doubt, randomize.

Consider a study in which two arthritis drugs are being compared (one might be a placebo). Then each subject can be described by his or her treatment sequence: AB (drug A first and drug B second) or BA. Patients are randomly assigned to a treatment sequence. A concern in such studies is carryover effects. These are dealt with in part by having a "washout" period between treatments. For each subject (1) a drug, based on the subject's treatment sequence, is administered for some period of time and outcome measures are recorded (this might be something as simple as the subject reporting the treatment as successful [S] in controlling symptoms or unsuccessful [U]); (2) a washout period intervenes; and (3) the second drug in the treatment sequence is administered and outcome measurements are recorded.

The analysis typically considers the effect of order and a comparison of outcomes between the two treatments (and carryover effects). In the example above there are two sequences (AB and BA) and associated with each are four outcomes: SS, SU, US, and UU (using only this simple dichotomous measure, in which SS refers to success in period 1 followed by success in period 2). A response profile contains the counts for each outcome (**Table 3-4**). The goal here is not analysis of these data. However, the data in Table 3-4 do suggest certain conclusions.

From the example it is easy to see that this design can be extended to more than two treatments (which results in longer treatment sequences), that the subjects can be stratified before assignment (e.g., in this example by gender), or that for more than

Table 3-4 Crossover Data					
	Response Profile				
Sequence	**SS**	**SU**	**US**	**UU**	**Total**
AB	4	15	5	6	30
BA	5	4	16	5	30

Note: S, successful; U, unsuccessful.

two treatments not all subjects are assigned to each treatment (e.g., suppose there is a placebo in the previously mentioned drug study, then one might assign subjects to any of six treatment sequences such as AP, BP, AB, and so on).

Factorial Designs

Below are the key attributes of a factorial design:

- Factors are variables that affect the outcome/response that one can set (control) during the experiment (study). One might think of these as design variables.
- Factors occur at levels (that is, they can be set at different values, which may be numerical or categorical). That is, factor A may be at i levels, factor B at j levels, and factor C at k levels. In this case there are $i \times j \times k$ factor level combinations. Setting (or deciding on) the factor levels is the manipulation part of the design—that is, they define the intervention.
- In a factorial study the effects of the factor levels on the response are investigated by setting the levels of all factors and then observing the response. In a *full factorial* responses are observed for each factor level combination. In a balanced design with n replicates there are then $i \times j \times k \times n$ observations in the sample. The number might be large, which is one of the drawbacks of full factorial designs.
- In factorial designs one examines what are called main effects and interactions. The fact that interactions can be studied explains why factorials are superior to "one factor at a time" studies.

The last bullet mentions interaction. Interaction occurs when the effect of factor A on the response is influenced by the level of factor B. Interaction is often interesting and always (when present) complicates the description of the relationship between the factors and the response.

When one adopts a factorial design, there is some number (M) of distinct factor level combinations. In the case of three factors described above, there are $M = i \times j \times k$ factor level combinations and the $N = i \times j \times k \times n$ subjects are randomly assigned to factor level combinations (random assignment is essential for this to be an experimental design). For example, suppose that diabetes control is the focus of a nurse-administered diet/exercise study that involves three diets and four exercise programs. There are 12 combinations of diet/exercise. If 60 subjects are enrolled in the study, then 5 subjects can be randomly assigned to each treatment combination (leading to a balanced 3×4 factorial design). Suppose the outcome measure is HbA_{1c}. If the subjects are measured at baseline and at end of study (e.g., 6 months), then this is really just a somewhat fancy RCT. It is worth noting that if the outcome measure were a dichotomous variable with values "in control" and "not in control," then it is unlikely that a study with 60 subjects would have enough power to make the study worth conducting.

The benefit derived from the factorial design is that interaction between diet and exercise can be examined (and quantified). When interaction is absent, then the main effects of diet and exercise program can be evaluated independently of one another.

The example above is a full factorial. There are designs called fractional factorials from which one can gain important information with less experimental effort (N less than 60). Authors such as Montgomery (2009) provide a thorough discussion of these approaches. One type of factorial design that could be a great value in clinical studies (it is quite commonly used in industrial applications) is screening designs. In screening designs several factors (sometimes as many as seven or eight) are set at only two levels (such as high or low or yes or no), leading to what are called 2^k designs (there are k factors). The goal is to identify "active" factors (that is, ones that influence the outcome).

In principle, factorial designs are separate from post-hoc stratification using several factors in as far as these factors (factors other than the design factors) are not subject to random assignment and are not "design variables," the levels of which are set by the researcher with the design. Analyses of this type are often conducted using analysis of variance (ANOVA). For example, in the previous study one might simultaneously look at the effects of gender and race on the outcome using two-factor (unbalanced) ANOVA (actually a general linear model)—the exact role of the two design factors (diet and exercise) in the model might complicate the analysis but does not obscure the point. In this case association of gender and race with HbA_{1c} can be established, but a causal argument such as the diet/exercise one is more tenuous.

QUASI-EXPERIMENTAL DESIGNS

As the name suggests, quasi-experimental designs share some of the characteristics of true experimental designs. The purposes (primarily to investigate cause-and-effect relationships) are similar to those motivating true experimental designs. One or more characteristics of true experimental designs are missing, either because they cannot be achieved or because there are valid reasons why a quasi-experimental design might be superior.

Nonequivalent Control Group Design

The fundamental difference between this design and the classic RCT is that there is no random assignment to treatment groups. There are still comparison groups and experimental control still needs to be exercised (apart from randomization). Most frequently, the treatment groups arise naturally, for example, they may be different hospitals, different nursing facilities, different practices, and so on. **Figure 3-8** contains a schematic for this design. It is important to note the following:

- Sampling is going on, that is, the subjects in the two groups came from somewhere. This is true for experimental designs also. This impacts on external validity—generalizability—regardless of whether random assignment takes place.
- The most convenient "assumption" is that the two groups are similar/comparable at baseline. This should be investigated (confirmed) using statistical methods. Sadly, this implies that only known confounding factors can be examined (or, worse yet, using only factors on which data can be collected). For comparison, consider that in designs in which random assignment is used it is often assumed that baseline differences in key (active) variables (as well as unknown variables) have been averaged out. In practice this may not occur,

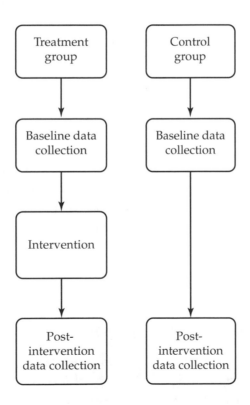

FIGURE 3-8 Nonequivalent control group design.

and in the context of the number of studies actually conducted, many will fail to be properly randomized.

In circumstances in which the groups are different, statistical methods (such as analysis of covariance) may be used to control for this. The remarks in the preceding bullet regarding known versus unknown factors apply here also. It is with regard to unknown or unanticipated factors that nonequivalent control group designs may lead to incorrect conclusions.

This design can be appropriately used when contamination is a danger. In a nursing setting, for example, the intervention can be used in one ward/hospital/unit and the comparison treatment in another so that nurses and patients in the two arms do not interact.

Consider the following example based on the research question: Does an additional "hands-on" session regarding baby care with a nurse while music is played improve a new mother's belief that she is ready to take care of her baby? A (hypothetical) validated instrument (BC10) consisting of 10 Likert (ordinal) scale questions is used to measure the mother's belief in her readiness. Note that the nurses will have to be trained and prepared for the hands-on session. To avoid "contamination" the researchers decided not to randomize patients within a unit, so two units were used for the study: One unit was randomly chosen to be the intervention unit. The nurses on that unit were trained to perform the intervention. The instrument (BC10) was administered after the "standard" baby care instructions were given to the mothers (usually day 2 of their hospital stay). In the intervention group the mothers were given the hands-on session. Before discharge the instrument was readministered to all subjects.

If the researcher wants to separate the "hands on" and music effects, four groups (units) are needed. Defined how? If one is concerned about a test–retest effect, then one could modify the Solomon design (without randomization) to suit this situation.

Selection bias is a major concern with this design. One method for detecting this is to have multiple (two or more) preintervention tests (measurements) to allow the analyst to detect trends in the measurements (and assess maturation threats). When there are differential preintervention maturation effects (different trends), that is suggestive of selection bias.

After-Only Nonequivalent Control Group Design

For the after-only nonequivalent control group design (**Figure 3-9**), no baseline data are collected (on the outcome variable). Because there are no baseline measurements, only the treatment groups can be compared postintervention, which makes it analo-

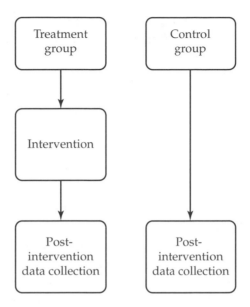

FIGURE 3-9   After-only nonequivalent control group design.

gous to its after-only experimental counterpart. The groups must be similar, or one must control for these differences to make valid comparisons and conclusion regarding the effect of the intervention/treatment. Consider an example based on the following research question: Does a nurse manager in a medical home plan produce better outcomes in adolescent diabetes patients? Two medical practices agree to participate in the study, and one is randomly chosen to have a nurse manager. The treatment group has 22 patients and the control group has 27 patients. After 6 months HbA_{1c} levels are measured for the 45 patients available for follow-up. Would this design be improved with pretest (baseline) measurements? In what way? Validity? Power?

Single-Group Designs

Single-group designs do not include a comparison group. For designs in which measurements on the outcome variable are made once preintervention and once postintervention, each subject is his or her own control and the design is frequently described as a single-group pretest posttest design. This is just a two-time point repeated measures design. If there are multiple postintervention time points at which outcome measurements are made, then this is single-group repeated-measures design. The key point is that repeated measurements on the same subject are likely to be nonindependent, which complicates the analysis. In this type of study interest is in the evolution of the outcome measures over time.

In a design in which there is a single group with after-only measurement (that is, there are no preintervention measurements), the researcher can make comparisons with respect to the intervention that are external to the study. For example, 5-year survival rates (actually proportions) for a treatment can be compared with published survival rates. Ascribing the observed survival rates to the treatment is tenuous because the outcomes may be solely attributable to characteristics of the treatment group or, worse yet, the result of some exogenous event. For example, in a study on sexual behavior in teens, behavior is measured baseline (how?), a nurse-based educational intervention is administered, and subsequently behavior is measured again. Between the pre- and postmeasurements there was a television series on the danger of sexually transmitted infections. Exogenous events such as this can contaminate the study. Minimally, critics can argue that unknown events induced the outcome (e.g., there was a full moon). Single-group after-only studies are typically exploratory and are useful for estimating characteristics of a population of interest but are unlikely to produce convincing cause-and-effect arguments unless supported by follow-up studies with a comparison group.

REPEATED-MEASURES (TIME SERIES) DESIGNS

Time series designs can be repeated-measures designs when the experimental unit is a human subject. In modeling some epidemiological measurement over time (e.g., infant mortality), what are frequently referred to as time series methods might be used. Modeling of this type is not the subject here.

Repeated-measures designs are sometimes referred to as longitudinal studies. The essential idea is that measurements are taken over time, perhaps at regular intervals of time or perhaps not. Because the repeated-measures design is so frequently used, it is useful to summarize some of its features even though some of this repeats previous discussions in this chapter.

- Repeated-measures designs may be experimental, quasi-experimental, or nonexperimental.
- Repeated-measures designs may have an intervention or not. If there is an intervention in which only some subjects receive the intervention, then the intervention groups define a between-subjects effect. There may be more than two treatment groups.

- Often, there is interest in a time effect. That is, the measurements evolve over time (even when there is no intervention and hence a single group). This is sometimes referred to as "maturation" but is more often referred to as a within-subjects effect (a statistician's characterization).
- When there is more than one arm/group (e.g., a treatment and a control arm), the interaction between time and group is often the focus of the study. That is, is the evolution of the repeated measurements of the outcome variable the same for the treatment group and the control group? This idea extends to more than one treatment group.
- The pretest–posttest design is a simple example of repeated measures. When there are only baseline and end of study measurements, then change = baseline – end of study is often used to measure the time effect.

STUDIES OF STUDIES: LEVELS OF EVIDENCE

In advanced nursing practice one is often interested in "degrees of proof" or levels of evidence. Once a design has been chosen (or even when not consciously chosen) and a study completed, the study will result in claims regarding the nature of some process or phenomenon. In our case some disease- or exposure-related conclusion will be offered. The truth offered will usually be supported by statistical and other arguments. What level of belief should be attached to these conclusions? And if there is belief, to whom (that is, to what population of subjects) do they apply? The practitioner asks, "can I use this knowledge in my practice?" Assessment of internal validity of a study offers a partial answer. That focuses on design. Generally, RCTs are thought to have high internal validity. Next, one might examine effect sizes. That is, given statistical significance, what are expected effects associated with a particular intervention? Recall that statistical significance is an artifact of three things: true effect size, sample size, and luck. The latter appears in two contexts: (1) a small (or nonexistent) true effect in the population produced through randomization a large observed effect in the treatment group and statistical significance and (2) a large effect through randomization leading to roughly equivalent treatment groups and hence lack of significance. Examination of a single study, no matter how carefully designed, never allows one to know whether luck has intervened in a manner that leads to false conclusions. Observe that published studies with false conclusions tend to be those of type 1. If 5% level of significance is used, then inevitably type I errors will arise and the practitioner will never know whether the study under consideration is a type 1.

Apart from the preceding concerns, having belief in good luck and observing a clinically significant effect size (perhaps by examining a confidence or tolerance interval), the practitioner must still ask to whom does this apply? That is, does this apply to my patients? Questions of external validity are even thornier than those of internal validity, and one must rely on the description of the study population (typically a sample with certain characteristics) to address this. Very seldom are studies based on random samples from some well-defined population. More typically, they are some sort of convenience sample.

One approach to the problems raised here is to engage in a systematic review. That is, one critically examines papers relating to the research question. Finding published papers if they exist is usually relatively easy. But what about studies that were not published? Of special interest are those not published because the findings were not statistically significant. And what is their role in an overall assessment of the "truth" regarding some intervention (or more generally a description of some disease phenomenon)? In general, there is belief that a systematic review (if properly conducted) offers a higher level of evidence regarding the truth than a single study. There is no doubt that it is more nuanced. When statistical methods (as opposed to clerical or ethnographic methods) are used to "combine results," the result is called meta-analysis. Meta-analytic studies are often considered to offer the highest level of evidence regarding the truthfulness of claims and are sometimes referred to as a "state-of-science" assessment. Meta-analytic methods are quite popular, but combining results from different studies is a nontrivial undertaking; given the same set of studies, different researchers might reach somewhat different conclusions regarding "the truth." Therefore, some caution should be exercised in interpreting meta-analytic results.

KEY POINTS

- Study design can be viewed from two perspectives. First, from the point of view of the primary researcher, careful consideration of study design is needed to ensure that methods and resources are combined in a manner that facilitates answering the research question motivating the study—that is, will the study provide answers to the research question in a manner that will convince scientists and practitioners that the conclusions of the study are useful and valid? Second, from the point of view of the practitioner (e.g., someone engaged in advanced nursing practice) who might implement findings from a study, critical examination of the research design is essential in evaluating the findings with respect to effects and validity. Put more bluntly, can these research findings be put to use in serving the needs of the people to whom I wish to apply them?

- Although there is a general consensus that the strongest causal evidence arises from true experimental designs (the gold standard being RCTs), the designs discussed in this chapter have meaningful roles and are often the best or only approach available either because of dollar/resource constraints or practical or ethical considerations.
- Cohort studies are the basis for classical epidemiological studies. They are expensive, and prospective ones take a very long time to conduct. Being observational studies, it is quite difficult to develop convincing cause-and-effect arguments based on them. However, cohort studies do offer clear opportunities to order events in time so that relationships between exposure and disease can be discovered and elucidated upon in ways experimental designs cannot offer.
- With respect to their frequency of use, case-control studies have turned out to be quite useful despite limitations regarding what can be estimated (inferred) with this design. These designs are the easiest way to study disease that either develops slowly or is relatively rare.
- Intervention studies, both experimental and quasi-experimental, have been invaluable sources of scientific information and knowledge. The essential methodology used in well-designed intervention studies is comparative and strives to answer the question, did the intervention work when compared with some other treatment? Comparison of this type is a fundamental part of the scientific method. Design principles, along with appropriate statistical analysis and modeling, are what make comparative studies effective in discovering truth. Aspects of design such as (random) selection, (random) assignment, blinding, experimental control through a carefully worked out protocol, pretesting, and fidelity are the major influences on validity.

CRITICAL QUESTIONS _____

1. Odds ratios can be appropriately calculated for data from exposed cohort, case-control, and cross-sectional studies. In which of these can one calculate (estimate) relative risk? Which of these measures of risk is easier to explain to a patient (odds ratio versus relative risk)? In which of these can one calculate attributable risk? Which of these measures of risk is easier to explain to a patient (relative risk, attributable risk, or the odds ratio)?
2. Create three scenarios for studies in which it is not feasible or prudent to collect "pretest" data.

3. Why is it okay to compare after-only outcomes in an experimental study but not in a quasi-experimental study?
4. Conduct a mind experiment in which your research question cannot be answered using cohort study data. Repeat this for an experimental study.

REFERENCES

Garson, G. D. (updated 2010). Research design. In Statnotes: Topics in multivariate analysis. Retrieved from http://faculty.chass.ncsu.edu/garson/PA765/design.htm

Montgomery, D. C. (2009). *Design and analysis of experiments*. Hoboken, NJ: John Wiley & Sons.

Rothman, K. J. (2002). *Epidemiology: An introduction*. New York: Oxford University Press.

Schlesselman, J. J. (1982). *Case control studies: Design, conduct and analysis*. New York: Oxford University Press.

Shindler, E. (updated 2010). Framingham Heart Study. Retrieved from http://www.framingham-heartstudy.org/index.html

Trochim, W. M. (updated 2006). Research methods knowledge base. Retrieved from http://www.socialresearchmethods.net/kb/design.php

CHAPTER 4

Nursing Resources for Epidemiology

"As our circle of knowledge expands, so does the circumference of darkness surrounding it."
—Albert Einstein

Kiran Macha
John P. McDonough
Lillia M. Loriz

OBJECTIVES

- Explain the role of information and technology in the field of epidemiology.
- Describe the role played by health data in the field of epidemiology.
- Know how to access vital statistics essential to influencing community health policy.
- Describe how the Internet improves the communication process in epidemiology.
- Identify Web-based resources for use in epidemiological research.

Data collection and analysis is one of the core areas of epidemiology. To make better health decisions for the community, a battery of quantitative data from a variety of sources must be analyzed. Epidemiologists gather data from physicians, laboratories, clinics, public health organizations, other public health departments, and automated surveillance systems. Public health organizations conduct community epidemiological research studies to answer, investigate, and sometimes formulate questions.

PUBLIC HEALTH INFORMATICS

Public health informatics is defined as the "systematic application of information and computer science and technology to public health practice, research, and learning" (Yasnoff, O'Carroll, Koo, Linkins, & Kilbourne, 2000, p. 68). This discipline is demanding because of constantly emerging public health emergency situations. There is a growing need for the establishment of national public health information systems to enhance communication activities during bioterrorist attacks, hurricanes, earthquakes, and other emergency relief operations.

Surveillance reporting systems alert public health professionals in the shortest possible time. Rapid dissemination of data is made possible among healthcare professionals with the adaptation of new technologies. In recent years technology-friendly environments have been successfully created in public health departments, with automated surveillance systems allowing the constant monitoring of health and disease in the community. Reportable disease and laboratory information is collected 24 hours a day. Analysis of incoming data is automated, with options set up to alert public health system professionals at all levels (Kukafka, 2007).

The establishment of information systems developed by public health informatics has contributed greatly to the globalization of public health. Conversion to the use of electronic medical records in hospitals is a perfect example of the efficiency of public health informatics in promoting better health care while better protecting the public. Electronic medical record software stores health information, and data can be used to initiate a public health action. The Medical Electronic Disease Surveillance Information System, Electronic Laboratory Reporting, Early Warning Infectious Disease Surveillance, and the Centers for Disease Control and Prevention's BioSense System are examples of public health informatics in use for surveillance. Major challenges involving the use of information and technology in epidemiology include the maintenance of data quality, access to monitoring systems, issues of Internet dependency, ethics, security, and the durability of monitoring systems.

MAJOR DATABANKS IN THE UNITED STATES

Public health services in the United States are offered primarily through the U.S. Department of Health and Human Services. The department's secretary oversees the functioning of agencies within his or her purview to keep Americans healthy. The following agencies and centers under the Department of Health and Human Services (in alphabetical order) are good resources for epidemiological data.

Administration on Aging

The Administration on Aging (http://www.aoa.gov/) is responsible for promoting the health and independence of the elderly through home and community-based activities.

Agency for Healthcare Research and Quality

The Agency for Healthcare Research and Quality (http://www.ahrq.gov/) is responsible for the delivery of quality health care to citizens through designing healthcare policies, researching evidence-based practices, and identifying ways to reduce health-care costs. The Agency for Healthcare Research and Quality offers grants for research related to its priority areas and conducts surveys on healthcare costs, medical expenditures, and health practices promoting quality outcomes.

Agency for Toxic Substances and Disease Registry

The Agency for Toxic Substances and Disease Registry (http://www.atsdr.cdc.gov/) is responsible for the identification, assessment, planning, research, monitoring, and evaluation of the effects of toxic material on the general population, initiating public health action in response to emergencies. The agency website offers a wide range of information on toxic materials, medical management guidelines, training, tool kits, and other resources. Information about recent investigations conducted in the community and related public health actions is available to the public.

Centers for Disease Control and Prevention

The CDC (http://www.cdc.gov/) coordinates activities of many agencies, including Environmental Health and Injury Prevention, Health Information and Services, Center for Health Promotion, Center for Infectious Diseases, Global Health, Terrorism Preparedness and Emergency Response, and the National Institute for Occupational Safety and Health. CDC is the major public health organization responsible for the surveillance of infectious diseases and bioterrorism and for the implementation of immunization programs. CDC collects health data, performs data analysis, establishes and maintains surveillance systems, and monitors safety at their respective institutions. CDC is responsible for the planning and implementation of effective public health actions, notifying the public, and coordinating activities with other nations to protect the public's health.

Centers for Medicare & Medicaid Services (http://www.cms.hhs.gov/)

The Centers for Medicare & Medicaid Services (http://www.cms.hhs.gov/) function in healthcare financing administration, managing the Medicare, Medicaid, and Children Health Insurance programs offered by the federal government. The Centers for Medicare & Medicaid Services also oversees healthcare administration standards, such as those established under the Health Insurance Portability and Accountability Act (HIPAA). HIPAA regulations address the security and privacy of health data and ensure the monitoring of standards for electronic healthcare transactions.

Food and Drug Administration

The Food and Drug Administration (http://www.fda.gov/) is responsible for monitoring the safety of human and veterinary drugs and drug research, food and food additives, medical devices, biological material such as blood products and vaccines, cosmetics, and radiation-emitting products and oversees the implementation of regulations to protect the public's health. In 2008, for example, the public was concerned about melamine contamination in milk after many infants in China died from consuming their milk products. The Food and Drug Administration addressed the concerns of the public by testing milk products, ensuring Americans that U.S. milk products meet safety standards with a chance of melamine contamination only from Chinese milk products.

Health Resources and Services Administration

The Health Resources and Services Administration (http://www.hrsa.gov/) is responsible for promoting the delivery of quality healthcare services, improving access to health care, eliminating health disparities, and providing a culturally competent healthcare environment. The organization focuses its resources on underserved areas and uninsured and underinsured populations, providing a safety net for those who do not have access to health resources.

Indian Health Services

The Indian Health Services (http://www.ihs.gov/) agency is responsible for promoting the health of Native Americans and Alaskan Natives. The Indian Health Services oversees health services such as primary care, preventive care, public health programs, and rehabilitation and facilitates establishment of partnerships with other public health organizations to improve the quality of care for all Native Americans.

National Institutes of Health

The National Institutes of Health (http://www.nih.gov/) is composed of 27 institutes and centers that conduct and support medical research benefiting the public. Some areas of current research include development of pain-free imaging techniques, human immunodeficiency virus (HIV) vaccines, and infectious organism rapid diagnostic tool kits, as well as extensive genetics research. Many researchers supported by the National Institutes of Health have earned Nobel prizes.

Office of Public Health and Science

The Office of Public Health and Science (http://www.hhs.gov/ophs/) supports many initiatives, campaigns, and programs that promote public health goals. The Office of Public Health and Science offices include, among others, the Office of the Surgeon General, Office of Minority Health, Office of Disease Prevention and Health Promotion, National Vaccine Program Office, and the Commissioned Corps of the U.S. Public Health Service.

Substance Abuse and Mental Health Services Administration

The Substance Abuse and Mental Health Services Administration (http://www.samhsa.gov/) is responsible for the quality improvement of programs, prevention, treatment of conditions, rehabilitation, and research related to substance abuse and mental illness. The agency implements select public health laws in the community, such as regulation of the sale of tobacco and alcohol products to minors.

NATIONAL SURVEYS AND DATA COLLECTION SYSTEMS IN THE UNITED STATES (http://www.cdc.gov/nchs/index.htm) _____

National Health Care Surveys

National Health Care Surveys are designed to gather information on different healthcare settings that can influence health policy changes. National Ambulatory Medical Care Survey, National Hospital Ambulatory Medical Care Survey, and National Survey on Ambulatory Surgery are conducted to gather information on, respectively, the provision and use of ambulatory medical services in physician offices and emergency hospital departments, and ambulatory surgical services. The National Hospital Discharge Survey is designed to collect data on inpatients discharged from nonfederal short-stay hospitals. The National Nursing Home Survey, the National Home and Hospice Care Survey, and the National Survey of Residential Care Facilities are conducted in long-term healthcare facilities.

National Health Interview Survey

The National Health Interview Survey is designed to gather information on health status, access to care, disability, and illnesses of the noninstitutionalized general population in the United States. Results help us gauge the achievements of national health objectives and identify barriers to access to health care while helping to identify needed policy changes to promote public health.

National Health and Nutrition Examination Survey

The National Health and Nutrition Examination Survey is designed to gather information on the health and nutritional status of the population. Participating subjects are interviewed, and a physical examination is conducted in a mobile examination center equipped with medical and laboratory equipment. The results of surveys are helpful in the development of pediatric growth charts, identifying disease risk factors (such as cholesterol as a risk for cardiovascular disease), and providing information to promote healthy practices.

National Immunization Survey

The National Immunization Survey is designed to obtain data on childhood, teenage, and adult immunization numbers in the United States. This information helps us understand the reasons for noncompliance with vaccination schedules.

National Survey of Family Growth

The National Survey of Family Growth gathers information on family life, marriage, divorce, pregnancy, infertility, use of contraception, and men's and women's health. Information on various related risk factors is also explored.

National Vital Statistics System

The National Vital Statistics System (http://www.cdc.gov/nchs/data_access/VitalStats Online.htm) collects, maintains, and analyzes data on births, marriages, divorces, and deaths. The System recognizes changes in the above data patterns, identifies links between different vital statistics, and reports results. Vital statistics data are made available online by state and county. "CDC WONDER" is an online database (http://wonder.cdc.gov/) providing acquired immune deficiency syndrome (AIDS), births, cancer, infant mortality, population data, and sexually transmitted disease morbidity statistics.

THE INTERNET: MANTRA OF THE MODERN AGE _____

The Internet is a complex global networking system created to improve communication and networking. Running on the Internet, the World Wide Web functions like a databank that holds information and links documents. Web browsers such as Internet Explorer, Safari, Opera, and Mozilla are used to retrieve and exchange information through the Web. The Internet, the Web, and web browsers together function as a unit. Search engines such as Google help us connect to knowledge/research databanks, enabling the retrieval of documents and website information based on keyword searches. The published research of many authors is available on the Web, allowing us not only to organize health information but also to use research findings. The Internet allows the timely exchange of information through a reduction in the gap of space and time to the shortest limit humanly possible. Information can be transferred through e-mails almost instantaneously.

Health education programs can be created online and help us provide up-to-date health information and guidelines to potentially millions of people. Complete information on diseases, treatments, alternative treatment methods, and research references are available on websites. The Internet is also being effectively used for health promotion and communication and for marketing various products, research and software tools, and healthcare plans.

In the cases of public health emergencies, action and alternate plans can be accessed through emergency information websites that can be continuously updated. In a short time surveys can be deployed, health data collected or monitored, and public health decisions can be made. Partnerships can be developed with multiple organizations, allowing the sharing of data online.

Issues associated with risk involving use of the Internet include increases in risky behavior, emotional disorders related to the frequency of Internet use, the questionable reliability or completeness of information, challenges involving adaptation to changing technology, and expenses related to computer/Internet use.

WEBSITES FOR EPIDEMIOLOGICAL RESEARCH _____

- **International Public Health Organizations:**
  Canadian Society for Epidemiology and Biostatistics
    http://www.cseb.ca/resources.php
  European Centre for Disease Prevention and Control
    http://ecdc.europa.eu/en/Pages/home.aspx

World Health Organization
   http://www.who.int/en/
- **U.S. Public Health Organizations:**
   Centers for Disease Control and Prevention
      http://www.cdc.gov/
   Centers for Medicare & Medicaid Services
      http://www.cms.hhs.gov/
   U.S. Census Bureau
      http://www.census.gov/
   U.S. Department of Health & Human Services
      http://www.hhs.gov/
   National Cancer Institute
      http://resresources.nci.nih.gov/categorydisplay.cfm?catid=666
   National Mental Health Information Center
      http://mentalhealth.samhsa.gov/
   Pan American Health Organization
      http://new.paho.org/
- **Research Databases:**
   CINAHL (Cumulative Index of Nursing and Allied Health Literature)
      http://www.ebscohost.com/cinahl/
   International Epidemiologic Databases to Evaluate AIDS
      http://www.iedea-hiv.org/
   Medline Plus
      http://medlineplus.gov/
   Medscape
      http://www.medscape.com/
   Oxford Journals, Oxford University Press
      http://www.oxfordjournals.org/
   Public Health Reports
      http://www.publichealthreports.org/index.cfm
   Science Direct
      http://www.sciencedirect.com/
   SpringerLink
      http://www.springerlink.com/home/main.mpx
   Surveillance Epidemiology and End Results
      http://seer.cancer.gov/
   The Cochrane Collaboration
      http://www.cochrane.org/

University of California, San Francisco, The WWW Virtual Library:
   Medicine and Health: Epidemiology
   http://www.epibiostat.ucsf.edu/epidem/epidem.html#DAT
U.S. National Library of Medicine and the National Institutes of Health
   http://www.ncbi.nlm.nih.gov/pubmed/

- **Public Health Journals:**
American Journal of Epidemiology
   http://aje.oxfordjournals.org/
American Journal of Public Health
   http://www.ajph.org/
BMC Public Health
   http://www.biomedcentral.com/bmcpublichealth/
Disaster Medicine and Public Health Preparedness
   http://www.dmphp.org/
Emerging Infectious Diseases
   http://www.cdc.gov/ncidod/EID/index.htm
The European Journal of Public Health
   http://eurpub.oxfordjournals.org/
Global Public Health
   http://www.informaworld.com/smpp/title~db=all~content=g915842079
Journal of Environmental and Public Health
   http://www.hindawi.com/journals/jeph/
Journal of Public Health
   http://jpubhealth.oxfordjournals.org/
Journal of Public Health
   http://www.palgrave-journals.com/jphp/index.html
Journal of Public Health Management and Practice
   http://journals.lww.com/jphmp/pages/default.aspx
Journal of Public Health Nursing
   http://www.wiley.com/bw/journal.asp?ref=0737-1209

- **Search Engines:**
Google
   http://www.google.com/
Bing
   http://www.bing.com/
Yahoo
   http://m.www.yahoo.com/
Altavista
   http://www.altavista.com/

NATIONALLY NOTIFIABLE INFECTIOUS DISEASES, UNITED STATES, 2010

The U.S. list of Nationally Notifiable Infectious Diseases is compiled and updated regularly by the CDC and state public health departments (http://www.cdc.gov/ncphi/disss/nndss/PHS/infdis2010.htm).

- Acquired immune deficiency syndrome (AIDS)
- Anthrax
- Arboviral neuroinvasive and non-neuroinvasive diseases
  - California serogroup virus disease
  - Eastern equine encephalitis virus disease
  - Powassan virus disease
  - St. Louis encephalitis virus disease
  - West Nile virus disease
  - Western equine encephalitis virus disease
  - Botulism
    - Botulism, foodborne
    - Botulism, infant
  - Botulism, other (wound and unspecified)
- Brucellosis
- Chancroid
- *Chlamydia trachomatis*, genital infections
- Cholera
- Coccidioidomycosis
- Cryptosporidiosis
- Cyclosporiasis
- Diphtheria
- Ehrlichiosis/Anaplasmosis
  - *Ehrlichia chaffeensis*
  - *Ehrlichia ewingii*
  - *Anaplasma phagocytophilum*
  - Undetermined
- Giardiasis
- Gonorrhea
  - *Haemophilus influenzae*, invasive disease
  - Hansen disease (leprosy)
  - Hantavirus pulmonary syndrome
  - Hemolytic uremic syndrome, postdiarrheal
  - Hepatitis, viral, acute
    - Hepatitis A, acute
    - Hepatitis B, acute
    - Hepatitis B virus, perinatal infection
    - Hepatitis, C, acute
  - Hepatitis, viral, chronic
    - Chronic Hepatitis B
    - Hepatitis C virus infection (past or present)
  - HIV infection
    - HIV infection, adult ≥ 13 years)
    - HIV infection, pediatric (<13 years)
- Influenza-associated pediatric mortality
- Legionellosis
- Listeriosis
- Lyme disease
- Malaria
- Measles

- Meningococcal disease
- Mumps
- Novel influenza A virus infections
- Pertussis
- Plague
- Poliomyelitis, paralytic
- Poliovirus infection, nonparalytic
- Psittacosis
- Q Fever
- Rabies
  - Rabies, animal
  - Rabies, human
- Rocky Mountain spotted fever
- Rubella
- Rubella, congenital syndrome
- Salmonellosis
- Severe acute respiratory syndrome-associated Coronavirus (SARS-CoV) disease
- Shiga toxin-producing *Escherichia coli* (STEC)
- Shigellosis
- Smallpox
- Streptococcal disease, invasive, group A
- Streptococcal toxic-shock syndrome
- *Streptococcus pneumoniae*, drug resistant, invasive disease

- *Streptococcus pneumoniae*, invasive disease non–drug resistant, in children < 5 years of age
- Syphilis
  - Syphilis, primary
  - Syphilis, secondary
  - Syphilis, latent
  - Syphilis, early latent
  - Syphilis, late latent
  - Syphilis, latent, unknown duration
  - Neurosyphilis
  - Syphilis, late, non-neurological
  - Syphilitic stillbirth
- Syphilis, congenital
- Tetanus
- Toxic-shock syndrome (other than Streptococcal)
- Trichinellosis (trichinosis)
- Tuberculosis
  - Tularemia
  - Typhoid fever
  - Vancomycin, intermediate *Staphylococcus aureus* (VISA)
  - Vancomycin, resistant *Staphylococcus aureus* (VRSA)
- Varicella (morbidity)
- Varicella (deaths only)
- Vibriosis
- Yellow fever

INTERNATIONAL DATA BANKS AND RESOURCES

European Centre for Disease Prevention and Control

The European Centre for Disease Prevention and Control, a well-known replica of the U.S. CDC, focuses on the health of European Union nations. The European Centre for Disease Prevention and Control website (http://ecdc.europa.eu/en/Pages/

home.aspx) posts information on health topics, research, surveillance, and professional bodies of European nations. Current issues (such as pandemic H_1N_1 status) are updated on the website, and the public is informed through recorded videos and publications. Core activities of the organization include disease surveillance, identification of health threats, formulation of responses to public health emergencies, training of health professionals, health communications, and technical assistance to participating nations.

Public Health Agency of Canada

The Public Health Agency of Canada (http://www.phac-aspc.gc.ca/index-eng.php) focuses on Canadian health issues, conducting surveillance activities, food safety testing, immunizations, injury prevention, and planning to respond to health emergencies. The Public Health Agency of Canada is also responsible for aboriginal health and oversees health programs designed specifically for them.

Health Protection Agency, United Kingdom

The Health Protection Agency (http://www.hpa.org.uk/HPA/) protects the public from infectious and environmental hazards and works with the National Health Scheme and national and local government health authorities, providing information and training and identifying and responding to health emergencies. The Centre for Emergency Preparedness and Response, the Centre for Infections, the Centre for Radiation, Chemical and Environmental Hazards, and the National Institute for Biological Standards and Controls are all part of the Health Protection Agency.

Other International Public Health Organizations

Institut De Veille Sanitaire, France
   http://www.invs.sante.fr/
Public Health Foundation of India
   http://www.phfi.org/home.asp
Centre for Health Protection, Hong Kong
   http://www.chp.gov.hk/

KEY POINTS

- The collection, maintenance, analysis, and storage of health data are vital for planning effective public health action.

- Public health organizations play an important role in conducting research while also providing services to promote the public's health.
- Health policy and law can be influenced through epidemiological research.
- Surveillance systems in the community continuously update health status information and provide us with feedback on community medical services.
- Epidemiologists use many types of technology for effective communication. Automation of information systems allows public health professionals to be alerted at all levels.
- Ethical issues, data privacy, quality of data, and storage are some of the challenges associated with the use of information and technology in the field of epidemiology.

CRITICAL QUESTIONS

1. What might be needed to accomplish change in community health policy and law?
2. To measure the quality of community medical services, which websites provide infant mortality information?
3. Describe the use of automated surveillance and alert systems in the field of epidemiology.
4. How can we use available data and technology to prevent an epidemic from developing into a pandemic?
5. How do national surveys help the community?
6. Discuss issues involved in the use of information and technology in epidemiology.

REFERENCES

Kukafka, R. R. (2007). Public health informatics. *Journal of Biomedical Informatics, 40*(4), 365–369.

Yasnoff, W. A., O'Carroll, P. W., Koo, D., Linkins, R. W., & Kilbourne, E. M. (2000). Public health informatics: Improving and transforming public health in the information age. *Journal of Public Health Management and Practice, 6*(6), 67–75.

CHAPTER 5

Emerging Infectious Diseases

"Natural forces within us are the true healers of disease."
—Hippocrates

Kiran Macha
John P. McDonough

OBJECTIVES

- Explain the factors responsible for emerging infectious disease.
- Describe various survival adaptation mechanisms of microorganisms.
- Identify pathways of disease transmission and pathogen survival opportunities.
- Describe infectious disease outbreaks in the United States.

EMERGENCE OF INFECTIOUS DISEASE

Emerging infectious disease is caused by pathogens identified in a human population for the first time or by pathogens occurring previously but now increasing in incidence or expanding into areas where they had not previously been reported (World Health Organization [WHO]). Microbes are the major cause of death in developing countries. In developed countries they can pose a threat as biological weapons. Our greater ability to manipulate genes contributes to the potential for microbes to transform into pathogens, resulting in infectious disease. Pathogens of today are more capable than ever of adapting to a changing environment. Changing climactic factors can also enable microbes in their survival.

Factors Affecting Disease Emergence

The inherent mechanisms of bacteria to evolve in ways that can decrease their exposure to antibiotic concentrations can help them survive and multiply in a changing environment. Bacteria that produce biofilms are well protected, because the matrix in the biofilm slows down the penetration of antibiotics. Some bacteria such as *Escherichia coli* have fimbriae, which allow bacteria to become intracellular in the urethral epithelium (Normark, 2002). The recurrence of urinary tract infection occurs when these rapidly multiply.

Efflux is one mechanism that allows bacterial resistance to antibiotics. Gram-negative bacteria have efflux pumps integrated within cell membranes that expel intracellular antibiotics through active transport. Bacteria can also undergo chromosomal changes to adapt to a changing environment through deletions, inversions, and point mutations. However, few bacteria produce the beta-lactamase enzyme essential to inactivating the antibiotic molecule by breaking the bonds in the beta-lactam ring.

Climate change plays an important role in the emergence of infectious diseases. Global warming, El Niño/South Western Oscillations, and deforestation are causing alternating flood and drought conditions. Changes brought about by dams built across rivers significantly alter ecosystems and affect microorganism survival. The incidence of waterborne diseases increases with the rise in sea surface temperature. Rising temperatures because of global warming favor the survival of the mosquito-borne infections such as malaria, dengue fever, and West Nile virus (**Figure 5-1**) (Epstein,

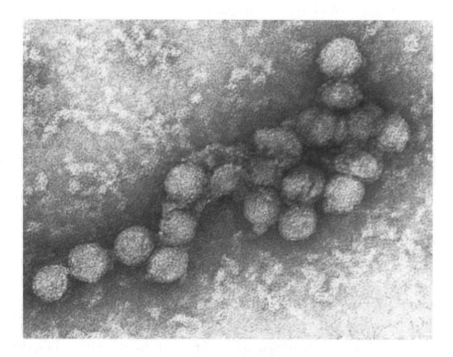

FIGURE 5-1   West Nile Virus that causes meningitis and encephalitis in humans was not known in the United States before 1999.
Source: Picture courtesy of the Centers for Disease Control and Prevention. Retrieved March 20, 2010, from http://phil.cdc.gov/phil/details.asp

2001; Patz, 1996). Changes in agricultural practices, the introduction of genetically modified plants, and the use of pesticides all have effects on the biosphere. Pathogens are capable of quickly adapting to changing temperatures and acidity. Darwin's theory of natural selection plays an important role in the survival of these organisms (Altekruse, Cohen, & Swerdlow, 1997).

An incidence of *Coccidioides immitis* yeast infection in San Joaquin Valley, California, was reported in 1936. Flu-like symptoms later associated with skin eruptions such as erythema nodosum or multiforme were classified as "San Joaquin fever," "San Joaquin Valley fever," "valley fever," "desert fever," or "desert rheumatism." Epidemiological studies in this area revealed that the rise in incidence was not the result of a change in health status of individuals but rather environmental changes. The surge in construction of houses in this area as well as mass migration into San Joaquin Valley were believed responsible for the higher incidence of fungal infection (Smith, 1940; Walsh & Groll, 1999).

The growing human population, overcrowding, and urbanization facilitate easy transmission of infectious diseases. Wars and conflicts displace large numbers of people, leading to the breakdown of public health systems. Human behavioral aspects are also known to contribute in the spread of pathogens. The increase in the incidence of irresponsible sexual behavior and abusive intravenous drug use encourage the spread of pathogens in the blood as well as those that are sexually transmitted, such as human immunodeficiency virus (HIV) and hepatitis. The production of pathogens for use as biological weapons is also cause for great concern.

Globalization is one of the reasons for increasing transmission of the once-considered endemic diseases. Modern transportation systems have not only shortened time for the spread of pathogens but have also increased the risk of suffering. Airborne infections affect passengers traveling in airplanes, where each passenger acts as a reservoir aiming to reach various destinations. This closed environment together with human contact distance and time comprise high risk factors for disease transmission. In 2009 China strictly implemented new public health policies in major airports, screening people whom they suspected to be suffering from flu and isolating all those who tested positive. Such public health efforts have reduced the incidence of influenza. Researchers are constantly searching for new viruses and bacteria that have the potential to cause epidemics and pandemics.

Zoonotic diseases (those that can be transmitted from nonhuman animals to humans) are also successfully adapting to the human environment. An analysis of studies suggests that zoonotic pathogens are more likely to emerge than nonzoonotic pathogens. The process of such emergence is influenced by the pathogen's taxonomy and its transmission routes (Taylor, Latham, Mark, & Louise, 2000). Continued surveillance of these organisms is warranted because their nature and progression of illness is unknown, yet they are potentially capable of starting a pandemic.

Modern technology is constantly evolving to satisfy our needs. Today's foods are often structured in texture, color, and taste to satisfy our visual or sensory ideals. In this process we have been introducing many food additives without knowing the long-term effects of these chemicals. Canned food usually contains preservatives and can sometimes contain bacteria or other contaminants. Great quantities of food are often prepared from ingredients that come from other countries with no record of origin, making it difficult to trace and contain the primary source of a pathogen.

Organ transplantation has gained importance in the world because of a rise in the number of donors, facilities capable of storing this tissue, availability of trained surgeons, and extensive research and experiences that are helping us succeed in this process. As organ transplantation expands, efficient methods and trained personnel should be increasingly available for infectious disease screening of tissues (**Figure 5-2**). The use of immunosuppressive drugs with transplantation is enabling certain

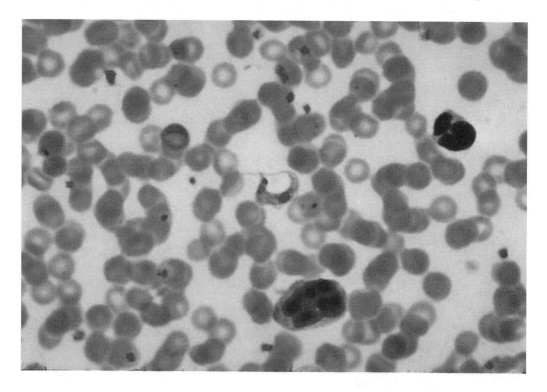

FIGURE 5-2   Blood smear showing *Trypanosoma cruzi*. Chagas disease was reported in organ transplant patients whose donor was endemic to Latin America.
Source: Picture courtesy of the Centers for Disease Control and Prevention. Retrieved March 25, 2010, from http://phil.cdc.gov/phil/details.asp

microorganisms, such as cytomegalovirus, to establish successfully in the human system.

Pharmacological research is focused on the discovery of new drugs to replace antibiotics that are no longer effective. Antigenic drift and antigenic shift phenomena are responsible for much of the antibiotic resistance, with microbes adapting to new chemical structures within a short period of time. At the same time many "forgotten" antibiotics remain effective, and bacterial sensitivity to some of these may be growing. (For example, sulfamethoxazole and trimethoprim antibiotics seem to be working well after a long period of resistance.) In the developing world so-called quacks have been misusing antibiotics with little knowledge on the consequences of misuse. (Misuse refers to the administration of wrong antibiotic for the disease and/or in wrong dosages.) With the constant adaptation of bacteria and viruses, vaccines need to be continuously updated. The time, research, and the amount of money invested in such activities are immense. However, an effective, timely response to an emerging infectious disease can prevent an epidemic or an epidemic evolving into a pandemic.

Most of the zoonotic diseases are transmitted indirectly and have either a human or animal reservoir (Taylor et al., 2000). Public health measures taken to control vectors of disease with insecticides have not been fruitful as vectors become increasingly resistant. Inadequate sanitation measures also contribute to the growing number and virulence of vectors. Vectors play an important role in disease transmission, acting within reservoirs for disease, with some microbes having ways to survive host systems without causing any harm to the reservoirs.

Proper functioning of the public health system is essential for the identification of infectious disease at an early stage, initiation of prompt investigation, involvement of necessary expert teams, and laboratory testing. Planning and implementation of an intervention, follow-up, and evaluation of outcomes of the process are other forward steps. Any breakdown in the public health surveillance system or communication process can lead to disastrous outcomes.

Our Losing War Against Pathogenic Microorganisms

Since the discovery of penicillin, many more antibiotics have been discovered (such as cephalosporins, aminoglycosides, monobactam, carbapenems, and macrolides). Antibiotics are continually modified to create new forms to counteract growing bacterial resistance. Bacteria develop antibiotic resistance using three mechanisms: (1) chromosomal mutation, (2) inductive expression of a latent chromosomal gene, or (3) exchange of genetic material through transformation, transduction, or conjugation (Neu, 1992). Antibiotics generally interfere with bacterial cell wall synthesis, protein synthesis, and DNA replication. Bacteria can resist these effects by altering the anti-biotic target site or attachment protein and can also produce enzymes such as beta-lactamase to inactivate antibiotics.

Staphylococcus aureus exemplifies the ability of the bacterium to resist and evolve to such an extent that it is responsible for millions of deaths (**Figure 5-3**). As an example, methicillin-resistant *S. aureus* is highly resistant to many antibiotics. Bacteria within the *Staphylococcus* family can produce lipase, which breaks down lipids in cell membranes to help bacteria penetrate the skin. The superantigens of *S. aureus* activate T cells and can produce toxic shock syndrome. Necrotizing fasciitis is a posttraumatic infectious fatal condition that includes the destruction of skin, fat, and muscles caused by the release of exotoxins from the bacteria. Severe gastroenteritis can result within 6 hours of eating food contaminated with *S. aureus*. Multiple toxic effects can proceed to shut down the human system.

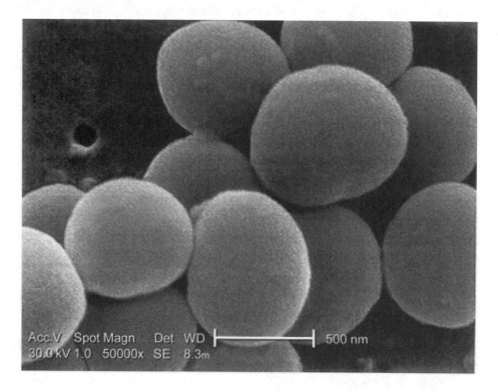

FIGURE 5-3 *Staphylococcus aureus* are gram-positive cocci that are seen in clusters like grapes under microscopy.
Source: Picture courtesy of the Centers for Disease Control and Prevention. Retrieved March 21, 2010, from http://phil.cdc.gov/phil/details.asp

Once they become resistant to one antibiotic, bacteria are capable of becoming resistant to other available antibiotics as well. The process of reversal of this acquired sensitivity may take a long time. For example, for the treatment of urinary tract infection, a sulfamethoxazole and trimethoprim drug combination known as Bactrim was used. Resistance to the drug had been observed, but after several years of study researchers found the bacteria to be susceptible to this drug combination once again. Another factor in bacterial resistance in the United States has proven to be American military deployment to other countries. Military personnel have unknowingly brought many penicillin-resistant bacteria to the United States. The addition of a bacterial antibiotic enzyme inhibitor to antibiotics (such as adding clavulanic acid to penicillin) to boost their effectiveness has not had an impact as bacteria continue to evolve and survive.

Certain medical practices have also had an effect on bacterial resistance. The treatment of infections in Ayurvedic medicine (an ancient Asian Indian medical system practiced widely in India) is different from that of allopathic medicine. Ayurveda stresses the importance of cleansing procedures called *panchakarma* and uses herbs to treat infections both internally and externally. These practices are known to boost our natural immunity to pathogens.

The collaborative efforts of the Centers for Disease Control and Prevention (CDC), the U.S. Food and Drug Administration (FDA), and U.S. Department for Agriculture have resulted in an action plan toward reducing the level of antibiotic resistance in the community. Strategies to be potentially undertaken include continuous surveillance of antibiotic resistance of pathogens of public health importance, investment in resources and hygienic practices education, increased vaccination programs in the community, and monitoring of antibiotic usage in the veterinary and agriculture industries. These efforts need to be extended globally through collaboration with international organizations to promote sharing of information to better understand the dynamics behind emergence of antibiotic resistance. Goossens' study (2005) on antibiotic usage and bacterial resistance noted that differences in antibiotic use in European countries were a result of variations in the incidence of community-acquired infections, culture and education, differences in drug regulations, and variations in the structures of national pharmaceutical markets.

Emerging Food- and Waterborne Pathogens

Epidemiological investigations of outbreaks in the United States have revealed that new pathogens have been imported from other countries. Some of these have evolved to cause severe food- and waterborne infections.

In 1990 *Cyclospora cayetanensis*, a coccidian protozoan, caused gastroenteritis in a group who ate cake made with raspberries. Epidemiological investigation and polymerase chain reaction studies of samples revealed that the raspberries were imported from Guatemala and identified *Cyclospora*. Since then, similar incidents have been reported in the United States and are easily identified in association with past experiences. *Cyclospora* is now known to cause serious infection in immunocompromised individuals (Ho et al., 2002; Tauxe, 1997). Pathogens of low incidence in the past are gaining momentum in their race to survive.

A massive recall of hamburger patties was ordered under the directions of Washington State Health Department in 1993. They discovered *E. coli* O157:H7 to be the cause of bloody diarrhea in patients who ate hamburgers (Bell, 1994). This pathogen is generally detected in the stools of cows and calves. The pathogen was able to survive because of inadequate cooking temperatures, causing infection in humans. (The detection of cases in high numbers led to the inclusion of *E. coli* O157: H7 in the list of notifiable diseases.) This contaminated meat caused multistate outbreaks because hamburger patties were supplied to many restaurants from a single facility.

Vibrio cholerae is an example of a waterborne emerging pathogen that causes diarrhea. Anyone infected with cholera may die because of dehydration and shock. This bacterium has caused several pandemics, usually starting in south Asia. India is one of the countries most affected. *V. cholerae* O1 and *V. cholerae* O139 are strains that have caused pandemics, with alternating virulence (Sharma, Sachdeva, & Virdi, 2003). *V. cholerae* O1 epidemic that started in 1991 ended with 1,041,422 cases and 9,642 deaths. The incidence of cholera is low in the United States because of more advanced sewage systems and sanitation. *V. vulnificus* and Norwalk virus live normally in oysters but have recently been found to be the cause of gastroenteritis in humans, with symptoms including shock and bullous skin lesions, often leading to death.

Guillain-Barré syndrome and Miller Fischer syndrome are demyelinating diseases known to cause paralysis. Ascending paralysis is noted in the Guillain-Barré syndrome. Miller Fischer syndrome causes facial muscle paralysis, ophthalmoplegia, ataxia, and areflexia. Studies identified the association of the pathogen *Campylobacter jejuni* with these immunological syndromes. The pathogen is transmitted through poultry products, with *C. jejuni* found in the stool specimens of most patients suffering from these syndromes. Researchers also found that antibodies produced against the glycolipids of *C. jejuni* cross-react with the nerve gangliosides to cause paralysis (Jung, 2005). Depending on the severity, most patients do recover slowly from the signs and symptoms of this disease.

Listeria monocytogenes is a foodborne, gram-positive bacterium that produces toxins such as hemolysin and listeriolysin O. These toxins enable the bacteria to infect and establish themselves successfully within host cells. *Listeria* is known to cause meningitis and usually is detected in pregnant women, neonates, and the immunocompromised, with many cases leading to death. The recent growing number of foodborne outbreaks caused by *Listeria* have led to the observation of strict sanitation, temperature control, and refrigeration methods by the meat industry (Farber & Peterkin, 1991).

Emerging Pathogens in the Immunocompromised

Conditions involving compromised immunity include neutropenia, immunoglobulin deficiency, HIV/acquired immune deficiency syndrome, cancer, many chronic conditions, corticosteroid use, increasing numbers of host/parasitic conditions, and organ transplantation. These conditions are enabling pathogen survival that would normally exist at lower incidences in communities.

Mycobacterium tuberculosis has infected 2 billion people worldwide (**Figure 5-4**). Other species of mycobacteria, such as *avium*, are gaining importance in their ability to infect the immunocompromised. These pathogens are developing resistance to an-

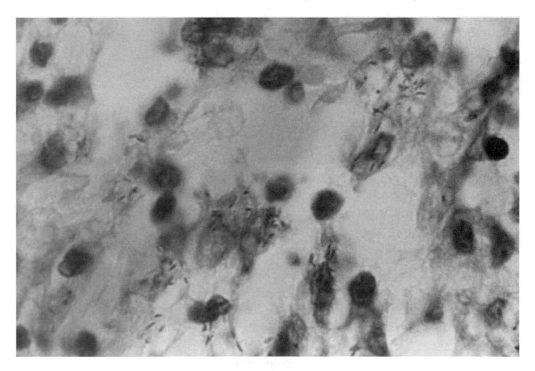

FIGURE 5-4 Specimen containing *Mycobacterium tuberculosis* after applying Ziehl-Neelsen stain appears red.
Source: Picture courtesy of the Centers for Disease Control and Prevention. Retrieved March 21, 2010, from http://phil.cdc.gov/phil/details.asp

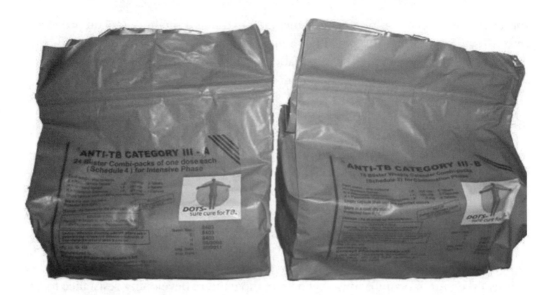

FIGURE 5-5   To avoid drug resistance and to increase patient compliance "Direct Observed Therapy Shortcourse (DOTS)" protocol is followed in countries such as India for the treatment of *Mycobacterium tuberculosis*.
Source: Picture courtesy of Dr. Suvarna Vemula, Medical Officer, India.

tibiotics, and a second line of drugs is not yet able to successfully combat them. A lack of culture equipment and antibiotic sensitivity tests essential to early identification of the disease symptoms in nonendemic places, limited access to health care, the expense of medication, misuse of antibiotics, the vulnerabilities of old age, and delayed treatments have all contributed to the current incidences of tuberculosis (McCormick, 1998).

Candida albicans, *Aspergillus fumigates*, and *Cryptococcus neoformans* are some of the opportunistic fungal pathogens causing increased damage to HIV-infected individuals. These fungi generally cause inflammation of mucosa, lungs, and meninges, respectively (Walsh, 2004). HIV virus is known to be associated with cancers such as Kaposi's sarcoma (**Figure 5-6**), high-grade B-cell lymphoma, and cervical carcinoma (Levine, 1993).

Epstein-Barr virus is a human carcinogen involved in the pathogenesis of lymphoid and epithelial malignancies and is commonly seen infecting organ transplant recipients (Ho et al., 1988). Incidences of such cases have been on the decline since patients have been treated with cyclosporine. Cytomegalovirus causes life-threatening

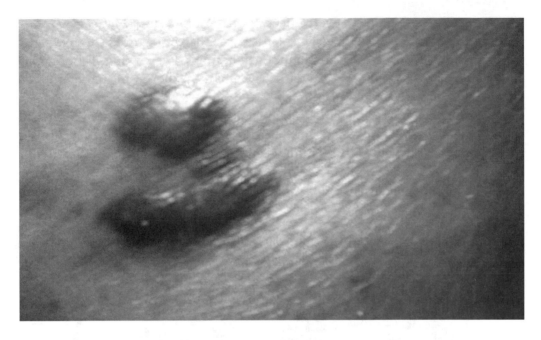

FIGURE 5-6 Kaposi sarcoma.
Source: Picture courtesy of the Centers for Disease Control and Prevention. Retrieved March 20, 2010, from http://phil.cdc.gov/phil/details.asp

pneumonia in patients treated with immunosuppressive drugs and stimulated granu-locyte transfusions from unscreened donors (Nguyen et al., 2001).

Vector-borne Emerging Infectious Diseases

Vector-borne diseases are an increasingly threatening group of infectious diseases that we are working to eliminate. WHO has been working closely with countries to which these diseases are endemic to implement prevention, control, and eradication pro-grams and to conduct surveillance activity. Resistance of vectors to insecticides and drugs, changes in public health policy, emphasis on emergency response combined with a deemphasis on prevention programs, demographic and societal changes, and genetic changes in pathogens are contributing to prevent reasonable success in com-bating vector-borne diseases (Gubler, 1998).

Malaria is one of the most common vector-borne diseases coming into the United States, with more than 300 million people infected worldwide each year. Malaria pre-vention, control, and eradication programs exist in African and south Asian countries.

The Anopheline mosquito is a very effective carrier of malaria (**Figure 5-7**). Approaches to end its survival with the use of insecticides have not proven effective given the mosquito's developed resistance to these applications. Even with malaria causing millions of deaths, we cannot predict the behavior of the pathogen and mosquito with time because of their ongoing adaptability.

Lyme disease is caused by the bacterium *Borrelia burgdorferi* and is transmitted by ticks belonging to the *Ixodes* species. In 2008, 28,921 confirmed cases of Lyme disease were reported in the United States, with the highest incidence noted in Connecticut, Delaware, Washington, DC, Maine, Michigan, Minnesota, and New York (**Figure 5-8**). The most common signs and symptoms include erythema migrans (rash), ar-

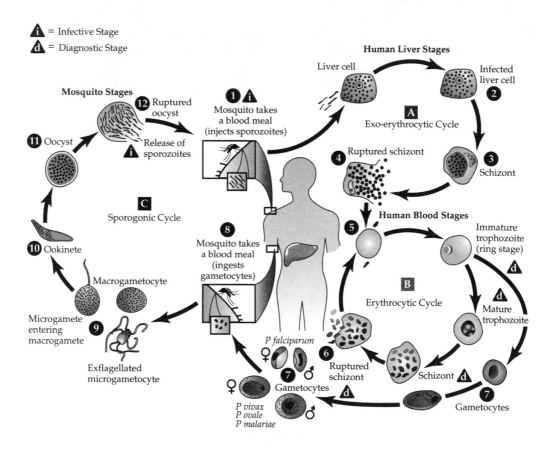

FIGURE 5-7   The life cycle of malaria.
Source: Picture courtesy of the Centers for Disease Control and Prevention. Retrieved March 21, 2010, from http://www.cdc.gov/malaria/biology/life_cycle.htm

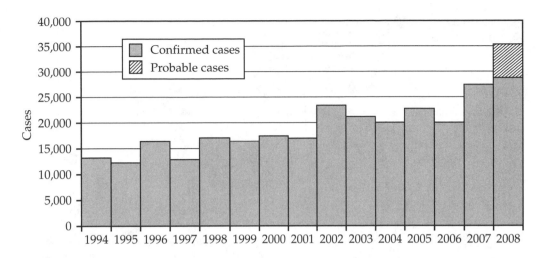

FIGURE 5-8   The incidence of Lyme disease from 1994 to 2008 in the United States. *Source:* Picture courtesy of the Centers for Disease Control and Prevention. Retrieved March 21, 2010, from http://www.cdc.gov/ncidod/dvbid/Lyme/ld_UpClimbLymeDis.htm

thritis, facial palsy, radiculopathy, meningitis, and heart block. The chronicity and severity of symptoms is of concern.

Dengue hemorrhagic fever is caused by dengue virus, transmitted by a mosquito called *Aedes aegypti.* The virus is responsible for several epidemics in southeast Asian countries with the introduction of new virus strains (DENV 1, DENV 2, DENV 3, and DENV 4). Dengue is prevalent in almost 100 countries and is responsible for 50-100 million cases each year worldwide. In 1996 a major outbreak was reported in northern India as a result of dengue virus type 2 and has since caused severe intermittent outbreaks. Dengue fever is also endemic to the southern United States. A major concern with this disease is a lack of immunity among U.S. populations.

Parasites That Survive Within Us

Strongyloides stercoralis is an intestinal nematode that is endemic to the temperate southern United States. The infective larval form of the parasite makes its way into the human body by piercing skin and by autoinfection (**Figure 5-9**). Larval forms then migrate to the lungs and other systems, with the adult worm living in the intestines. The parasite causes gastrointestinal symptoms such as abdominal pain and diarrhea and is detected in the stool. When the larval forms are in the lungs, they cause eosinophilia (called Loeffler's syndrome). The parasite is readily disseminated in the

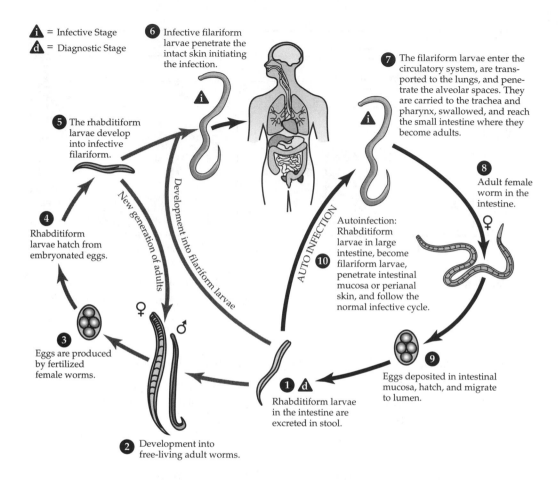

FIGURE 5-9   Life cycle of *Strongyloides stercoralis*.
Source: Picture courtesy of the Centers for Disease Control and Prevention. Retrieved March 21, 2010, from http://www.dpd.cdc.gov/DPDX/HTML/ImageLibrary/Strongyloidiasis_il.htm

immunosuppressed. In some cases intestinal obstruction and abdominal pain, shock, septicemia, and other symptoms depending on the organ may be present. The infection is treated with ivermectin drugs.

Taenia solium, also known as the pork tapeworm, infects the human gastrointestinal tract. This parasite is generally transmitted to humans by eating undercooked pork infected with the larval parasite. Autoinfection in humans is another reason for its survival. This parasite is mostly seen in southwestern United States because of widespread consumption of pork by immigrants. The adult tapeworm lives in the small intestine with the help of hooks (**Figure 5-10**) and causes intestinal obstruc-

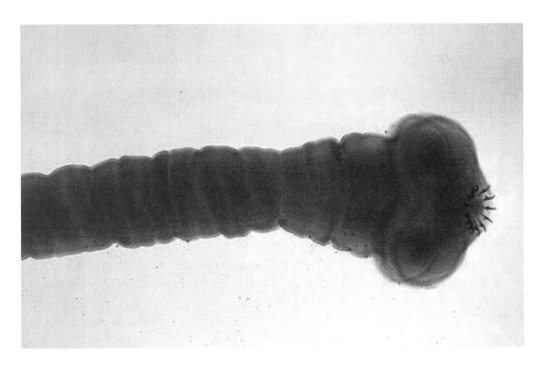

FIGURE 5-10 *Taenia solium* with scolex (head), hooks, neck, and body.
Source: Picture courtesy of the Centers for Disease Control and Prevention. Retrieved March 21, 2010, from http://phil.cdc.gov/phil/details.asp

tion, abdominal pain, and diarrhea. The larval forms (cysticerci) migrate to different tissues in the human body to cause cysticercosis. Neurocysticercosis is common because of deposition of cysticerci in the human brain, causing increased intracranial pressure, seizures, and altered mental status. Adult tapeworms are detected in stools and through radiography. Enzyme-linked immunosorbent assay (ELISA) technique may help in the detection of cysticerci. Tapeworm is treated with albendazole drugs.

Giardiasis is a caused by *Giardia lamblia*, an intestinal parasite transmitted through food and water contaminated with human or animal feces. Signs and symptoms include greasy stools, diarrhea, abdominal pain, and nausea. This parasite has caused outbreaks all over the United States—most commonly in child care centers. Recently, a surge in incidence has been noted in HIV-infected individuals, causing colitis. The parasite can be detected by the microscopic examination of stool samples. The disease can be treated with the antibiotic metronidazole, and hygiene precautions reduce the chances of parasite transmission.

Vaccinations yet to crunch numbers.....

Polio virus once caused widespread infection in many countries. After the launch of global eradication efforts with the help of many organizations, polio is now endemic only to Afghanistan, India, Pakistan, and Nigeria. Polio virus causes irreversible paralysis of lower limb muscles and in 5% to 10% of cases may affect respiratory muscles. Whenever an acute flaccid paralysis case is reported, an epidemiological search is conducted in the community to identify and detect unreported cases. According to WHO statistics, 1,663 acute flaccid paralysis cases were reported in the United States, with none confirmed as polio. Had these cases been caused by the polio virus, a massive vaccination campaign would be conducted to cover large populations. Vaccination has decreased polio-infected individuals from 350,000 cases in 1988 to 125 cases worldwide in 2008. Because there is no treatment available, mass vaccination in the community seems to be the only way to interrupt transmission of the wild virus.

Rabies virus was known as early as 3,500 B.C. A vaccine for rabies (a member of the *Lyssavirus* genus) was prepared in the 18th century by Louis Pasteur (**Figure 5-11**). Even though the process of developing a vaccine has improved, the disease has

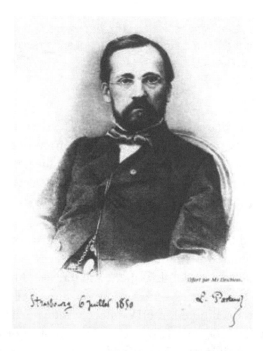

FIGURE 5-11   Louis Pasteur, Father of Microbiology.
Source: From National Library of Medicine. Retrieved April 5, 2010, from http://ihm.nlm.nih.gov/luna/servlet/view/search?q=B020595

not been contained because there is no specific treatment. The incidence of disease transmission is very low with occurrence only in certain parts of the world. Dogs, cats, bats, raccoons, skunks, foxes, and coyotes seem to be principal hosts of the virus (**Figure 5-12**), which is transmitted to humans through an animal bite. Rabies is detected in the saliva and central nervous system in both humans and animals. Patients die as a result of paralysis of respiratory muscles and may present with gastrointestinal, central nervous system, and constitutional symptoms. In 2008 in the United States 6,481 cases of rabies in animals and 2 human cases were detected.

Hepatitis B is a virus that can cause fatal liver disease during its acute stage. In the chronic stage those affected may develop hepatic cell carcinoma. Almost 2 billion people are infected with this virus, with the highest incidence in Asian countries (**Figure 5-13**). In the United States 1.2 million persons are estimated to suffer from chronic Hepatitis B infection. Hepatitis B virus is transmitted through blood products, sharing needles, mother to child, and unsafe sexual practices. Global prevalence

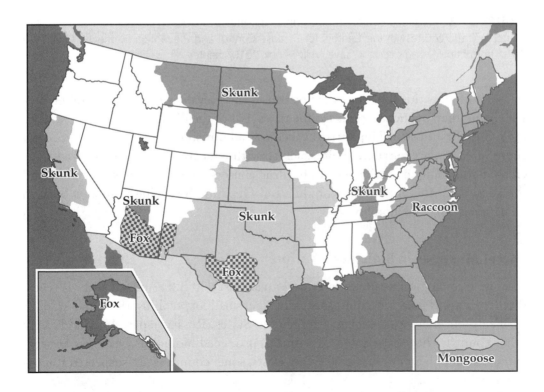

FIGURE 5-12 Geographic distribution and cause of rabies in the United States, 2008. *Source:* Picture courtesy of the Centers for Disease Control and Prevention. Retrieved March 21, 2010, from http://www.cdc.gov/rabies/epidemiology.html

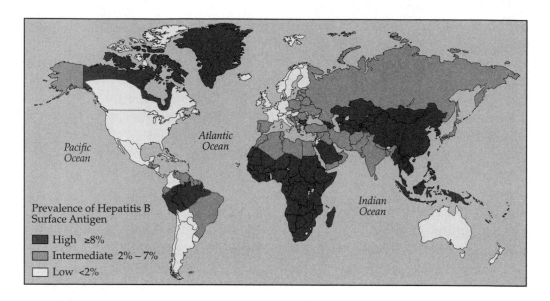

FIGURE 5-13   Global prevalence of chronic Hepatitis B, 2006.
Source: Picture courtesy of the Centers for Disease Control and Prevention. Retrieved March 21, 2010, from http://wwwnc.cdc.gov/travel/yellowbook/2010/chapter-2/hepatitis-b.aspx

statistics of Hepatitis B is almost equivalent to the prevalence statistics of tuberculosis. Chemotherapeutic solutions for the treatment of the disease are yet to be discovered. The first dose of Hepatitis B vaccine is administered at birth. Incidences of acute infection are currently being tackled with education, safer sex practices, increased availability of sterile needles for drug abusers, blood products screening, and the administration of immunoglobulins and Hepatitis B vaccine to infants born to Hepatitis B–infected mothers.

Use of Microbes in Biological Warfare

The use of biological weapons dates back to at least 600 B.C. Ancient records reveal that civilizations used venomous snakes, plague, smallpox, syphilis, ricin, and ergot to weaken their enemies. Germany, the United States, Russia, Japan, Iraq, and many other countries have experimented with and produced biological weapons. At present, even though an international treaty exists, some countries are suspected to possess such material.

Past actions involving the proliferation of biological weapons led to a 2001 bioterrorist attack, when terrorists mailed envelopes containing anthrax spores to several offices in the United States. The U.S. Public Health Service was not anticipating such an event. Gaps in national preparedness, such as a lack of laboratory resources and inter- and intradepartmental cooperation and communication and an inadequate surge in the form of emergency response to the situation, are now recognized and are being addressed.

Anthrax and smallpox are potentially some of the deadliest biological weapons. *Bacillus anthracis* is a facultative anaerobe found in soil rich in organic matter. This bacterium is naturally occurring in the soil and can be produced on a mass scale in a short time. *B. anthracis* produces dehydrated spores that are resistant to heat, radiation, chemicals, and enzymes. Anthrax is a zoonotic disease typically transmitted to humans from infected animals through cutaneous, gastrointestinal, and respiratory routes. Infection causes fever, chills, gastrointestinal symptoms, shortness of breath, and meningitis. The likelihood of fatality if untreated is 20% (and with antibiotics is 1%) within 48 hours of contact. After 48 hours the mortality rate is greater than 95%. Rapid diagnostic methods such as polymerase chain reaction and ELISA tests are available. Penicillin G, ciprofloxacin, and doxycycline are some of the antibiotics used to treat anthrax, and vaccines are now available. All U.S. soldiers received anthrax vaccinations before the Gulf War, because Iraq had in the past used anthrax as a biological weapon. The weapon poses a serious challenge because although diagnostic tests, chemotherapeutic solutions, and vaccines are available, the bacteria are so lethal that massive decontamination measures must be taken immediately to prevent widespread fatalities. Resources for such mass activities are limited at any given time.

Variola virus causes smallpox and is responsible for millions of deaths worldwide over thousands of years (**Figure 5-14**). Signs and symptoms include fever, headache, vomiting, and rash that spreads to all parts of the body. Smallpox is transmitted from human to human through respiratory droplets and does not require involvement of animals and insects. A vaccine is available, and many chemotherapeutic agents such as cidofovir are under investigation. In 1980 WHO declared that smallpox had been successfully eradicated, and the laboratories that had smallpox samples around the globe were moved to CDC headquarters in Atlanta and to the Institute of Viral Preparations in Moscow, Russia. However, after the fall of the Union of Soviet Socialist Republics, many feared that samples of the virus might have fallen into the hands of terrorists because of a lack of funds and maintenance. CDC has classified this virus as a potential biological warfare agent.

Ebola virus is a zoonotic disease native to Africa that causes hemorrhagic fever (**Figure 5-15**). The incubation period is 2 to 21 days. Signs and symptoms of *Ebola* include fever, headache, muscle aches, rash, and bleeding—both internally and externally. The

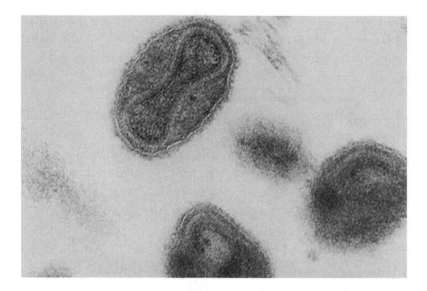

FIGURE 5-14   Smallpox virus can be used as a weapon as most of us are not immune to it. *Source:* Picture courtesy of the Centers for Disease Control and Prevention. http://phil.cdc.gov/phil/details.asp; Picture ID: 1849. Accessed March 21, 2010.

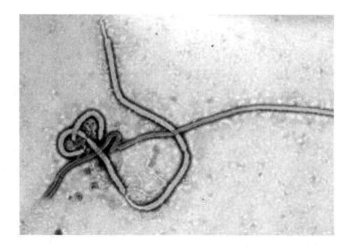

FIGURE 5-15   Ebola virus.
Source: Picture courtesy of the Centers for Disease Control and Prevention. Retrieved March 21, 2010, from http://phil.cdc.gov/phil/details.asp

virus is transmitted from animal to human and between human to human through contact with blood and body fluids. (The exact animal host is not yet known.) Polymerase chain reaction and ELISA tests are available to diagnose the disease. There is no specific treatment available; patients are treated symptomatically. Patients should be isolated, and healthcare professionals involved in patient care should wear protective clothing, gloves, and goggles to avoid direct contact with the patient's body fluids.

Hepatitis C Virus

Hepatitis C is a contagious viral disease that causes liver problems. Acutely infected patients present with fever, body aches, vomiting, jaundice, and abdominal pain. About 80% of patients on average develop chronic liver disease that may end up as liver cell carcinoma. The disease is transmitted through contact with blood, needle stick injuries, sharing of contaminated needles by drug abusers, transfusion of contaminated blood and clotting factors, infected mother to child transmission at birth, and by sexual contact. In the United States 27,000 newly infected cases were detected in 2007 alone (**Figure 5-16**), with 3.2 million estimated to be suffering from chronic

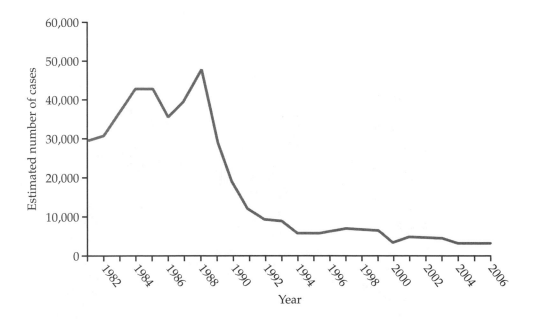

FIGURE 5-16   Incidence of Hepatitis C from 1980 to 2007 in the United States.
Source: Courtesy of the Centers for Disease Control and Prevention. Retrieved March 21, 2010, from http://www.cdc.gov/hepatitis/HCV/StatisticsHCV.htm#section1

Hepatitis C. Preventive measures include avoiding the sharing of needles, using protective barriers during sexual intercourse, and screening blood products. Drugs such as interferon and ribavarin are used to treat patients with Hepatitis C.

OUTBREAKS IN THE UNITED STATES

H_1N_1 Influenza Virus (Swine Flu)

H_1N_1 flu is thought to have originated in Mexico in April 2009. By June 2009 WHO declared it a pandemic. Some of the genes involved in H_1N_1 virus (swine flu; **Figure 5-17**) are similar to those of the influenza virus in pigs. In the United States, CDC reported 1,779 deaths and 38,455 hospitalizations of patients with confirmed cases of H_1N_1 (April 2009 to January 2010) (**Figure 5-18**). According to WHO, as of January 10, 2010, there were 13,554 deaths reported involving laboratory-confirmed cases worldwide. H_1N_1 flu vaccine was developed in 2009 and was made available initially to those considered most susceptible to the virus and later to the remainder of the population. CDC has worked closely with local public health departments, and WHO has established the Global Influenza Surveillance network to monitor the situation

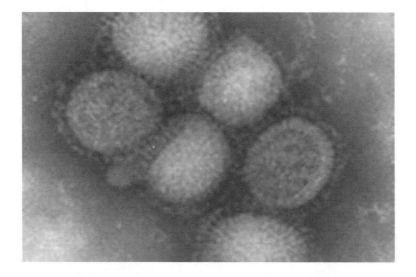

FIGURE 5-17 H_1N_1 virus.
Source: Picture courtesy of the Centers for Disease Control and Prevention. Retrieved March 21, 2010, from http://www.cdc.gov/h1n1flu/qa.htm

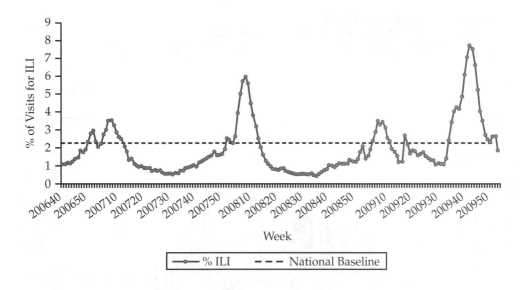

FIGURE 5-18 The U.S. H_1N_1 flu monthly incidence data.
Source: Courtesy of the Centers for Disease Control and Prevention. Retrieved March 21, 2010, from http://www.cdc.gov/h1n1flu/updates/us/#iligraph

and track incidence data all over the world. Viral resistance of H_1N_1 virus to oseltamivir (Tamiflu) has been reported in some cases.

Salmonella Outbreaks

A multistate *Salmonella typhimurium* outbreak was reported in the United States in November 2008 (**Figure 5-19**). The FDA identified the *Salmonella* strain as identical in all outbreaks reported. *Salmonella* causes gastroenteritis, the signs and symptoms of which include bloody or mucous diarrhea that lasts 24 to 72 hours, abdominal cramps, fever, dehydration, nausea, vomiting, and muscle aches. From its investigation of the outbreak at three facilities, the Minnesota Department of Health found the source to be peanut butter supplied in bulk by a brand-name company. FDA found the company's facility in Georgia to be the source of contamination, and all peanut butter traced to that plant was recalled. The outbreak had affected 529 people, causing 116 hospitalizations and 8 deaths.

In another outbreak, more than 1,000 cases were detected involving *Salmonella enterica*, with the victims suffering from severe gastroenteritis. The cause of this

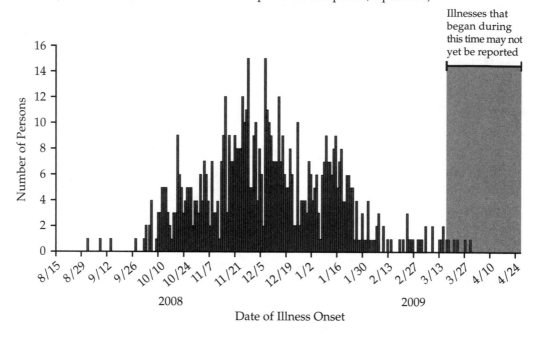

Infections with the outbreak strain of
Salmonella Typhimurium, **by date of illness onset**
(n = 696 for whom information was reported as of April 20, 9 pm EDT)

FIGURE 5-19   *Salmonella* outbreak.
Source: Courtesy of the Centers for Disease Control and Prevention. Retrieved March 21, 2010, from
http://www.cdc.gov/salmonella/typhimurium/update.html

outbreak was reportedly contamination of raw tomatoes, jalapeno peppers, and cilantro imported from Mexico. The food industry for a certain period stopped using tomatoes because of the reported outbreak.

Measles Outbreak in 2008

In 2000 the United States declared that measles had been eliminated within its boundaries. Yet, an outbreak of measles was reported in 15 states from January 2008 to July 2008, with an incidence of 131 cases. Measles causes cough, runny nose, conjunctivitis, and maculopapular rash. The long-term complications are much worse and may include pneumonia, myocarditis, and encephalitis. There is no treatment for the disease, though it can be prevented through measles, mumps, and rubella vaccination. None of the patients involved in the outbreak had been previously immunized. Because globalization had led to transport of the measles virus from another endemic region, immunization for this disease needs to be encouraged and sustained.

Statistics in Infectious Disease Outbreak

An outbreak of *E. coli* was reported in a Latino community. An epidemiologist conducted an investigation and reported the following descriptive statistics:

Total population in the community: 96
Males: 49
Females: 47
Culture: 100% Latinos
Children: None
Age: 23 to 44 years old
Number of cases infected with *E. coli*: 23 (male, 16; female, 7)

Twenty-three cases infected with *E. coli* were admitted to the hospital, and 3 persons died as a result of the severity of the infection. The incidence proportion (percent) can be calculated for this outbreak and is referred to as the attack rate (AR). That is,

$$AR = \frac{\text{new cases reported during a time period}}{\text{total population at risk}} \times 100$$

For this example,

$$AR = \frac{\text{new cases reported during a time period}}{\text{total population at risk}} \times 100 = \frac{23}{96} \times 100 = 23.95$$

This is strictly speaking a percentage and could be reported as 23.95% or, equivalently, as 23.95 cases per 100. The AR is frequently reported as cases per thousand (or on some other basis). That is, in this example, it would be 239.5 cases per thousand.

Gender-specific ARs (or ARs for any stratification for which data are present) can also be calculated:

$$\text{Male-specific AR} = (16 / 49) \times 100 = 32.65$$
$$\text{Female-specific AR} = (17 / 47) \times 100 = 14.89$$

The severity of the disease can be described by the case fatality rate, which is the proportion of identified cases that result in death. Expressing this as a percentage, the definition is as follows:

$$\text{Case fatality rate} = \frac{\text{number of deaths from specific cause}}{\text{number of cases identified}} \times 100$$

Which for this example is

$$\text{Case fatality rate} = \frac{\text{number of deaths from specific cause } (\textit{E. coli})}{\text{number of cases identified } (\textit{E. coli})} \times 100$$

Leading to a case fatality rate of $(3/23) \times 100 = 13.04$.

KEY POINTS

- Pathogens have caused a major loss of human life without human interference and are still causing damage even with human interference. Their rapid evolution challenges us in our war against them.
- Genes are strong pillars for the existence and survival of bacteria. Bacterial genes are responsible for the production of enzymes, biofilms, deregulation of receptors, and formulation of counter mechanisms against our endeavors to combat disease within humans or the environment. Climatic changes, globalization, research, and modern technology are also contributing to the survival of pathogens.
- The growing population of immunocompromised individuals because of HIV, organ transplantation, and corticosteroids is enabling the survival of many pathogens whose incidence used to be less of a public health concern.
- Reasons for the incidence resurgence of pathogens vary by disease. Public health action taken for a particular endemic disease may be insufficient to contain and eradicate disease. Globalization seems to be playing a key role in changing the ecology of the modern world, opening the door for new pathogens to emerge.
- Even though infections are not the primary cause of death in the United States, they are a major burden to the healthcare system. A series of multistate outbreaks have been reported, and new diseases are being detected that are not endemic to the United States.

- Vaccinations are playing an important preventive role in the community. The preparation, administration, and analysis of the body's response to a vaccine call for time and money. An infectious disease emergency cannot be contained with vaccination alone.
- Eradicated diseases such as smallpox, to which few people are immune, are a major threat to the population. Such pathogens in the hands of terrorists are a potential biological weapon.

CRITICAL QUESTIONS

1. How do you define emerging infectious disease? What factors enable the virulence of pathogens?
2. How can we live in harmony with pathogens? How can we stop bacterial mutation?
3. List the organizations responsible for tracking outbreaks and maintaining data on such incidences.
4. What are the implications for pathogen eradication when samples are preserved in laboratories?
5. What strategies need to be used to counter an infectious disease emergency?

REFERENCES

Altekruse, S. F., Cohen, M. L., & Swerdlow, D. L. (1997). Emerging foodborne diseases. *Emerging Infectious Diseases, 3*(3), 285–293.

Bell, B. B. P. (1994). A multistate outbreak of *Escherichia coli* O157:H7-associated bloody diarrhea and hemolytic uremic syndrome from hamburgers: The Washington experience. *Journal of the American Medical Association, 272*(17), 1349–1353.

Epstein, P. R. (2001). Climate change and emerging infectious diseases. *Microbes and Infection, 3*(9), 747.

Farber, J. M., & Peterkin, P. I. (1991). *Listeria monocytogenes*, a food-borne pathogen. *Microbiology Review, 55*(3), 476–511.

Goossens, H. H. (2005). Outpatient antibiotic use in Europe and association with resistance: A cross-national database study. *The Lancet (British Edition), 365*(9459), 579–587.

Gubler, D. (1998). Resurgent vector-borne diseases as a global health problem. *Emerging Infectious Diseases, 4*(3), 442.

Ho, M., Jaffe, R., Miller, G., Breinig, M. K., Dummer, J. S., Makowka, L., et al. (1988). The frequency of Epstein-Barr virus infection and associated lymphoproliferative syndrome after transplantation and its manifestations in children. *Transplantation, 45*(4), 719–727.

Ho, A. Y., Lopez, A. S., Eberhart, M. G., Levenson, R., Finkel, B. S., da Silva, A. J., & Herwaldt, B. L. (2002). Outbreak of cyclosporiasis associated with imported raspberries, Philadelphia, Pennsylvania, 2000. *Emerging Infectious Diseases, 8*(8), 783–788.

Jung, S. S. (2005). Lipooligosaccharide of *Campylobacter jejuni* prevents myelin-specific enteral tolerance to autoimmune neuritis—a potential mechanism in Guillain-Barré syndrome? *Neuroscience Letters, 381*(1–2), 175–178.

Levine, A. A. M. (1993). AIDS-related malignancies: The emerging epidemic. *Journal of the National Cancer Institute, 85*(17), 1382–1397.

McCormick, J. B. (1998). Epidemiology of emerging/re-emerging antimicrobial-resistant bacterial pathogens. *Current Opinion in Microbiology, 1*(1), 125.

Neu, H. H. C. (1992). The crisis in antibiotic resistance. *Science, 257*(5073), 1064–1073.

Nguyen, Q., Estey, E., Raad, I., Rolston, K., Kantarjian, H., Jacobson, K., et al. (2001). Cytomegalovirus pneumonia in adults with leukemia: An emerging problem. *Clinical Infectious Diseases, 32*(4), 539–545.

Normark, B. B. H. (2002). Evolution and spread of antibiotic resistance. *Journal of Internal Medicine, 252*(2), 91–106.

Patz, J. J. A. (1996). Global climate change and emerging infectious diseases. *Journal of the American Medical Association, 275*(3), 217–223.

Sharma, S., Sachdeva, P., & Virdi, J. S. (2003). Emerging water-borne pathogens. *Applied Microbiology and Biotechnology, 61*(5), 424.

Smith, C. C. E. (1940). Epidemiology of acute coccidioidomycosis with erythema nodosum ("San Joaquin" or "valley fever"). *American Journal of Public Health (1971), 30*(6), 600–611.

Tauxe, R. V. (1997). Emerging foodborne diseases: An evolving public health challenge. *Emerging Infectious Diseases, 3*(4), 425.

Taylor, H., Latham, S. M., Mark, E., & Louise, L. H. (2000). Risk factors for human disease emergence. *Philosophical Transactions in the Biological Sciences, 356*(1411), 983–989.

Walsh, T. T. J. (2004). Infections due to emerging and uncommon medically important fungal pathogens. *Clinical Microbiology and Infection, 10*(s1), 48–66.

Walsh, T. J., & Groll, A. H. (1999). Emerging fungal pathogens: Evolving challenges to immunocompromised patients for the twenty-first century. *Transplant Infectious Disease, 1*(4), 247–261.

CHAPTER 6

Screening and Prevention of Diseases

"The only purpose for which power can be rightfully exercised over any member of a civilized community, against his will, is to prevent harm to others."

—John Staurt Mill

Jan Meires
Carol Ledbetter

OBJECTIVES

- Appreciate the natural history of common diseases and the relationship of the disease states to levels of prevention.
- Describe important similarities and differences between screening and diagnostic tests.
- Develop practical knowledge of the common statistics used in screening tests, diagnostic tests, guidelines, and evidence useful for clinical practice.
- Discuss the advanced practice nurse's role as it relates to levels of prevention, screening tests, diagnostic tests, guideline use, and evidence-based care.

INTRODUCTION

This chapter is organized into two parts. Part 1 presents the concepts and contexts related to the natural evolution of disease, prevention, screening tests, diagnostic tests and common statistics used in screening and diagnosing a variety of conditions, disorders, and diseases. Part 2 provides an opportunity for the advanced practice nurse to apply these concepts to a set of carefully crafted exercises designed to meet the chapter objectives.

PART 1: CONTEXTS AND CONCEPTS

Advanced practice nurses for the purpose of this chapter are advanced practice registered nurses who may be nurse practitioners (NPs), clinical nurse specialists, certified nurse midwives, certified registered nurse anesthetists, or specialists in nursing administration. The content is written for clinicians, but those in administration may find the knowledge valuable as well. The terms "clinician" and "practitioner" may be used interchangeably throughout the chapter.

TERMINOLOGY

- Natural history of disease
- Prevention
- Levels of prevention
- Primary, secondary, and tertiary prevention
- Screening, screening principles, and screening tests
- Screening guidelines and evidence ratings
- Diagnostic tests and evidence ratings
- True-positive and false-positive results
- Validity and reliability
- Probability
- Sensitivity and specificity
- Predictive values, positive predictive value, and negative predictive value
- Prevalence and incidence
- *p* value
- Confidence interval
- Statistically significant and clinically significant
- Odds ratio (OR), likelihood ratio (LR), relative risk (RR), and risk reduction

Take a few moments to think about the terms listed above. Can you define them? Can you use them in a clinical scenario? As an advanced practice nurse seeking a doctor of nursing practice (DNP) degree, you are being asked to develop knowledge and skills in an area that has traditionally been the domain of physicians and epidemiologists. As you continue to grow into the DNP role, you may discover a new you! The way you think about prevention, screening, and diagnosing may change. Embrace this change with an open heart and mind. Today more than ever, our country's healthcare system needs the advanced practice nurse to master many new skills. Let's begin the transformation by looking at the natural history of disease from an epidemiological viewpoint.

Natural History of Disease

Although nursing has historically been about promoting and restoring health, nurses are also adept at understanding disease states and how the course of the disease affects a person, family, group, or population. The natural history of disease recounts the nature of the disease and how the disease progresses. Disease progression may depend on a variety of factors, such as genetics (gender, ethnicity, predilections) and genomics (how the host's lifestyle and environment influences genes). Epidemiologists describe the natural history of disease simply as a process in the human host. The process involves the interaction of three factors: the causative agent, the susceptible host, and the environment (**Figure 6-1**).

Health is maintained as long as the process is in a state of equilibrium. Conversely, health may be jeopardized if an imbalance occurs with the process or with any of its factors. For example, the risk for disease increases if host susceptibility is negatively influenced by conditions such as chronic insomnia, inadequate nutrition, aging, or significant stress. Frequent exposures to a causative agent found in the environment such as a potent carcinogen or contagion increase the risk for cancer or infection.

Most nurses recognize Florence Nightingale's footprint in the above description. Nightingale was one of the first persons to acknowledge that a healthy environment and lifestyle were important adjuncts to the healing process. As student nurses we learned that the hospital wards under her influence were expected to be clean. Injured soldiers were bathed, placed in clean gowns, and given adequate nutrition (**Figure 6-2**). Care was taken to promote rest and minimize the stressors that hindered the patient's recovery. Nightingale's knowledge of health and disease led her to test inter-

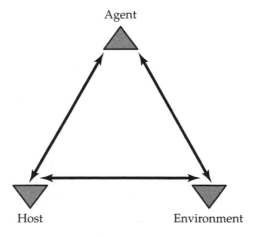

FIGURE 6-1 The interaction between agent, host, and environment.
Source: Picture courtesy of Dr. Kiran Macha.

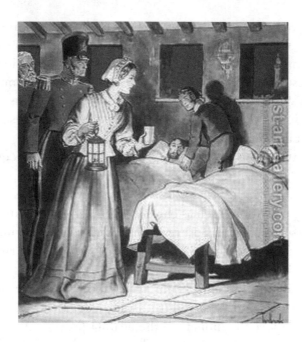

FIGURE 6-2 Florence Nightingale's hospital rounds. Note the hosts (injured soldiers) are convalescing in a well-ventilated, clean hospital ward. An effort is being made to limit agents of harm (contagion) and to decrease (environmental) stressors by promoting rest and providing measures of comfort.
Source: Picture courtesy 1st art gallery, 1997–2010.

ventions aimed at promoting health as well as limiting the natural course of the diseases affecting her patients. Her approach to care has been woven into the fabric of modern-day nursing regardless of whether care is administered in hospitals or in community settings.

We hope this brief introduction, with its roots embedded in epidemiology and the philosophy of nursing, has prompted you to think about the natural history of disease and how it fits into your practice paradigm. To that end, take a moment and think about the following question: *Does nursing care alter the natural history of disease?* Before committing to an answer, consider the following narratives expressed over the years by a few of our graduate students. If your background is hospital based, then your thoughts may be similar to these answers:

> *"Hospital-based nursing care is very specific. Nursing treatments are intended to stabilize patients with acute illnesses. The overall goal is to discharge patients in stable and improved*

condition. Minimal thought is given to preventing disease progression beyond initial treatments and a brief explanation of how the treatments soothe disease processes."

"There is limited time, energy, and money for nurses to undertake much more than managing the acute illness requiring admission."

"Nurses may limit disease through patient referrals to an appropriate national organization. For example, patients with heart failure may be referred to the American Heart Association while patients with lung cancer may be referred to the American Cancer Society."

If your background is community based, your sentiments may be more in tune with one of these statements:

"Home health nurses may be consulted to help care for the patient and family after hospital discharge. The goal is to continue therapy as needed and to facilitate progress toward regaining health. Limiting the natural progression of disease? Maybe indirectly, but not directly."

"Public health nurses may work with a person, a family, a group, or a population and may provide interventions and education useful to limiting the long-term disease course. An example of this service might be group therapy for type 2 diabetics or group consults with a nutritionist to learn the new food pyramid guidelines."

It is clear that as a registered nurse you used interventions that limited the natural course of disease. As an advanced practice nurse, you can do much more by actively screening for diseases, diagnosing disease states, and counseling persons receiving care. As a DNP you will need knowledge and skills that heretofore were the purview of medical doctors and epidemiologists but is now deeply rooted in the education and practice of advanced practice nurses.

Levels of Prevention

The natural history of a disease can be interrupted through carefully planned interventions aimed at preventing the condition, disorder, or disease altogether (primary prevention); detecting it early in its course (secondary prevention); or limiting the effects once it is established (tertiary prevention) (**Figure 6-3**). Knowledge of levels of prevention is an important aspect of planning, rendering, and evaluating care for persons, families, groups, and populations.

An example of *primary prevention* is the practice of providing recommended immunizations to healthy, asymptomatic persons of any age or stage. The vaccinations would likely occur during the prepathogenesis period where the host is exposed to the causative agent and has time to adapt (e.g., recognize the antigen, make antibodies). Screening for a variety of conditions, disorders, and diseases is accomplished at this

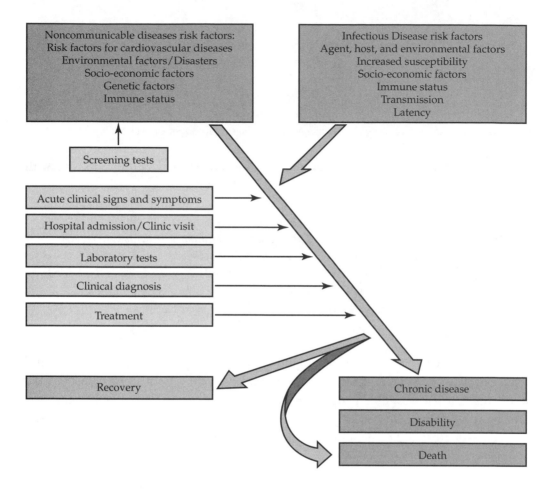

FIGURE 6-3   History of a disease.
Source: Picture courtesy of Dr. Kiran Macha.

level for those with risk or potential risk. Factors such as age, stage, gender, health history, physical findings, family history including genogram results, lifestyle, environment, and/or exposure to a causative agent or agents must be considered before screening. Primary prevention strategies also include screening initiatives on a large scale. Contemporary immunization programs recommend vaccinations for the population at risk and also for those caring the population. For example, a nurse should receive an annual flu vaccination for self-protection as well as to protect coworkers and those receiving care.

Secondary prevention occurs during the pathogenesis period. Those at risk may develop symptoms heralding the onset of pathology, but the disease state may not be recognized until care is sought. Clinicians may discover pathology during office visits for illnesses or during visits scheduled for health maintenance. The early detection of disease allows the practitioner to provide appropriate treatments to limit its course. An example of this level occurs when a certified nurse midwife uncovers risk factors for osteoporosis and obtains a screening test for osteoporosis. If the results are positive, the practitioner will likely treat with medication, weight-bearing exercises, and enhanced nutrition. If the results are negative, he or she may not provide the medication but will instruct the person in the same nonpharmacological treatments.

Tertiary prevention also occurs during the pathogenesis period and differs from secondary prevention in that the disease under question has obvious advanced clinical manifestations. The goal in tertiary prevention is to preserve capacity, maintain or improve capabilities, and limit disability. A person after stroke or after myocardial infarction may receive rehabilitative services as a form of tertiary prevention.

Prevention

As children we learned the wise words of Benjamin Franklin: *an ounce of prevention is worth a pound of cure*. Despite the proven benefits of preventive care, many preventive strategies have had limited effects. The U.S. Department of Health and Human Services is currently reviewing the lessons learned from the previous decade's Healthy People initiatives and is leveraging new scientific evidence, trends, and innovations to develop the next cycle's agenda. As an advanced practice nurse, you have first-hand knowledge of the barriers to preventive practices. The problems with prevention can be related to providers, patients, insurers, systems, and the media.

Providers

Healthcare providers complain they do not have sufficient time to implement preventive protocols and report substandard reimbursement rates for preventive services. Providers also report that preventive practices are fraught with implementation difficulties. To add to the confusion, the evidence for the best preventive practice may lack credibility or may be conflicting.

Patients

Refusal of the patient population to comply with recommendations even when the evidence is impressive is also a factor. Patients complain that preventive practices are time consuming, challenging to schedule, uncomfortable, costly, and confusing.

System

The system presents its own difficulties because payer sources require patients to receive preventive care in a specific insurance/reimbursement plan. Scheduling may present unique challenges for screening tests. How many patients "look forward" to a dental exam, a prostate exam, or a colonoscopy?

Media

The media may inadvertently confuse patients and providers as they erroneously report findings from the newest study. Media spokespersons may take findings out of context and use sensational sound bytes to lure consumers to stay tuned to boost ratings. For example, the consumer reaction to a poorly designed study reported by the media on a link between measles, mumps, and rubella immunization and autism created a fire storm, confusion, and under-immunized children.

The problems with prevention can be solved in part by providers, patients, and the media if everyone learns to think responsibly. Thanks to the World Wide Web, and now The Cloud, there is an unprecedented amount of information available to all of us. Recall that information is only useful when it is relevant, valid, and reliable. An advanced practice nurse at the doctoral level must know the difference between information and knowledge. Additionally, he or she needs to be able to determine what is useful based on evidence. Because we cannot address all areas of prevention in this chapter, we place preventive practices under the umbrella of screening for disease (U.S. Department of Health and Human Services, 2010).

Screening

Knowledge of the natural history of disease and levels of prevention are prerequisite to appreciating the screening process. Nearly four decades ago Dr. J. M. Wilson published a pathology article on the principles of screening for disease in the *Proceedings of the Royal Society of Medicine* (Wilson, 1971). At the time screening tests were not well understood in western civilizations and there was a great debate over their usefulness. Dr. Wilson's article offered a thoughtful and scholarly view about screening tests:

> A recent useful definition of screening is "medical investigation which does not arise from a patient's request for advice for specific complaints" (Nuffield Provincial Hospitals Trust 1968). This screening differs from the usual form of clinical diagnosis in that the doctor is offering a benefit either to the general population or to some particular group, in contrast to patients with symptoms. For this reason, among others,

screening tests need to be especially justified to ensure that benefits outweigh drawbacks.

Screening tests differ from diagnostic tests in that a screening test is a justified investigation to benefit the asymptomatic population. Note that a justified screening test also needed to be valid and reliable.

Modern-day efforts related to health promotion and disease prevention have increasingly recognized the importance of screening and levels of disease prevention. Prevention strategies aimed at controlling disease by detecting it early in its course have led to a fundamental change in practice patterns in the United States and in the world. Practitioners across specialties and disciplines are not merely focusing on disease management but spend a considerable amount of time and effort in preventing the onset of disease in those who appear to be asymptomatic and healthy. Additionally, care is taken to limit the effects of the disease, particularly for disabling diseases such as diabetes mellitus, colorectal cancer, or chronic obstructive pulmonary disease because these diseases impair the quality of life by limiting participation in work and pleasurable activities.

Figure 6-4 demonstrates the natural history of diabetes type 1 may be related to a viral event such as the onset of Coxsackie virus in an infant with susceptibility

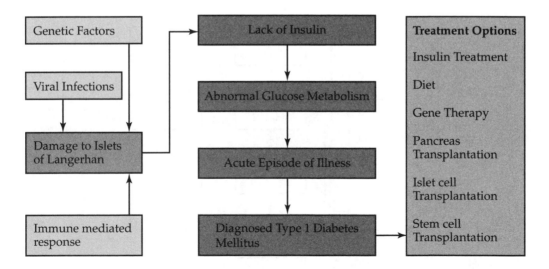

FIGURE 6-4 The natural history of immune-mediated diabetes mellitus type 1 and available treatments.
Source: Picture courtesy of Dr. Kiran Macha.

because of genetic predispositions and the lack of environmental protection from the immune system. Note early diagnosis and treatment with insulin and islet cell transplantation may limit the progression of the disease. Immunization against some viruses may prevent the disease.

The advanced practice nurse has an opportunity to interrupt the natural history of this disease through screening initiatives (**Figure 6-5**). Both primary and secondary prevention measures are effective during the adenoma and preclinical cancer states where the host is asymptomatic. Tertiary measures are used during the clinical cancer states.

Limiting the natural progression of chronic obstructive pulmonary disease by avoiding environment toxins (e.g., smoking, pollution) may slow the progression in some patients (**Figure 6-6**). Early diagnosis and treatment with oxygen therapy, medications, and pulmonary rehabilitation may hinder disease progression and limit the disability associated with advanced chronic obstructive pulmonary disease (**Figure 6-7**).

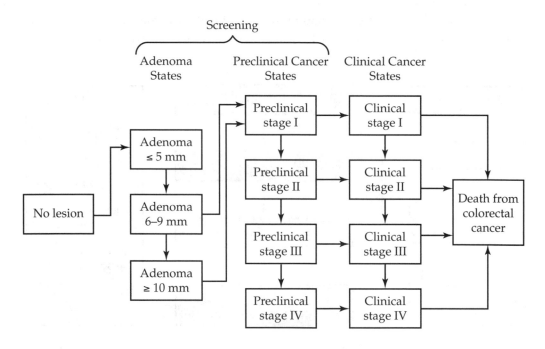

FIGURE 6-5   Depiction of the natural history of disease of colorectal cancer.
Source: From Zauber, A. G. (2008). Evaluating test strategies for colorectal cancer screening: A decision analysis for the US preventive services task force. *Annals of Internal Medicine, 149*(9), 659.

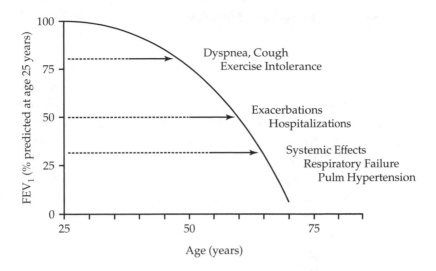

FIGURE 6-6 The natural history of chronic obstructive pulmonary disease (COPD). The relationship between the reduction of forced expiratory volume in 1 second (FEV1) and symptom onset and symptom severity is striking.
Source: From Hanania, N., & Martinez, F. J. (2007). Improving outcomes and awareness of COPD. Retrieved August 30, 2010, from http://cme.medscape.com/viewarticle/553196

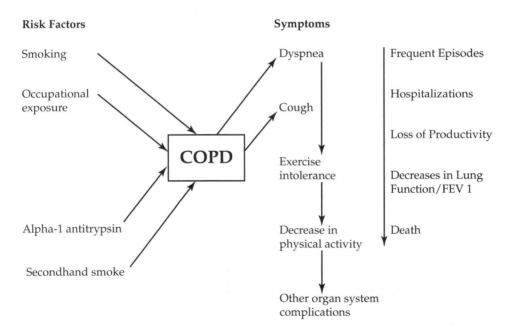

FIGURE 6-7 Consequences of disease progression in patients with chronic obstructive pulmonary disease (COPD).
Source: Picture courtesy of Dr. Kiran Macha.

In primary care settings, screening and disease-limiting strategies are part of health promotion/disease prevention plans. In acute care settings these strategies are a part of many protocols. For example, obtaining a prealbumin level may be one screening test for a malnourished patient undergoing elective surgery. Adequate protein stores are needed for healing, and low prealbumin levels correlate with a longer recovery time. A patient receiving chemotherapy for breast cancer undergoes pretreatment screening laboratory tests to determine if she has adequate values and a functioning hemopoietic system. Screening 12-lead electrocardiograms, echocardiograms, radiographs, pulmonary function tests, stress tests, and blood tests may be required for many patients before undergoing surgery.

There are also screening recommendations for all Americans. The current surgeon general recommends obtaining a genogram on each person going back three generations. Reviewing the person's lineage through a genogram may provide valuable insight into risks. The genogram should be on file in the person's medical record and needs to be reviewed and updated periodically (U.S. Department of Health & Human Services, 2010).

Healthcare professionals have known for a long time that common diseases (i.e., heart disease, cancer, and diabetes) and rare diseases (i.e., hemophilia, cystic fibrosis, and sickle cell anemia) can run in families. If one generation of a family has high blood pressure (BP), it is not unusual for the next generation to have high BP. Tracing the illnesses suffered by your parents, grandparents, and other blood relatives can help your doctor predict the disorders to which you may be at risk and take action to keep you and your family healthy.

Family health history is a powerful screening tool. "My Family Health Portrait" is a Web-based tool that helps users organize family history information and then print it out for presentation to their family doctor. In addition, the tool helps users save their family history information to their own computer and even share family history information with other family members. Access the My Family Health Portrait web tool at https:// familyhistory.hhs.gov/.

Determining the appropriate screening strategies beyond individuals and families is also necessary. Advanced practice nurses may use screening strategies within a practice, clinic, or geographic area. Thus, appreciating the intersection of practice and the principles of screening is useful knowledge for the advanced practice nurse.

Principles of Screening

Four principles of screening were derived from Wilson's 1971 seminal work. Note that the term "condition" can be interchanged with "disorder" or "disease." Interestingly, these principles are still appropriate and serve as the foundation for modern screening and diagnostic initiatives.

1. The condition sought should be important to public health, and a successful method to treat should be available. Before screening, the severity, incidence, and prevalence of the condition should be considered. Screening asymptomatic groups or populations for uncommon or rare diseases with minimal severity is probably not useful. Screening asymptomatic persons and families for rare and uncommon hereditary conditions may be warranted in some cases.
2. There should be a reasonable balance between the cost of screening and its consequences. In other words, the sensitivity, specificity, and predictive values of screening tests should be excellent to limit confusion, prevent delays in diagnosis, minimize misdiagnoses, and contain costs.
3. Before screening, the natural history of the disease needs to be understood. Knowledge derived from the disease course helps the practitioner to identify levels of prevention. The reliability and the validity of screening tests can be determined and the effectiveness of screening and early treatment can be acquired.
4. The ability of the screening test to reach the intended group or population must be known. Proper validation of screening techniques before adopting the technique is central for success.

A fifth principle is emerging and relates to early screening and early detection of disease. In Dr. Wilson's time the physician had the burden of decisions regarding screening. Today, the patient and his or her healthcare provider are encouraged to bear the burden together. They must also understand the consequences of screening. Let's consider the application of prostate cancer screening guidelines to dichotomous groups. Certainly there are high-risk groups of men who require early screening, early detection, and treatment to limit the course of the disease and restore health. However, some prostate cancers are less aggressive, and the natural progression of these types of cancers may not limit mortality. Screening programs may find groups of men with less aggressive, precancerous states or may identify men with these cancers early in their course. Treatments exist to eradicate these nonaggressive forms of cancer but may pose hazards. Is it best to treat or avoid treatment? Obviously, the aggressive cancers will be treated. What about the groups of men with "slow growing not likely to progress" prostate cancers? Time will tell, but in the interim men and their healthcare providers are left wondering about the best course of action. The new prostate cancer screening guidelines stress having a conversation between the provider and the patient about screening and screening consequences. Personalizing the plan according to the man's beliefs and desires in the context of risk is paramount (Mulcahy & Murata, 2010).

Screening Tests

Contemporary screening tests are designed to identify those who have a condition, disorder, or disease that adversely affects health, fertility, or longevity. Screening tests may require a person, family, group, or population to respond to a questionnaire/ survey or may require a procedure such as a history and physical exam. Many screening tests require a specimen from blood, urine, stool, mucus, or some other type of specimen for cellular analysis.

Screening tests vary according to accuracy, cost, accessibility and usefulness. Some screening tests are inexpensive, noninvasive, and pain free and can be administered by unlicensed personnel but may have limited accuracy for pinpointing a specific condition, disorder, or disease. Others are expensive, invasive, cause discomfort, are highly accurate, and can be administered only by licensed/credentialed professionals. Most screening tests have issues affecting their use and fall somewhere between these two extremes.

Screening programs can screen for one or multiple conditions, disorders, or diseases in a person, family, group, or population. *Multiphasic screening techniques* use two or more screening tests together among large groups or populations. Sometimes this screening technique is used along with a preemployment history and physical examination. The most obvious application of this practice is requiring a preemployment urine drug screening test commonly used to identify potential workers who use illicit drugs. Another application of this practice relates to large health maintenance organizations that routinely screen and collect data on employees with the goal of keeping their workforce healthy. *Mass screening* or population screening is a large-scale endeavor aimed at identifying those at risk for certain diseases requiring early identification for maximal success in treatment (limit morbidity/mortality). Regardless of type of screening, the problem under investigation should be important to the person and the community. There should be a mechanism in place to ensure diagnostic follow-up, and appropriate treatment should be available. An acceptable cost-to-benefit ratio is essential, and public, scientific, and ethical acceptance of the test is important (Friis & Sellers, 2009).

Recently, genetic testing became readily available through a variety of venues. Although testing high-risk persons, families, groups, or populations for specific genes related to selected diseases like breast cancer or colon cancer is likely to become more commonplace, screening for those with low or no risk may offer limited benefits. Using some of the available screening techniques may create confusion, result in misdiagnoses, delay diagnoses, and cause harm. The rationale behind this statement can be traced back to the basic principles of screening and the fact that preventive measures do not exist for all diseases. Therefore, it is best to avoid screening for diseases when no preventive measures (either genotypic or phenotypic) are available. As opportunities expand the availability of these types of tests, practitioners will need to ensure that the principles of effective and responsible screening are used.

Screening strategies may also vary according to the person's age and overall health status. An aging, frail person may be less willing to submit to screening tests. Additionally, the evidence related to screening in the older person may limit the usefulness of screening tests because of a person's age. Until there is good evidence from clinical trials, decisions regarding screening in older persons require insightful clinical judgment (Max & Lynn, n.d.)

Consider these different approaches to screening. What if screening recommendations involve guidelines that reflect scientific uncertainty and the recommendations are based on consensus, as is the case in the following examples:

1. The American College of Physicians and the American Society of Internal Medicine recommend against routine screening mammography for breast cancer in women older than 75 years of age.
2. The U.S. Preventive Services Task Force (USPSTF) states that evidence for or against routine screening in women over 70 years of age is insufficient to make recommendations.
3. The American Cancer Society and American Medical Association do not offer an upper age limit for routine screening.

The recommendations disagree and do not provide a clear pathway to best screening practices. When this occurs, it may be best to personalize the screening strategy by estimating the benefits and harms of screening. Knowing the person's feelings about a diagnostic work-up and treatment if the screening test result is abnormal is also prudent.

The decision to screen regardless of age and stage may require the advanced practice nurse or the physician to estimate life expectancy. Benefits from screening may not be realized if life expectancy is low. It is also important to consider the harms of testing. An elderly, kyphotic woman may not submit to mammography screening because the test is very uncomfortable and her body habitus precludes certain views. A homebound person may not have the energy to travel to a testing site. False-positive or false-negative test results can be traumatizing at any age and may cause duress. Results from screening tests may call for additional tests that may be expensive, invasive, and yield little data. Again, having a conversation with the patient and personalizing the approach to screening helps to minimize these issues and is central to success (Melnyk & Fineout-Overholt, 2010).

Screening Guidelines and Evidence Ratings

Many screening guidelines are available to clinicians, including the advanced practice nurse. The quality of screening guidelines varies considerably and needs to be evaluated before use. Some guidelines may be based solely on evidence or may be a mix of consensus statements and evidence. The evidence may be of high quality, poor quality, or somewhere in the middle. The consensus statements themselves may result from an expert panel voicing an opinion or they may be from a panel whose members painstakingly sift through the highest level of research on the topic before publishing their statements. The following is from the U.S. Preventive Services Task Force (USPSTF, 2008a):

> The USPSTF is an independent panel of non-Federal experts in prevention and evidence-based medicine and is composed of primary care providers (such as internists, pediatricians, family physicians, gynecologists, obstetricians, nurses, and health behavior specialists). The USPSTF conducts scientific evidence, reviews a broad range of clinical preventive health care services (such as screening, counseling, and preventive medications) and develops recommendations for primary care clinicians and health systems (**Figures 6-8** and **6-9**). These recommendations are published in the form of "Recommendation Statements."

Grade	Definition	Suggestions for Practice
A	The USPSTF recommends the service. There is high certainty that the net benefit is substantial.	Offer or provide this service.
B	The USPSTF recommends the service. There is high certainty that the net benefit is moderate or there is moderate certainty that the net benefit is moderate to substantial.	Offer or provide this service.
C	The USPSTF recommends against routinely providing the service. There may be considerations that support providing the service in an individual patient. There is at least moderate certainty that the net benefit is small.	Offer or provide this service only if other considerations support the offering or providing the service in an individual patient.
D	The USPSTF recommends against the service. There is moderate or high certainty that the service has no net benefit or that the harms outweigh the benefits.	Discourage the use of this service.
I Statement	The USPSTF concludes that the current evidence is insufficient to assess the balance of benefits and harms of the service. Evidence is lacking, of poor quality, or conflicting, and the balance of benefits and harms cannot be determined.	Read the clinical considerations section of USPSTF Recommendation Statement. If the service is offered, patients should understand the uncertainty about the balance of benefits and harms.

FIGURE 6-8   Grade definitions after May 2007.
Source: From USPSTF, 2008.

Level of Certainty	Description
High	The available evidence usually includes consistent results from well-designed, well-conducted studies in representative primary care populations. These studies assess the effects of the preventive service on health outcomes. This conclusion is therefore unlikely to be strongly affected by the results of future studies.
Moderate	The available evidence is sufficient to determine the effects of the preventive service on health outcomes, but confidence in the estimate is constrained by such factors as • The number, size, or quality of individual studies. • Inconsistency of findings across individual studies. • Limited generalizability of findings to routine primary care practice. • Lack of coherence in the chain of evidence. As more information becomes available, the magnitude or direction of the observed effect could change, and this change may be large enough to alter the conclusion.
Low	The available evidence is insufficient to assess effects on health outcomes. Evidence is insufficient because of • The limited number or size of studies. • Important flaws in study design or methods. • Inconsistency of findings across individual studies. • Gaps in the chain of evidence. • Findings not generalizable to routine primary care practice. • Lack of information on important health outcomes. More information may allow estimation of effects on health outcomes.

FIGURE 6-9 Levels of certainty regarding net benefit.
Source: From USPSTF, 2008.

Diagnosis and Diagnostic Tests

A clinical diagnosis in advanced practice nursing requires the practitioner to reach a conclusion based on evidence gained through deliberate and thoughtful processes. The steps for accurate diagnosing require one to collect data, determine potential problems, develop differential diagnoses, prioritize the differential diagnoses, test hypotheses, and so on until a final diagnosis is reached and supported (Stern, Cifu, & Altkorn, 2010). Data from the history, physical examination, and diagnostic tests are used to "rule in or rule out" a variety of conditions.

A diagnostic test is designed to directly measure and predict. Often, a "cutoff value" for a diagnostic test's outcome is used to determine if the test result is positive or negative. Positive results for a diagnostic test exceed the cutoff value, whereas negative results do not. According to Elavunkal and Sinert (2009), it is important to limit error of test interpretation by measuring the test's accuracy against a criterion standard. Diagnostic tests may cause harm to the person or family member when they create undue stress and lead to unnecessary procedures that may be costly and confusing.

Principles of Diagnostic Tests

There are four principles of diagnostic tests. Similar to the principles of screening, the principles of diagnostic tests serve as the foundation for modern diagnostic initiatives.

1) The natural history of the condition needs to be known before making a diagnosis. Information gained from studying the natural history of the disease is useful for identifying the levels of disease prevention. Throughout this process the reliability and the validity of diagnostic tests can be determined and the effectiveness of diagnosis and early treatment regimens related to the disease can be acquired.

2) Before using the test for diagnostic purposes, the severity, incidence, and prevalence of the condition should be considered. Diagnostic tests should be used to confirm or eliminate a disorder, condition, or disease after a careful history and physical exam is conducted and differential diagnoses are considered. Sometimes the practitioner will have results of screening tests and other objective "pieces" of data before committing to a diagnosis. Other times the diagnosis is based on the history, physical examination, insightful knowledge related to the natural history of the disease, and an understanding of the disease patterns for the geographic area. In some situations a diagnostic test may not be readily available or treatment may need to ensue before the results are available.

3) There should be a reasonable balance between the cost of diagnostic tests and the tests' sensitivity, specificity, predictive values, and likelihood ratios to limit confusion and minimize misdiagnoses. Clinicians should use diagnostic tests with the best evidence related to sensitivity, specificity, predictive values, and likelihood ratios.

4) Practitioners need to use reason, informed judgment, and the best evidence before ordering a test to rule in or rule out a particular disorder, condition, or disease.

Currently, there is a trend toward personalizing the diagnostic test to the patient based on many factors, including genetic testing. As the benefits from the human genome project become more fully realized, diagnostic testing may reach a new level with greater predictive values. We may maximize the therapeutic effect of the medication while limiting adverse effects (Mikail, 2008).

False and True Test Results

Results of tests can be positive or negative. Test results can be further categorized into true and false positives or negatives. A *false-positive test* result occurs when the person being tested is disease free but the test result is positive. A *false-negative test* occurs when a person has the disease but the diagnostic test classifies the person as disease free or negative. The accuracy of test results is represented by measuring validity, reliability, sensitivity, and specificity. Both screening and diagnostic tests may render false-/true-positive and false-/true-negative results. It may be easier to think about this concept with a group or population using a 2×2 table. Add the counts of each in **Table 6-1** to determine the results.

The advanced practice nurse must weigh in the possibility of a false-positive or false-negative test. Remember, screening and diagnostic tests are just part of the picture. Sometimes more than one screening or diagnostic test is used to help rule in or rule out a disease process (Elavunkal & Sinert, 2009).

Validity and Reliability

A synonym for validity is accuracy. The accuracy of a screening or diagnostic test is the test's ability to produce the correct results (no false positives, no false negatives, only true positives and true negatives). The reliability of a test means the test will perform the same way time after time; in other words, the test is consistent and repeatable. The selection of screening and diagnostic tests with adequate validity and reliability is crucial because decisions regarding treatment are often based on test results (Elavunkal & Sinert, 2009).

Table 6-1 Criterion Standard Test		
	Disease Positive	**Disease Negative**
Test positive	True +	False +
Test negative	False −	True −

Probability

Organizing and summarizing data related to a person, group, or population is a common task for the advanced practice nurse. Weighing the probability or chance that an event will occur prompts the practitioner to order either a screening test in a healthy asymptomatic person or a diagnostic test in a symptomatic person. As the practitioner uses tests to rule in or rule out a set of differential diagnoses, he or she is thinking about the differentials in terms of "certainty." For example, the advanced practice nurse may ask, "How certain am I of this diagnosis?" Is the pretest probability or certainty of the disease high enough or low enough that a diagnosis can be made or eliminated? What is the probability of acute myocardial infarction in an adolescent male who complains of one brief episode of sharp chest pain while reaching for a book on a shelf compared with a nauseated, diaphoretic, 65-year-old man with metabolic syndrome presenting to the emergency department with acute, crushing anterior chest pain with a 12-lead electrocardiogram demonstrating ST segment elevation in the inferior leads? The pretest probability of acute myocardial infarction in the adolescent is probably very low, whereas the pretest probability in the 65-year-old man with significant risk factors, classic pain, and a positive electrocardiogram is very high.

A "threshold model" helps conceptualize the probabilities for these two cases. A threshold can be thought of graphically as a line where one end of the line is 0% probability for the disease and the other end is 100% probability for the disease. Somewhere between 0% and 100% is the test's threshold. The adolescent's probability of acute myocardial infarction is so low the number on the line falls below the threshold, close to 0%. The number for the 65-year-old should plot above the threshold on the high end of the line. Confirmatory diagnostic tests such as cardiac enzymes are likely to be positive on the 65-year-old (Stern et al., 2010).

Probability can also be looked at in terms of detecting true-positive and true-negative test results. The probability of detecting a true positive refers to sensitivity, whereas the probability of a true negative refers to specificity.

Sensitivity and Specificity

The most useful screening and diagnostic tests have high ratings for sensitivity and specificity. Sensitivity refers to the tests' ability to yield a positive result when the person actually has the condition, disorder, or disease. Specificity refers to tests' ability to yield a negative result when the person does not have the condition, disorder, or disease. Most screening and diagnostic tests have sensitivity and specificity ratings expressed in percents. Tests with 100% sensitivity and specificity are referred to as meeting the gold standard for tests because they have perfect sensitivity and specificity.

Elavunkal and Sinert (2009) report the following:

> The more sensitive a test is for a disease, the higher its false-positive rate, lowering its specificity. A test with a higher specificity will usually sacrifice sensitivity by increasing its false-negative rate. This makes a highly sensitive test ideal for a screening examination while highly specific tests are best in a confirmatory role. The mnemonics SnOut and SpIn provide some guidelines on how to interpret sensitivity and specificity. SnOut helps physicians to remember that a highly Sensitive test with a negative result is good at ruling-out the disease. SpIn reminds physicians that a highly Specific test with a positive result is good at ruling-in the disease.

Consider the information in **Table 6-2**. Which of the following is the best test? If we used the criteria for best sensitivity and specificity, we would choose B. A 100% value for both means we do not have to worry about false-positive and false-negative results. With this knowledge, we might be prompted to ask another question: What are some other things to consider when selecting a screening test?

There are many things to consider, such as ease of obtaining sample, ease of storing supplies for test, cost, and predictive values. Consider the following questions: What if test A in Table 6-2 could be stored at room temperature and a sample for this test can be obtained by mouth swab and test B needs to be stored at 2 to 8°C and required a blood draw? Most of us would select test A because it is easier to obtain and store and the sensitivity and specificity is comparable with B.

What if test C was the least expensive, easiest to store, and could be done in the privacy of one's home? Testing at home is convenient, but tests done at home may not be accurate. Before ordering a test, a history and physical exam needs to be obtained. Omitting this step increases the chance for a misdiagnosis, a delay in diagnosis, or a delay in treatment. False-positive or negative-test results can occur, necessitating the need for predictive values.

Table 6-2 Sensitivity and Specificity of Three Rapid Tests		
Test	**Sensitivity (%)**	**Specificity (%)**
A	97.9–100	100
B	100	100
C	99.2	87.3

Predictive Values or Pretest/Posttest Probability

Predictive values are useful for a variety of reasons. First, predictive values take into account false-positive and false-negative results and estimate probability. The positive predictive value is the probability of the person actually having the disease when the screening or diagnostic test result is positive. The negative predictive value is the probability of the person being free of disease when the screening or diagnostic test result is negative. Although these values are useful clinically, they have one major deterrent related to usefulness. The positive predictive value and the negative predictive value depend on the prevalence of the disease among the population of interest. The positive/negative predictive value is also referred to as the pretest and posttest probability (Elavunkal & Sinert, 2009). (See Chapters 2 and 3 for a more in-depth discussion on prevalence, incidence, p value, confidence intervals, OR, and RR.)

Statistically Significant and Clinically Significant

Evidence-based practice requires the clinician to understand the difference between statistical and clinical significance. Sometimes study results may have statistical significance (significance levels at 0.05, 0.01, and 0.001) but little or no clinical significance. In others words, the study may have relevance to a scientific endeavor but little or no application to a patient clinically.

Likelihood Ratio

The LR combines data (sensitivity/specificity) and helps the clinician quantify how much the odds of disease change based on a positive or a negative test result. To calculate the LR, first determine the pretest odds. Multiply the pretest odds by the LR to get the posttest odds (Statsdirect, n.d.).

Examples in Advanced Nursing Practice

A. The concepts related to the natural history of disease, levels of prevention, screening tests, and diagnostic tests are demonstrated in the scenario of a young woman presenting with possible pregnancy.

> *Chief Complaint:* "I am concerned that I may be pregnant."
>
> *History and Physical Exam:* A young woman presents to the urgent care center worried she may be pregnant **(condition)** because she has had repeated exposures to unprotected sexual intercourse **(risk)**. Her last menstrual period was 4 weeks ago and she is a few days late. She states she is very regular. A home **pregnancy screening test** was negative, but she wants a more reliable **pregnancy test** and a **diagnosis** as soon as possible.

Review of Systems: A review of systems indicates that her BP on two separate occasions was 140/90. Her body mass index (BMI) is 31%. Her primary care provider ordered recent screening labs tests. She reports the results as a slightly elevated fasting blood glucose level of 110 mg/dL **(disorder)** and an elevated cholesterol level of 300 mg/dL **(risk)**. She is undergoing daily physical therapy for a torn meniscus of the left knee **(condition)**.

Allergies: No known allergies to medications or other substances.

Medications: She is not on any regular medications but takes ibuprofen 600 mg po prn.

Family History: Her family history is positive for obesity, diabetes, and heart disease **(risks)**.

Diet: She is following a low-salt, low-sugar, low-cholesterol diet. A 24-hour diet recall indicates that she is limiting these nutrients in her diet.

Vital Signs: BP, 144/80; P, 80; R, 20; Temp, 98.6°F; BMI, 31%; waist circumference, 35 inches.

Physical Exam: alert, oriented, slightly anxious; skin pink, warm and dry, no lesions. Lungs are clear to auscultation; heart rate and rhythm are regular without murmur; abdomen soft, nontender, obese. There is slight swelling and limited range of motion in left knee.

Assessment: think about pretest and posttest probability as the diagnoses emerge:

- The pretest probability of pregnancy is high related to exposure and the positive at-home test by history, but the pregnancy test is negative and reports 100% sensitivity and 100% specificity.
- She has a history of elevated BP so her pretest probability for elevated BP result is also high. A posttest confirms this as her BP recheck was 142/70 mm of Hg.
- Her history of hypercholesterolemia, elevated blood sugar, elevated BMI (obese) with waist circumference of 35 inches, prompts a **new disorder/disease** of "metabolic syndrome" and a **new diagnosis** of "hypertension."

Diagnoses: (1) Not pregnant, but at risk for unplanned pregnancy and sexually transmitted infections because of unprotected sexual encounters; (2) hypertension; (3) obesity; (4) hypercholesterolemia; (5) hyperglycemia, at risk for continued impaired glucose secondary to obesity and insulin resistance; (6) metabolic syndrome; (7) torn meniscus left knee; (8) education deficits regarding risks and diagnoses.

Plan: The plan needs to address her chief complaint, risks, diagnoses, education, counseling, and follow-up care. The **primary screening** activities for this visit included (1) BP readings, (2) waist circumference, (3) 24-hour diet recall, (4) skin check, and (5) BMI. **Primary prevention counseling** for the visit included reinforcing methods to (1) prevent pregnancy and sexually transmitted infections; (2) limit salt, sugar, and fats; and (3) visit primary care provider for BP medication. It is important to discuss this patient's cardiovascular risks and the need to follow-up her abnormal labs with her primary care provider. Preventive counseling should also stress safety (use seat belts, avoid alcohol, avoid drugs, avoid smoking) and reinforce the prevention efforts related to physical therapy/rehabilitation of left knee injury.

There are some important things to consider regarding this case:

1. The ratings/grades for the above recommendations should be known. The latest evidence-based guideline for diagnosis and treatment of hypercholesterolemia, hypertension, obesity, and metabolic syndrome should be considered. The latest guidelines on preventive services/counseling for safety, pregnancy prevention, and sexually transmitted infection prevention should be applied as well. The practitioner should determine if there is an applicable guideline for knee damage related to injury.

2. This case demonstrates the need for the clinician to remain current with evidence-based guidelines, including decision to treat rules. Remember to listen to patients. Take time to discuss the rationale for your recommendations, especially when the patient's requests and recommendations are discordant.

3. Screening strategies are not always successful. If primary prevention fails, then secondary prevention strategies should be used to identify unrecognized disorders as with our case (metabolic syndrome) or undiagnosed disease (hypertension) before onset of signs/symptoms. When primary and secondary screening efforts fail, tertiary strategies aimed at preserving function and quality of life should be sought. Regular health maintenance visits to a primary care provider for an annual history and physical examination can help the practitioner uncover risk related to family history (genetics) and the person's environment and lifestyle (genomics). Symptom analysis and findings from the physical examination may reveal a pathogenic process. Disease detection can be aided by judicious use of both screening and diagnostic tests. Additionally, the practitioner can find ways to praise and reinforce positive health habits during an office visit or during an annual review. Together the practitioner and the person can discuss options and review evidence. A similar scenario can be accomplished for family members, groups, and populations. Ultimately, a plan of care can be collaboratively determined with specific and pertinent endpoints and outcomes for success.

B. What is the best way to use guidelines and evidence ratings?

Advanced practice nurses use guidelines and evidence ratings to help select the best tests and treatments related to a particular condition, disorder, or diagnosis. Similar to screening guidelines, the integration of research findings into diagnostic and treatment guidelines is an ongoing process with many challenges. There is a plethora of readily available evidence-based guidelines. The problem is finding the best guideline and matching the guideline to the need. Hansen, Hoss, and Wesorick (2008, pp. 186) describe guidelines and their uses for nurses as a "collection of practical information that assists with clinical decision making." They further state that guidelines have evolved in the last few decades, moving away from expert opinion and consensus to evidence-based guidelines useful for practice. The rationale for this argument against opinion/consensus is logical because experts may be wrong.

This last section provides the advanced practice nurse with tables for applying statistics to clinical situations. The definitions of key terms and formulas for a variety of standard tests are described. **Tables 6-3** and **6-4** may be useful to the advanced practice nurse in practice and may be helpful for the exercises in Part 2 of this chapter.

Table 6-3 Terms, Formulas, and Definitions		
Term	**Calculation**	**Plain English**
True positive (TP)	Counts in 2×2 table	# Patients with the disease who have a positive test result
True negative (TN)	Counts in 2×2 table	# Patients without the disease who have a negative test result
False positive (FP)	Counts in 2×2 table	# Patients without the disease who have a positive test result
False negative (FN)	Counts in 2×2 table	# Patients with the disease who have a negative test result
Sensitivity = True positive rate (TPR)	TP / (TP + FN)	The probability that a patient with the disease will have a positive test result
1 - Sensitivity = False-negative rate (FNR)	FN / (TP + FN)	The probability that a patient with the disease will have a negative test result

(continues)

Table 6-3 Terms, Formulas, and Definitions *(continued)*

Term	Calculation	Plain English
Specificity = True negative rate (TNR)	TN / (TN + FP)	The probability that a patient without the disease will have a negative test result
1 - Specificity = False-positive rate (FPR)	FP / (TN + FP)	The probability that a patient without the disease will have a positive test result
Positive predictive value	TP / (TP + FP)	The probability that a patient with a positive test result will have the disease
Negative predictive value	TN / (TN + FN)	The probability that a patient with a negative test result will not have the disease
Accuracy	(TP + TN) / (TP + TN + FP + FN)	The probability that the results of a test will accurately predict presence or absence of disease
Bayes' theorem	Posttest odds = pretest odds × likelihood ratio	The odds of having or not having the disease after testing
Likelihood ratio of a positive test result (LR+)	Sensitivity / (1 - specificity)	The increase in the odds of having the disease after a positive test result
Likelihood ratio of a negative test result (LR−)	(1 - Sensitivity) / Specificity	The decrease in the odds of having the disease after a negative test result

Source: From Elavunkal and Sinert (2009) and Merck Online manual home edition (n.d.).

Table 6-4 Qualitative Strength of the Test by Likelihood Ratio

Qualitative Strength	LR(+)	LR(−)
Excellent	10	0.1
Very good	6	0.2
Fair	2	0.5
Useless	1	1

LR, likelihood ratio.

Source: From Elavunkal and Sinert (2009).

PART 2: APPLICATION

Exercise 1: Applying Concepts Related to Screening, Test Sensitivity and Specificity

Marilyn Newby, a recently divorced 55-year-old banker, presented to her family NP for an annual well woman visit. Ms. Newby has no significant family history or medical concerns. Her past medical history is negative, and her parents and both sets of her grandparents are alive and well. The only disease that runs in her family is hypertension. The medical assistant noted Ms. Newby's initial BP reading as 150/94. Ten minutes later, the medical assistant rechecked the BP and recorded 154/92. Previous BP readings were documented on the electronic medical record as 144/88, 140/90, and 146/90.

The family NP completed the well woman exam, including a Pap smear, breast exam, and full skin exam. The family NP ordered a panel of screening tests (comprehensive metabolic panel, thyroid-stimulating hormone, and lipid levels). The diagnosis of hypertension, stage 1, was made.

Ms. Newby's case demonstrates the use of several common, valid, and reliable screening tests. Screening for high BP is relatively inexpensive and easy to perform by technical or professional personnel. Although it takes a clinician to make the diagnosis, the screening test was administered and the results were recorded by an unlicensed person schooled in proper BP technique. Screening was initiated when the family NP reviewed Ms. Newby's records, conducted the interval history, and completed the physical exam, including the Pap smear and bimanual pelvic exam.

Name three screening tests other than BP that can be done by unlicensed personnel:

1.

2.

3.

Assistive personnel can perform a number of screening and diagnostic tests and record findings, but the diagnosis must be made by a licensed professional. Fingerstick labs such as cholesterol, iron screen, enzyme, urine analysis, urine specific gravity, height, weight, BMI, vital signs, and skin mapping are a few of the tests performed by assistants. The family NP followed evidence-based screening guidelines when caring for Ms. Newby.

Other than the Pap smear, what other screening tests were performed? According to the latest evidence, what should be performed for Ms. Newby?

Other tests performed included a complete skin exam looking for precancerous or cancerous lesions. Fasting blood tests were ordered to screen for hyperlipidemia, elevated glucose levels, and thyroid disease. According to the latest evidence, Ms. Newby should receive a screening mammogram and a screening colonoscopy. She should be referred to a dentist if she has not had a recent oral exam and should see an eye doctor for an evaluation.

Ms. Newby's screening tests were performed and all were negative. She was placed on medication for hypertension and will be seen regularly by the family NP. The family NP has plans to address other screening needs and will provide preventive counseling for a variety of needs during future visits.

Ms. Newby's case demonstrated several important aspects about screening tests. Some of her tests were inexpensive, easy to obtain, and obtained by unlicensed assistive personnel. Other tests were expensive, invasive, caused discomfort, and were administered and interpreted by highly skilled, licensed, and certified clinicians. For example, the advanced practice nurse is qualified to order a screening mammogram or colonoscopy but is not able to perform the test. A referral must be made to appropriately credentialed specialists—a radiologist for mammography and a gastroenterologist for colonoscopy.

Are there other screening tests for colon cancer that are just as good as colonoscopy but are less invasive and less expensive?

Currently, a screening colonoscopy is recommended by most. There are promising, less invasive, and less expensive tests available, but they have not achieved the preferred test status and are not considered the gold standard.

Exercise 2: Use Your Knowledge to Determine the Screening Level of the Following Scenarios. Use: P = primary; S = secondary; T = tertiary.

_____ A family NP looks for evidence of acanthosis nigricans in an obese adolescent with a family history of type 2 diabetes mellitus.

_____ As part of an evidenced-based project, a DNP student identifies those with elevated BP readings and elevated fingerstick cholesterol screens on 20 obese adolescents with parents who died of acute myocardial infarction at a young age. The group's results will be sent to a primary care NP for review and follow-up.

_____ A certified nurse midwife performs pregnancy tests on a population of young, healthy, married women.

_____ A pediatric NP orders annual immunizations for toddlers.

_____ The adult NP orders annual flu immunizations for her clients with lung cancer.

_____ A clinical nurse specialist supervises a group of post–myocardial infarction patients receiving complimentary Brain Natriuretic Peptide (BNP) and inflammatory marker analyses screening in a hospital-based cardiac rehabilitation program.

_____ A family NP works with the medical team to provide tuberculosis screening tests for a group of healthy, asymptomatic college students.

_____ A DNP resident determines which group of tests for breast cancer yields the greatest accuracy for the lowest cost per test for a study population with metastatic cervical cancer.

_____ A DNP-prepared geriatric NP studies the evidence regarding the sensitivity, specificity, and costs of a cadre of tests before determining which test is best for a study population with colon polyps.

Remember primary prevention strategies are for persons, families, groups, and populations who are asymptomatic and have no evidence of the disease. The following are examples:

- A family NP works with the medical team to provide tuberculosis screening tests for a group of healthy, asymptomatic college students.
- A certified nurse midwife performs pregnancy tests on a population of young, healthy, married women.
- A pediatric NP orders annual immunizations for toddlers.

All these examples can be categorized as primary prevention because the population is healthy and asymptomatic.

Primary screening tests are frequently ordered in these situations. Other forms of evidence-based primary prevention may be offered to these groups, including counseling for prevention of pregnancy, sexually transmitted disease, and drug and alcohol use/abuse along with other health issues common to young adults. Chemoprevention related to daily multivitamin/mineral and folic acid intake may be warranted to prevent anemia and neural tube defects in those at risk for pregnancy. Toddlers and their parents have many needs beyond immunizations, including counseling and anticipatory guidance related to growth/development, safety, nutrition, exercise, and rest among other things.

Secondary prevention strategies are reserved for those who are asymptomatic but are at risk for the condition, disorder, or disease. The risk factor may be related to family history, lifestyle, environment, or a disease that places them at greater risk than a person without the exposure to the risk factors.

A family NP looks for evidence of acanthosis nigricans in an obese adolescent with a family history of type 2 diabetes mellitus.

An obese adolescent with family history positive for diabetes mellitus is at risk for type 2 diabetes. In this example, there is a high probability that the acanthosis nigricans is related to insulin resistance, heralding the onset of diabetes. Screening in this case involved history and physical exam before performing the additional tests.

As part of an evidence-based project, a DNP student identifies those with elevated BP readings and elevated finger stick cholesterol screens on 20 obese adolescents who had parents who died of acute myocardial infarction at a young age. Based on the results the group is referred to a primary care NP.

The DNP student initially used primary screening techniques to uncover hypertension and hypercholesterolemia in an "at risk group" with a chronic disease: obesity. There is a high likelihood that the diagnoses will be confirmed in several persons in the group after the results of fasting lipid profiles and additional BP readings are reviewed.

A DNP-prepared geriatric NP studies the evidence regarding the sensitivity, specificity, and costs of a cadre of screening and diagnostic tests before determining which test is best for her patients with atypical colon polyps.

The DNP-prepared geriatric NP was using a more sophisticated technique to determine the best test for asymptomatic persons who have a risk factor for colon cancer: atypical colon polyps. Most likely, a primary screening test (colonoscopy) identified the atypical colon polyps. As a result of this finding, this population moved into a higher risk category because they have a chronic condition (atypical polyps) making them at greater than average risk for colon cancer.

These examples represent asymptomatic persons at risk who need secondary screening techniques to limit the harmful effects of disease.

Tertiary levels of prevention are generally reserved for those with chronic diseases. The following examples represent persons, groups, or populations with a significant chronic disease such as the post–myocardial infarction group at risk for heart failure, the population of persons with invasive cervical cancer, and a population of persons with lung cancer needing annual influenza immunizations. Note that the levels of prevention categories may overlap and the lines between the levels may be blurred. At times the situation seems to cover more than one level of prevention.

A clinical nurse specialist supervises a group of post–myocardial infarction patients receiving complimentary BNP and inflammatory marker analyses screening in a hospital-based cardiac rehabilitation program.

Knowing the natural progression of disease is helpful in ascertaining the appropriate level or levels of screening in these scenarios. In persons without chronic disease, screening for a disease such as BNP levels or providing an annual immunization may be considered primary. A BNP level and other inflammatory markers in a person with hypertension may be secondary prevention. However, a group with recent myocardial infarction is at greater risk for heart failure. In this case screening for BNP levels may alert the practitioner to obtain an interval history/physical exam and order additional tests for heart failure. The results may prompt a new diagnosis, whereas a delay in diagnosis may increase morbidity and mortality. Please note that this population is at risk for other atherosclerosis-related diseases such as stroke, peripheral artery disease, and hyperlipidemia. This population is at increased risk for other diseases as well such as depression and obesity. The advanced practice nurse along with members of the multidisciplinary team would consider these risks and many other aspects of care for this population.

A DNP resident determines which group of tests for breast cancer yields the greatest accuracy for the lowest cost per test in a study population with a history of invasive cervical cancer.

Those with invasive cervical cancer may not have palpable breast masses but may have risks above and beyond a population who is asymptomatic (e.g., those with normal breast exams and no evidence of cancer). Generally, diagnostic mammography differs from screening mammography in that more views of the breast—particularly areas where masses may be palpated—are obtained and reviewed. Additionally, those with invasive cancer may get more frequent mammography and other tests depending on a variety of factors. Does the above scenario fit best as a secondary or tertiary level of prevention? An argument might be made for both depending on one's interpretation of levels.

An adult NP orders annual flu immunizations for a study population with lung cancer.

Many would argue that this scenario is primary prevention because immunizations are always primary. Others may consider the setting and context. If the population has lung cancer, then administering the flu shot is necessary to prevent further lung damage or harm. Recall that those undergoing treatment for cancer are often immunocompromised, making them at greater risk for infections.

Exercise 3: Using the Concepts and Statistics in Practice

Calculate Probabilities

Some advanced practice nurses use the natural history of disease, levels of prevention, screening tests, diagnostic tests, and statistics daily. For example, as part of a multidisciplinary team, a nurse anesthetist was conducting a preoperative assessment and ordered a screening test on a person complaining of chest pain. Suspecting that the chest pain may be related to pulmonary embolus, the nurse anesthetist calculated the pretest probability of pulmonary embolism at 28%. The nurse anesthetist used the steps in **Table 6-5** to calculate the posttest probability of pulmonary embolus at 87.5%.

Although the above method is mathematically correct, it requires multiple steps and is inconvenient for bedside use. In 1975, Fagan published a nomogram based on Bayes' theorem (**Figure 6-10**). To use the nomogram, draw a straight line from the person's pretest probability through the appropriate likelihood ratio, connecting to the posttest probability (blue line).

LR+ was first calculated and is a measure of how much more likely a diseased person is to have a positive test result when compared to a non-diseased person. In this example a diseased person is 18 times more likely to test positive than a non-diseased person. LR− when calculated is 0.105, which is a measure of the relative likelihood

Table 6-5 Calculating Probability of Disease	
Steps	**Calculations**
1. Convert pretest probability to odds. Odds = Probability / (1 - Probability)	Pretest odds = 0.28 / (1 - 0.28) = 0.389
2. Calculate LR+. LR+ = Sensitivity / (1 - Specificity)	LR+ = 0.90 / (1 − 0.95) = 18.0
3. Calculate Bayes' Theorem. Posttest Odds = Pretest Odds × LR	Posttest odds = 0.389 × 18 = 7.0
4. Convert posttest odds to probability. Probability = Odds / (1 + Odds)	Posttest probability = 7 / (1 + 7) = 87.5%

The person had a positive screening test with a sensitivity of 90%, a specificity of 95%, and a calculated pretest probability of 28%. LR, likelihood ratio.

Source: From Elavunkal and Sinert (2009).

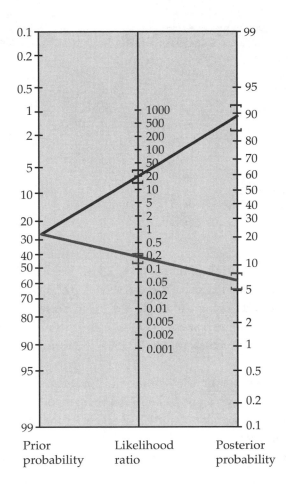

FIGURE 6-10 Fagan's nomogram is used to determine posttest probability of 87.5% for pulmonary embolism in a person with a pretest probability of 28%. Note that this nomogram has a likelihood ratio. What does the likelihood ratio of minus 0.2 mean?
Source: From Elavunkal & Sinert, 2009.

that a diseased person has a negative test result. In this example, a diseased person has about one-tenth the chance of a negative test compared to a non-diseased person. Hence one desires LR+ > 1 and LR– < 1 (**Tables 6-6** and **6-7**). If you read the nomogram, you can see that the posttest probability given a negative test result is 0.039. The two posttest probabilities tell a more complete story. This person had a

Table 6-6 Qualitative Strength of the Test by Likelihood Ratio		
Qualitative Strength	**LR(+)**	**LR(−)**
Excellent	10	0.1
Very good	6	0.2
Fair	2	0.5
Useless	1	1

LR, likelihood ratio.

Source: From Elavunkal and Sinert (2009).

positive test result; based on that, one can say there is a 87.5% risk of the disease event. Had the person tested negative, there is a small 3.9% chance of the disease being present. Since LR+ = 18 is high and LR− = 0.10, this test would typically be rated as very good to excellent. Some researchers look at the ratio LR+/LR− and like that to be larger than some cutoff such as 50. In this case the ratio is 171, which is perhaps excellent.

According to the nomogram, the likelihood of minus 0.2 (LR (−) is 0.105 when calculated) means there is a very good likelihood that the person has pulmonary embolus. Often, practitioners wonder about LRs and about the differences and similarities between ORs and RRs. Remember that LRs can be calculated from Bayes' theorem and sensitivity/specificity results. [Sensitivity and specificity are intrinsic

Table 6-7 Formulas for Likelihood Ratios		
Bayes' theorem	Posttest Odds = Pretest Odds × Likelihood Ratio	The odds of having or not having the disease after testing
Likelihood ratio of a positive test result (LR+)	Sensitivity / (1 - Specificity)	The increase in the odds of having the disease after a positive test result
Likelihood ratio of a negative test result (LR−)	(1 - Sensitivity) / Specificity	The decrease in the odds of having the disease after a negative test resultt

LR, likelihood ratio.

Source: From Elavunkal and Sinert (2009).

measures of the screening test and do not depend on prevalence. Since LRs are simple functions of sensitivity and specificity they are also intrinsic to the test. If one knows prevalence, the positive predictive value (PPV) and negative predictive value (NPV) can be calculated and these are typically what one is interested in clinically.]

Odds Ratios and Relative Risk

The following example may help you appreciate the difference between OR and RR and may offer a method to convert OR to RR. As part of a multidisciplinary team, the acute care NP was reviewing a published paper on the risk for developing heart failure in older adults on nonsteroidal anti-inflammatory drugs (NSAIDs). Her goal was to prevent heart failure in a person with heart disease on daily NSAIDs to control osteoarthritis pain. She happened upon a paper calculating the postexposure probability for developing heart failure where the RR was calculated from ORs using a modified nomogram. She wondered about the accuracy of this practice and mentioned it to her team during rounds.

Page and Attia (2003) described a method to convert OR to RR given a known baseline risk:

> Using a straight edge on the nomogram, line up the baseline probability of an event on axis A, with the OR on axis B, and read off the postexposure probability on axis C. The postexposure probability divided by the baseline probability then yields the RR. Thus, with available information on the OR from epidemiological studies and the baseline risk, Bayes' nomogram calculates the postexposure risk in the presence of the risk factor. Knowledge of the postexposure risk also allows easy and accurate calculation of the absolute risk difference and the number needed to treat (NNT) or the number needed to harm (NNH).

With the above in hand, the acute care NP found a peer-reviewed article in a respected journal estimating the "odds ratio of 10.5 for developing heart failure associated with the NSAID use in persons with a history of heart disease"(Page & Attia, 2003, p. 133). The team decided to apply the study findings to a person under their care. First, the team members estimated the baseline risk of heart failure using an equation derived by Kannel et al. (1999) based on the Framingham database.

The person was a 60-year-old man with "documented coronary artery disease who had a vital capacity of 2.5 L, systolic blood pressure of 160 mm Hg, heart rate of 85 beats per minute, evidence of left ventricular hypertrophy on electrocardiogram and cardiomegaly on chest radiogram" (Page & Attia, 2003). A 4-year risk of heart failure was calculated at 34%. His 1-year risk was approximately 8.5%.

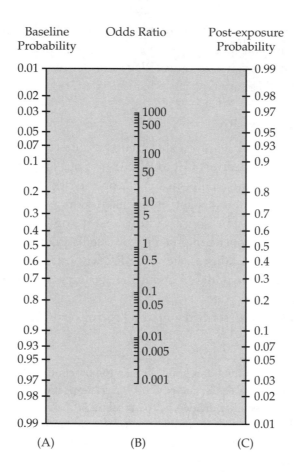

FIGURE 6-11   Nomogram to calculate postexposure probability given estimates of the OR and baseline probability. This nomogram is equivalent to the Bayes' nomogram, but with different labels.
Source: From Page & Attia, 2003.

Using Bayes' nomogram, a member of the team anchored a straight edge at 0.085 (baseline risk) on axis A and directed the edge through axis B at 10.5 (OR). The postexposure risk at axis C was determined as 0.49, or a 49% chance of developing heart failure over 1 year after starting NSAIDs.

The RR was then estimated by dividing the posttest probability, 49%, by the pretest probability, 8.5%, to get the RR of 5.8 (not an RR of 10.5 as some would misinterpret the OR). The absolute risk difference is 0.49 − 0.085 = 0.405.

The number needed to treat is the reciprocal of the absolute risk difference of 0.405, which is approximately 2.5. Thus, five such patients exposed to NSAIDs for a year would be expected to result in two new cases of heart failure.

ORs are used frequently in retrospective studies, whereas RR is commonly used in prospective studies. The study design matters. For example, in case-control studies only ORs can be calculated. In cross-sectional studies (or using data extracted from cohorts), either can be calculated. Clinicians frequently interchange the meanings of ORs with RRs. Although the two statistics may be close (when the risk in both groups is small), mistakes in judgment can occur if the clinician does not understand the differences between the two. [RR is much easier to understand because e.g., an RR = 4 says the risk is 4 times as great. This has the easy-to-understand property that if you have two groups of 100 each, there will be on average 4 times as many events in one of the groups. I would point out that RR can be quite deceiving when reported without reporting absolute risk. Note that in the case where the absolute risks are .1 and .4 respectively, RR = 4.0 and OR = 6.0; see Chapter 3]. One way to convert ORs to RR is by using the modified nomogram as described in the example above. Care must be taken to mark the nomogram appropriately because the axes are "logarithmic rather than linear." In other words, failure to accurately place the marks on the scale translates into error (Page & Attia, 2003).

Probability Values and Confidence Intervals

A primary care NP was asked to search the literature to find a way to increase annual flu immunization rates for staff with direct care responsibilities at the clinic. The NP found a study by Abramson, Avni, and Miskin (2010). The purpose of the study was to increase staff rates through an education program that included a lecture on the topic from a primary care physician, e-mails to remind the staff person to get immunized, and using a key figure in the clinic to encourage staff members to accept an annual flu shot. The results of the study are as follows (p. 293):

> Influenza immunization rate was 52.8% (86 of 163) in the intervention group compared with 26.5% (48 of 181) in the control group ($p < .001$). When compared with the rate of immunization for the previous season, the absolute increase in immunization rate was 25.8% in the intervention clinics and 6.6% in the control clinics. Multivariate analysis showed a highly significant ($p < .001$) independent association between intervention and immunization, with an odds ratio of 3.51 (95% confidence interval, 2.03–6.09).

Overall, the immunization rate for staff members improved. Based on the odds ratio, staff members who received the intervention were more likely to get immunized than those who were not in the intervention group. p Value results in the 0.001 range are highly significant. The confidence interval is fairly narrow and is also a measure of significance. [Because it does not contain 1, it shows significance at 5%.

Furthermore, the lower limit is well above 1.0. The width is more related to accuracy, which depends on the sample size.] The NP can be 95% confident that the population parameter of interest falls between 2.03 and 6.09. The NP can say with confidence that the strategies worked for the study population and that the strategies also have a very good chance of being successful in other work settings. This finding was statistically significant and clinically significant.

Exercise 4: Your Practice and the Natural History of Disease, Levels of Prevention, and Concepts Related to Statistics

Close your eyes, take a deep breath, exhale, and think back to your last day at work. How many patients did you see? Now, focus your thoughts on the most interesting one. You probably reviewed the person's chief complaint, wrote a SOAP (subjective, objective, assessment, plan) note, and provided counseling/education about the disease on the medical record. Did you think about the natural progression of the disease you treated? How about levels of prevention—did they apply to this case? Did you wonder about the patient's family and their risks for disease?

Next, think about your entire practice. Have you seen a higher incidence or prevalence of a particular disease or condition lately? Were you prompted to wonder about this phenomenon and ponder the effects of the disease on your community? Have you compared your care outcomes for the 10 most common diseases in your practice with those of your peer group?

Think about the past week. How many screening or diagnostic tests did you order? How many did you interpret? Did you use the results of these tests in planning or evaluating care for your patient? Did you contemplate the accuracy of the tests? How many false-positive/false-negative results did you encounter? Did the sensitivity or specificity of a screening/diagnostic test enter into your decision calculus?

At the last conference you attended, did you engage colleagues in conversation about your approval or disapproval of the latest evidence-based guideline? Did you dialogue with your peer group about the LRs or another statistic in the last article you read in your favorite peer-reviewed journal?

Did you attend the monthly local health planning council meeting? Did you get a chance to work with business groups to facilitate health promotion activities for your community?

Chances are good that you answered, "Yes, I did," to some of the questions and recalled utilizing some of these concepts. Furthermore, chances are good that you are not sure if you did or did not do some of these things. Most of us do not think too much about these things because the processes are ingrained in our practice patterns.

In other words, you don't think too much about these things, you just do them! Continue reading and see how one NP answered these questions.

Most Interesting Patient and Natural History of Disease

I am an NP and a cardiovascular clinical specialist. The most interesting person I saw last week is also a person representing the majority of the adults in my practice with chronic diseases. The gentleman, Mr. Vascularo, is 55 years old and is being treated for metabolic syndrome (central obesity, hypertension, hyperlipidemia), mild depression, mild anxiety, and sleep apnea. He had an ST segment elevated myocardial infarction (STEMI) 3 months ago. Currently, Mr. Vascularo is stable and on appropriate lifestyle modification prescriptions and medications (aspirin, beta-blocker, angiotensin-converting enzyme, niacin, and an omega 3 supplement). The recent STEMI "scared him," and he was motivated to change to regain a reasonable level of health. In a nutshell, his cardiac rehabilitation program helped him appreciate the need to limit daily salt intake to 1,500 mg per day, decrease fats, restrict calories to 2,200 per day, eat more frequent meals with smaller portion sizes, and eat more fresh fruits and more colorful vegetables each day. Last week he increased his 45-minute exercise sessions from three times a week to five times a week. The nutritionist told him that he should lose 1 to 2 pounds per week on this plan. He has already lost 10 pounds (BMI, 33) and 2 inches from his waist (45 to 43 inches).

Mr. Vascularo's desire to improve his health is paramount to limiting the natural history of a major disease process—atherosclerosis. The natural history of atherosclerosis and myocardial infarction is well known. The atherosclerotic process affects most small and medium-sized arteries. When the disease is not treated or is undertreated, it will progress. As a result, Mr. Vascularo is at risk for another myocardial infarction, heart failure, peripheral artery disease, and stroke. The atherosclerotic process has also been implicated as one of the major pathological disorders of those with metabolic syndrome. Additionally, there is a relationship between atherosclerosis and sleep apnea, depression, and anxiety. Limiting the progression of atherosclerosis is a primary endpoint. Certainly, the holistic plan for Mr. Vascularo's condition will include other treatments, but for the purposes of this exercise we focus on controlling atherosclerosis.

Levels of Prevention

In this case, we cannot evoke primary prevention strategies for Mr. Vascularo—he already has the disease. But we can search the literature and find the best evidence to limit further progression of the disease. The American College of Cardiology and the

American Heart Association issued a recent update to the 2004 guidelines related to current treatment for STEMI, including secondary prevention strategies. Because the STEMI is not recent, we need to focus our energies on the secondary and tertiary prevention strategies. We can also focus on primary prevention strategies for Mr. Vascularo's children who are healthy.

Many times a busy primary care practitioner cannot take the time to read the latest evidence from specialty groups. Fortunately, most of the peer-reviewed primary care journals update guidelines regularly, including guidelines from specialty groups like the American College of Cardiology or the American Heart Association. The journal, *American Family Physician*, is a great resource for updated guidelines. The June 15, 2009, issue published an update I can use for Mr. Vascularo (and many others in my practice). The update includes the latest evidence related to the intervention, recommendation, and level of evidence.

As I review the latest evidence-based guideline, I notice that my plan meets the secondary prevention recommendations for Mr. Vascularo. He is on appropriate prescriptions for medications and lifestyle modifications. He does not smoke and has a normal BP on his current medications. He has decreased his BMI and waist measurements and is following the nutritionist's recommendations for the daily intake of salt, fiber, fats, proteins, carbohydrates, calories, and trace minerals.

I make a note in the medical record to offer him an annual influenza vaccination in the fall. I document the need to discuss the recommendation to increase exercise frequency from five times per week to daily exercise with his next visit in 2 months. I wonder if he needs a daily multivitamin/mineral supplement and a pneumonia vaccination. I prescribe the daily vitamin. I make a mental note to look up the latest on adult immunizations.

A month later I see Mr. Vascularo's 17-year-old daughter for a sports physical. Although the primary purpose of the visit is to clear her to safely participate in sports, I take the opportunity to evoke the primary prevention strategies. My goal is to limit her risk for cardiovascular disease. After a complete cardiovascular risk factor assessment (smoking, diabetes, hyperlipidemia, age, gender, and family history) was completed, I refer her to the Surgeon General's website on genograms and give her a form to fill out documenting her family history for three generations. We talk about her risks for heart disease because heart disease is present on both sides of her family. I explain that she may have genetic risk factors for heart and blood vessel disease but remind her that lifestyle and environmental factors also play a role. My goal is to empower her to make changes that will limit her risks for heart disease. I think about other prevention strategies and use my counseling skills to encourage her to (1) wear seat belts while driving or riding in vehicles, (2) follow the new food guide pyramid, (3) take a multivitamin mineral supplement daily, and (4) say "no" to nicotine, alcohol, and drugs, among other things.

My last words during Mr. Vascularo's visit and his daughter's visit are how to reach me if they have questions or other health concerns. I also let them know they can see me as needed between scheduled appointments. Finally, I make a mental note to find the latest guidelines on tertiary prevention for those with advanced cardiovascular disease. I know that despite my best efforts, I will not always be able to alter the progression of atherosclerosis with medication or lifestyle/environmental modifications.

Have You Seen a Higher Incidence or Prevalence of a Particular Disease or Condition Lately?

The incidence and prevalence of obesity, hypertension, diabetes, atherosclerosis, heart disease, vascular disease, and STEMI in my county is higher than the national average and higher than the average for my state. The local health planning council has compiled these statistics for these diseases and along with the local health department has conveyed these concerns to all primary care and specialty care clinicians. Local community leaders have also been notified of the alarming statistics.

Were You Prompted to Wonder About This Phenomenon and Ponder the Effects of the Disease on Your Community?

Yes, I was prompted and felt compelled to ponder the effects of the disease on my community and the communities within my county. I am working with community partners to offer better access to free or low-cost fitness facilities along with low-cost access to nutrition counseling for children and adults who are at risk for disease.

Have You Compared Your Care Outcomes for the 10 Most Common Diseases in Your Practice With Those of Your Peer Group?

An independent group reviews my outcomes for several conditions, disorders, and diseases. Outcomes for health promotion and disease prevention strategies related to nutrition and obesity screens (BMI, diet counseling), osteoporosis screening (identifying high-risk persons, DEXA scans), cancer screening (mammography, Pap smears, Prostate Specific Antigen, skin), and disease management for depression, pain management, hypertension, diabetes mellitus, hyperlipidemia, and metabolic syndrome are computed for the clinic and for each clinician annually. The clinic staff reviews the results annually. We compare our outcomes with guidelines from our continuous quality improvement plan. There are so many expectations placed on us related to guideline implementation. The continuous quality improvement plan helps us focus and stay on track.

Think About the Past Week. How Many Screening or Diagnostic Tests Did You Order? How Many Did You Interpret?

In all honesty, I don't know the actual number of screening/diagnostic tests I ordered. Every person is measured and weighed. A BMI is calculated, recorded, and compared with previous readings. All my patients have their BP measured and recorded and comparisons are made to previous readings. If the person is presenting for an annual exam, he or she will probably receive a vision screen, waist to hip measurement/ratio, and some will have a urine analysis screen (e.g., those with diabetes, hypertension, etc.).

I think about each person's needs based on history, physical exam, age, stage, and gender. I focus on all the levels of prevention and think through a plausible plan for each one. It may take me several visits to come up with the health promotion plan because I have only a few minutes with each person.

The clinic's policy requires the documentation of the plan and timeline for each person receiving care. We also are expected to document counseling sessions and discussions regarding the plan of care.

Did You Use the Results of These Tests in Planning or Evaluating Care for Your Patient?

Of course, the results are used in planning care! It is important to note that sometimes the results are not always in the record. If a test is ordered, the clinician needs to follow up. I do a quick scan of each person's orders and test results before entering the examination room.

Did You Contemplate the Accuracy of the Tests? How Many False-Positive/False-Negative Results Did You Encounter? Did the Sensitivity or Specificity of a Screening/Diagnostic Test Enter Into Your Decision Calculus?

Matching the condition, disorder, or disease to the best test for accuracy is crucial. Sometimes the screening or diagnostic test has limited value, but it is all that is available. For example, I would recommend a colonoscopy for a person meeting the guidelines for colon cancer screening. The colonoscopy has the best sensitivity, specificity, predictive values, and confidence intervals—it is the gold standard. The colonoscopy allows direct visualization of the colon and provides an opportunity for biopsy if needed. Sometimes a person needs the colonoscopy but cannot afford it. I have to find a way to get him or her a complimentary one or one at a reduced rate. Or, I can offer alternative screening procedures even though they are less effective. I can recommend sigmoidoscopy or double-contrast barium enema. The overall costs for one of these tests may be less expensive, but the results are less valid and reliable. Another test I can offer is stools for occult blood × 3. The statistics related to this test are limited because of false-negative and false-positive results. Regardless of the test used, it is important to have a discussion with the person about his or her risks for colon cancer. The conversation should include the best evidence related to screening tests, costs, and which is most acceptable to the person. The conversation should be documented on the medical record.

Figure 6-12 shows an excerpt taken from the USPSTF website on July 6, 2010 (USPSTF, 2008b). Practitioners can access the website on a regular basis and use the evidence to help guide decisions related to screening

Exercise 5: Using Concepts Related to the Natural History of Disease, Screening, and Diagnosis

Mr. Bill Monroe, an 85-year-old retired engineer, is being evaluated for cognitive decline. His wife, Jane, has become too frail to care for him at home. Mrs. Monroe asks the geriatric NP to evaluate him for placement in a care facility. The geriatric NP documents the wife's chief complain on the medical record. Next, he obtains a history of the present illness and reviews and updates Mr. Monroe's past medical and surgical history. He performs a physical exam including a Mini Mental State Exam (MMSE). Mr. Monroe scored a 23 on the MMSE. Findings from the history, physical exam, and the medical record review prompt the NP to consider Alzheimer's type dementia (**Figure 6-13**).

The NP noted that Mr. Monroe's baseline MMSE score obtained 4 years ago was normal. The current score reveals a significant drop, indicating significant cognitive decline compatible with moderate dementia (**Figure 6-14**). Plot Mr. Monroe's course.

The NP orders several tests (complete blood count, free T3, T4, thyroid-stimulating hormone, comprehensive metabolic panel, B12, rapid plasma regain, and

You Are Here: AHRQ Home > Clinical Information > U.S. Preventive Services Task Force > Topic Index > Screening: Colorectal Cancer

---

U.S. Preventive Services Task Force

Screening for Colorectal Cancer

Release Date: October 2008

The U.S. Preventive Services Task Force recommendation on Screening for Colorectal Cancer was published on October 7, 2008, by the *Annals of Internal Medicine* and the Agency for Healthcare Research and Quality as an early online release. The print publication in *Annals* occurred on November 4, 2008.

Summary of Recommendations / Supporting Documents

Summary of Recommendations

The USPSTF recommends screening for colorectal cancer (CRC) using fecal occult blood testing, sigmoidoscopy, or colonoscopy, in adults, beginning at age 50 years and continuing until age 75 years. The risks and benefits of these screening methods vary.

Grade: A Recommendation.

The USPSTF recommends against routine screening for colorectal cancer in adults age 76 to 85 years. There may be considerations that support colorectal cancer screening in an individual patient.

Grade: C Recommendation.

The USPSTF recommends against screening for colorectal cancer in adults older than age 85 years.

Grade: D Recommendation.

The USPSTF concludes that the evidence is insufficient to assess the benefits and harms of computed tomographic colonography and fecal DNA testing as screening modalities for colorectal cancer.

Grade: I Statement.

FIGURE 6-12 Screening for colorectal cancer taken from the USPSTF website.
Source: From USPSTF, 2008b.

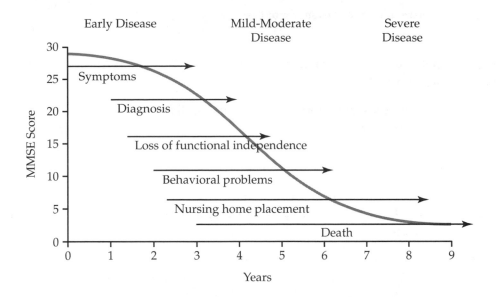

FIGURE 6-13 The natural history of Alzheimer's disease.
Source: From Tangalos, E. G. (2003). Transforming long-term care for Alzheimer's disease. Retrieved August 30, 2010 from http://cme.medscape.com/viewarticle/456034_2

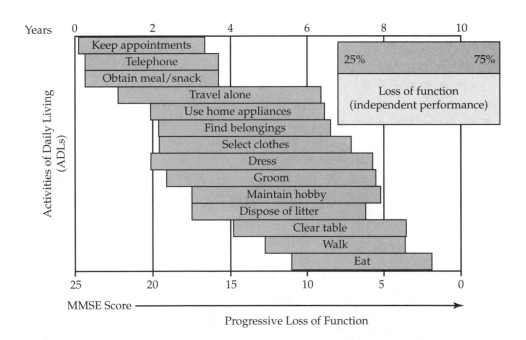

FIGURE 6-14 Relationship between MMSE score and activities of daily living (ADLs).
Source: From Tangalos, E. G. (2003). Transforming long-term care for Alzheimer's disease. Retrieved August 30, 2010 from http://cme.medscape.com/viewarticle/456034_2

brain computed tomogram) that may be affecting Mr. Monroe's cognitive decline and may indicate a reversible form of dementia.

1. Are Mr. Monroe's laboratory tests screening or diagnostic tests?
2. At this point, does Mr. Monroe need assisted care or nursing home care?
3. What is the probability that Mr. Monroe has a reversible form of dementia such as hypothyroidism or substance abuse?

Exercise 6: Define the Following Terms and Describe How You Use Them in Your Practice

- What is the natural history of disease?
- What is the natural history of the most common disease in your practice?
- What is primary, secondary, and tertiary prevention?
- List two examples of common primary, secondary, and tertiary prevention strategies in your practice.
- Is there a relationship between the natural history of the most common disease you selected and a primary, secondary, and tertiary prevention strategy? If yes, describe the relationship. If no, should there be?
- Compare and contrast the most frequently ordered screening and diagnostic tests in your practice. Is there a relationship among these tests and the natural history of the most common diseases in your practice? Is there a relationship between the screening and diagnostic tests and levels of prevention?
- Consider the sensitivity, specificity, predictive values, confidence intervals, ORs, LRs, RRs, and the like for the common screening and diagnostic tests and the evidence-based practices used in your practice. Have you grown more confident in the understanding of these concepts? Are you more confident in your role as an advanced practice nurse in ordering and interpreting these tests?

REFERENCES

1st art gallery. (1997–2010). Florence Nightingale. Retrieved from gallery.com/Trelleek/Florence-Nig

Abramson, Z., Avni, O., & Miskin, I. (2010). Randomized trial of a program to increase staff influenza vaccination in primary care clinics. *Annals of Family Medicine, 8*(4), 293–298.

Elavunkal, J., & Sinert, R. H. (2009). Screening and diagnostic tests. Retrieved from http://emedicine.medscape.com/article/773832

Fagan, T. J. (1975). Letter: Nomogram for Bayes theorem. *New England Journal of Medicine, 293*(5), 257.

Friis, R. H., & Sellers, T. A. (2009). *Epidemiology for public health practice* (4th ed.). Sudbury, MA: Jones and Bartlett.

Hansen, D., Hoss, B., & Wesorick, B. (2008). Evaluating the evidence: Guidelines. *AORN Journal*, *88*(2), 184–196.

Kannel, W. B., D'Agostino, R. B., Silbershatz, H., Belanger, A. J., Wilson, P. W., & Levy, D. (1999). Profile for estimating risk of heart failure. *Archives of Internal Medicine*, *159*(11), 1197–1204.

Max, M. B., & Lynn, J. (n.d.). Chapter 14: Tools for decision making. Retrieved from http://symptomresearch.nih.gov/index.htm

Melnyk, B. M., & Fineout-Overholt, E. (2010). *Evidence-based practice in nursing & healthcare: A guide to best practice*. Philadelphia: Lippincott Williams & Wilkins.

Mikail, C. N. (2008). *Public Health Genomics*. San Francisco: Jossey-Bass A Wiley Imprint.

Mulcahy, N., & Murata, P. (2010). Prostate cancer screening guideline updated by ACS. Retrieved from http://www.medscape.com/viewarticle/717875

Page, J., & Attia, J. (2003). Using Baye's nomogram to help interpret odds ratios. Retrieved from http://ebm.bmj.com/contant/85/132.full

Statsdirect. (n.d.). *P* Values. Retrieved from www.statsdirect.com

Stern, S. D., Cifu, A. S., & Altkorn, D. (2010). *Symptom to diagnosis: An evidence-based guide*. New York: McGraw Hill Medical.

U.S. Department of Health & Human Services. (2010). Surgeon General's family health history initiative. Retrieved from http://www.hhs.gov/familyhistory

U.S. Preventive Services Task Force (USPSTF). (2008a). Grade definitions after May 2007. Retrieved from http://www.uspreventiveservicestaskforce.org/uspstf/gradespost

U.S. Preventive Services Task Force (USPSTF). (2008b). Screening for colorectal cancer. Retrieved from http://www.uspreventiveservicestaskforce.org/uspstf/uspscolo.htm

Wilson, J. (1971). Principles of screening for disease. *Proceedings of the Royal Society of Medicine*, *64*(12), 1255–1256.

CHAPTER 7

Epidemiology of Chronic Diseases

"All diseases run into one, old age."
—Ralph Waldo Emerson

Kiran Macha
John P. McDonough

OBJECTIVES

- Identify chronic disease mortality and morbidity.
- Describe risk factors for chronic diseases.
- Describe disease surveillance and related metrics.
- Identify prevention strategies.

"THE CHANGE YOU LIKE TO SEE...."

The story starts in a country that is far away in the east. The man does not know the world of the microwave, canned food, and refrigerated food. He was happy living in tune with nature, eating from the fields, and enjoying the tastes of nature. He was not aware of created beverages and was satisfied with the miraculous divine drink, water. He played in the dirt and never complained about the sunshine. One day, the man was curious to look into the other side of the world and so was tempted to try human-made wonders. Years later, he was drinking beverages, riding in cars, shopping online, eating fried food, talking to himself, and surrounded with many phones. Alas, he complained to the doctor: "An apple a day does not help me!" "Oops—my friend, you have gone too far. Your cholesterol is rising, your testosterone levels are falling, and your heart says something is wrong." The man now listens to his heart and his intuition, saying, "an apple a day is not enough; a good habit a day is far better." He believes now that he knows how to survive today to see the sunshine tomorrow.

Introduction

Chronic diseases are the result of the prolongation of acute illness with periods of remission and exacerbation of signs and symptoms that lead to disability (**Figure 7-1**).

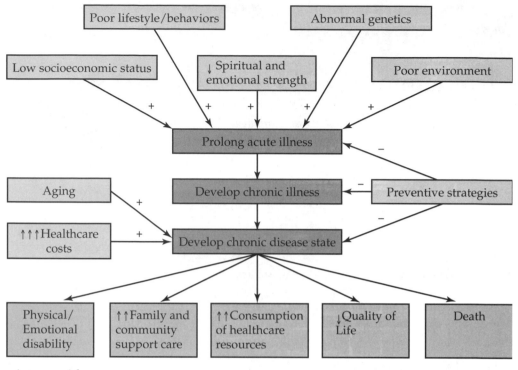

FIGURE 7-1   Chronic disease and risk factors.
Source: Picture courtesy of Dr. Kiran Macha.

Chronic diseases demand medical attention throughout the life span. Chronic diseases or illnesses are referred to globally as noncommunicable diseases. Chronic conditions include arthritis, heart disease, stroke, cancer, chronic obstructive pulmonary disease, hypertension, and diabetes mellitus. Several factors, such as low socioeconomic status, inadequate access to health care, poor lifestyle, abnormal genetics, poor environment, and decreased emotional strength, may contribute to the progression of acute illness to chronic conditions or diseases. Not all acute illnesses progress to chronic states. Chronic diseases are the leading cause of death in the United States and are associated with high morbidity and mortality, disability, and healthcare expenditures. Descriptive epidemiology has contributed to the surveillance of chronic disease mortality and morbidity among populations.

CHRONIC DISEASE MORTALITY AND MORBIDITY _____

Mortality data collected from death certificates, autopsies, hospital administrative records, patient information systems, physician offices, and public health tracking records provide information about the leading causes of death. Measures of mortality include a defined population (denominator), a time period, and the number of deaths occurring in a location/place (numerator) during that time period (see Chapter 2). A crude mortality rate can be derived and a comparison can then be made to total mortality or disease-specific mortality rates from one year to the next within a given population. However, when comparing among different regions or states, age-adjusted mortality rates should be used. A comparison of data for a state having an age distribution with more elders with those for a state where residents are younger is not possible without adjusting (standardizing) for age. One would expect the mortality rate to be higher as the population ages. Other considerations when interpreting mortality rates include gender, race and ethnicity, and socioeconomic (occupation, education, income) status. Chronic diseases accounted for almost 70% of deaths in the United States in 2007 (**Table 7-1**; **Figure 7-2**), with life expectancy reaching a record high of 77.9 years (Xu, Kochanek, Murphy, & Tejada-Vera, 2010).

Table 7-1 Total Deaths for the 10 Leading Causes of Death in the United States, 2007	
Cause of Death	**Total Deaths**
Heart disease	616,067
Malignant neoplasm	562,875
Cerebrovascular diseases	135,952
Chronic lower respiratory diseases	127,924
Accidents (unintentional injuries)	123,706
Alzheimer's disease	74,632
Diabetes mellitus	71,382
Influenza and pneumonia	52,717
Kidney disease	46,448
Septicemia	34,828

Source: http://www.cdc.gov/nchs/fastats/lcod.htm

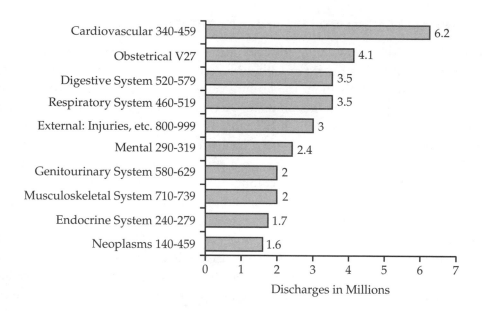

FIGURE 7-2 Hospital discharges for the 10 leading diagnostic groups (United States: 2006).
Source: CDC; NHDS/NCHS, and NHLBI.

Risk Factors for Chronic Diseases

A seminal study by McGinnis and Foege (1993) estimated that approximately 38% of all deaths that occurred in 1990 were related to behavioral or lifestyle choice: tobacco use, poor diet, poor physical activity patterns, and alcohol abuse. These risk factors continue to be identified as the underlying causes of major chronic illness mortality (McKenna & Collins, 2010). Tobacco, for example, has been implicated in cardiovascular, cancer, lung, and musculoskeletal diseases, whereas high cholesterol, high blood pressure, poor diet, and lack of physical activity are related to risk of cardiovascular disease and certain cancers. Recognition that a few key risk factors account for most of the chronic disease burden has led to global and national health agendas that specifically target risk factor and disease surveillance efforts in conjunction with prevention agendas (**Figure 7-3**).

Obesity

Dietary changes can be the result of affordability, availability, and access as well as to the choices we make to nourish our bodies. In the United States in the 1960s, Ameri-

Disease Risk Factors	Top 10 Leading Causes of Death	Prevention
Age Gender Genetics Tobacco Smoking Diabetes Mellitus Body Mass Index > 25 ↑ Blood Pressure ↑ Cholesterol ↑ Stress ↑ Alcohol consumption ↓ Emotional capacity ↓ Physical activity	Diseases of the heart Malignant neoplasms Cerebrovascular diseases Chronic obstructive 　pulmonary diseases Accidents Diabetes mellitus Alzheimer's disease Influenza and Pneumonia Kidney disease Septicemia	Quit Smoking Regular exercise Decrease alcohol consumption Regular physical examinations Immunizations Dietary changes Control of blood glucose 　levels in diabetic patients Yoga and meditation

FIGURE 7-3   Risk factors, leading causes of death, and prevention.
Source: Picture courtesy of Dr. Kiran Macha.

cans drank whole milk more than any other beverage; today, cola is the single most important product consumed in excess (**Figure 7-4**). Colas are acidic, with pH ranging from 3 to 6. The trend toward consumption of processed and fatty, sugar-laden foods and eating excess food, along with a lack of exercise related to comforts derived from modern technology, are increasing the incidence of obesity throughout parts of the world. Initially, obesity was thought to be a major problem primarily in the United States. However, according to the World Health Organization (WHO), obesity is now pandemic and has even been referred to as "globesity." Food companies are experimenting with genetically engineered food such as salmon to produce food in larger quantities in a short period of time. The public often resists such genetically modified food products because of rising fears of unknown consequences.

According to prevalence statistics collected through the National Health and Nutrition Examination Survey for 2007 and 2008, over one-third of the U.S. population is obese and two-thirds are overweight and obese (Flegal, 2010). The prevalence of obesity is higher among women. African Americans have the highest prevalence of obesity, followed by Hispanics and Whites. Obesity numbers are lower in Asian Americans (8.9%), whereas the incidence is surprisingly higher in Native Americans

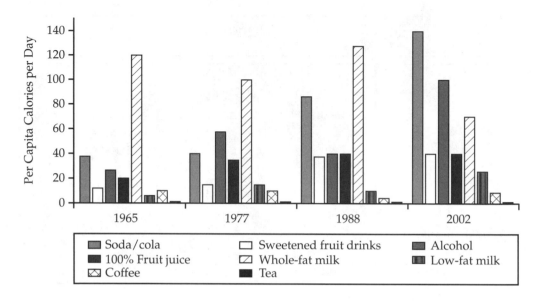

FIGURE 7-4   Per capita calories consumed from different beverages by U.S. adults (≥19 years of age) from 1965 to 2002.
Source: Centers for Disease Control and Prevention, Nationwide Food Consumption Surveys, and National Health and Nutrition Examination Survey.

and Alaskans (32%). The incidence of obesity increases with age, perhaps because of a decrease in physical activity (**Figure 7-5**).

Overweight and obesity lead to dyslipidemia and insulin resistance, increasing the risk of suffering from cardiovascular and cerebrovascular diseases as a result of the acceleration of atherosclerosis in the blood vessels. With the increase in weight, knee joints are affected, and subjects are prone to suffer from arthritis. Behavioral and environmental causes of obesity can be modified, but not contributing genetic factors. Pharmacological and surgical options are also available to halt the progression of obesity.

Cholesterol

Cholesterol is an important lipid required for the formation of cell membranes, bile acids, and vitamin D. Sex hormones are synthesized from cholesterol in the human body. Low-density lipoprotein carries cholesterol from the liver to the tissues, including the artery wall. High-density lipoprotein transports cholesterol from tissues to the liver. Lipoproteins play an important role in the transportation of the cholesterol because lipids are not soluble in water. Cholesterol is synthesized in the liver and also

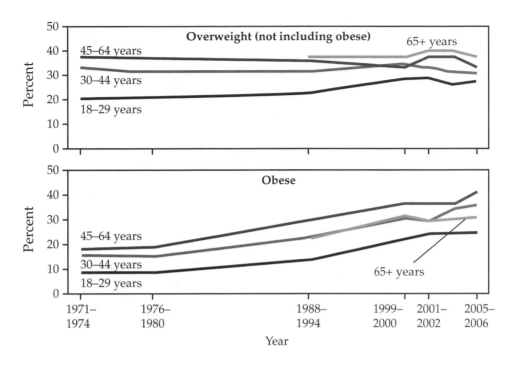

FIGURE 7-5   Overweight and obesity statistics based on age.
Sources: Centers for Disease Control and Prevention/NCHS, Health, United States, (2008). Data from the National Health and Nutrition Examination Survey. Retrieved September 21, 2010, from http://www.win.niddk.nih.gov/statistics/index.htm

absorbed from food. When cholesterol exceeds normal amounts, the physiology of the human body is affected. Deposition of oxidized low-density lipoprotein in the artery wall triggers inflammatory reaction and results in the formation of atherosclerotic plaque. High-density lipoprotein protects us from experiencing cardiovascular events because it collects cholesterol from the tissues and transports it to the liver for excretion.

A total cholesterol level of at least 240 mg/dL in the plasma for a prolonged time increases the risk of heart disease. According to Centers for Disease Control and Prevention (CDC, 2010), 16.3% of the U.S. adult population has high total cholesterol levels in the blood. Statistics indicate that a greater percentage of women (16.9%) than men (15.6%) have higher levels of cholesterol, with cholesterol levels increasing with a woman's age. Postmenopausal women deprived of the protective effects of estrogen are at higher risk of suffering from cardiovascular events (**Figure 7-6**).

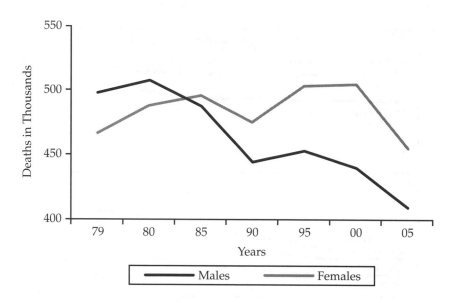

FIGURE 7-6   Deaths from cardiovascular diseases based on gender.
Source: CDC.

Tobacco Smoking

According to the CDC (2010), tobacco smoking rates in the United States have gradually declined as of 2006 (20.6%) compared with 1965 (40%). Nicotine is one of the most potent addictive chemicals present in tobacco smoke along with hundreds of harmful chemicals and toxins. Research has shown that secondhand smoke can also cause diseases. Public health regulations have been formulated in recent years to restrict smoking in public places as states begin to enact Smoke Free Air laws. Some of the harmful effects of tobacco smoking include myocardial infarction, stroke, and cancers (**Figure 7-7**). Smoking also affects reproductive health and alters hormonal physiology in the brain. The most common reasons for not quitting tobacco smoking are nicotine addiction and withdrawal symptoms.

A significant number of multiorgan system disease conditions have also been detected in those who work in the tobacco industry and handle tobacco manually, such as beedi workers (Yasmin, Afroz, Hyat, & D'Souza, 2010). (Beedi involves rolling and tying the tobacco leaf with a small thread.) The tobacco industry invests money in research, but at the same time it influences the decisions and regulations that may affect the progress of the industry. Each individual has the responsibility to keep away

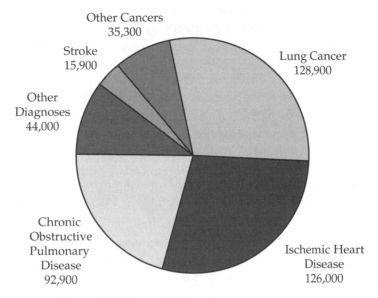

**About 443,000 U.S. Deaths Attributable
Each Year to Cigarette Smoking***

Other Cancers
35,300

Stroke
15,900

Other
Diagnoses
44,000

Lung Cancer
128,900

Chronic
Obstructive
Pulmonary
Disease
92,900

Ischemic Heart
Disease
126,000

*Average annual number of deaths, 2000–2004.
Source: MMWR 2008;57(45): 1226–1228.

FIGURE 7-7 Cigarette smoking is injurious to health.
Source: CDC. Retrieved September 21, 2010, from http://www.cdc.gov/tobacco/data_statistics/tables/health/attrdeaths/index.htm

from such addicting agents, to seek help with a firm will to quit smoking, to use all community resources available, and to embrace behavioral modifications to conquer nicotine addiction.

Physical Activity

CDC guidelines currently recommend that one should get involved in activities (such as walking, bicycling, and gardening) that increase heart rate and breathing for at least 30 minutes/day, 5 days a week, or participate in 20 minutes of vigorous exercises 3 days a week (see resource for CDC/Physical Activity, 2010). Overcrowded places, poor air quality, low socioeconomic conditions, high crime activity neighborhoods, and a lack of recreational places impact daily physical activity plans for many (WHO/

Physical Activity, 2010). Age, disability, and medical problems can also impact levels of physical activity. The benefits of increased physical activity include a decrease in the incidence of many diseases, including type 2 diabetes mellitus, hypertension, obesity, osteoporosis, tumors of the large intestine, breast and prostate cancer, and depression (Helmrich, Ragland, Leung, & Paffenbarger, 1991; Sobieszczanska, Kalka, Pilecki, & Adamus, 2009).

Alcohol Use

Alcohol is used in the field of medicine as an antiseptic, anesthetic, and preservative. In those who consume alcohol, it affects judgment and prolongs reaction time. With an increase in alcohol consumption, consciousness, respiration, and motor skills are affected, potentially leading to death. The risk of suffering from a motor vehicle accident is higher with the increase in the levels of alcohol in the blood. Alcohol is also linked to the crimes in society. According to the National Highway Traffic Safety Administration in 2008, 10,679 of the reported accidents were alcohol related. In the United States, law enforcement can take action against a person with blood alcohol concentration of more than 0.10 (and in some states the limit is 0.08). Sobriety checkpoints have been established in some areas to assess blood alcohol levels and impairment in drivers.

Pancreatitis, cardiomyopathy, cancers, cirrhosis of the liver, and stroke can result from drinking alcohol in excess for a prolonged period of time. Pregnant women should avoid alcohol because the fetus is at risk of developing fetal alcohol syndrome. The Behavioral Risk Factor Surveillance System, Youth Risk Behavior Surveillance System, National Health Interview Survey, Pregnancy Risk Assessment Monitoring System, and Alcohol Epidemiologic Data Directory are some of the national surveys that collect data on alcohol drinking in the United States. In addition to the alcohol screening test shown in **Table 7-2**, other tests include the Michigan Alcohol Screening Test and the Alcohol Use Disorders Identification Test.

Emotional Disorders

According to the National Institute of Mental Health (2010), one-fourth of adult Americans suffer from one or more mental disorders. Mental illnesses include mood disorders, depression, schizophrenia, anxiety disorders, eating disorders, and personality disorders. Mental illness may be caused by genetic factors, brain injury, brain infections, alcohol and substance abuse, nutritional deficiencies, and injury to the fetal brain during pregnancy. Work-related stress, unemployment, poverty, social isolation, war, discrimination, and chronic medical diseases may also lead to mental

Table 7-2 Alcohol Screening Test, CAGE Questionnaire	
1. Have you ever felt you should *cut down* on your drinking?	Yes/no
2. Have people *annoyed* you by criticizing your drinking?	Yes/no
3. Have you ever felt bad or *guilty* about your drinking?	Yes/no
4. Have you ever had a drink first thing in the morning to steady your nerves or get rid of a hangover (*eye*-opener)?	Yes/no
Answering "yes" to two or more of the above questions is clinically significant.	

disorders. Many veterans suffer from posttraumatic stress disorder. Child abuse and organized rapes during war experiences are also highly damaging actions. Education, family support, community resources, social interactions, reduction of substance abuse, learning skills to manage adverse situations, and good diet are some protective factors. Because depression is common in the elderly, the psychological status of these individuals should be regularly evaluated.

Diet and Nutrition

It has long been known that nutrition is a preventable risk factor for chronic diseases. Green leafy vegetables supply vitamins, folates, and iron. Dietary fiber not only improves digestion but also decreases the absorption of harmful substances. Fruits are rich in antioxidants and offer some protection from cancers and heart disease. Milk provides calcium and helps to prevent osteoporosis. Spices can boost our immunity, and garlic is known to reduce cholesterol levels. Proteins essential for building muscles and for reducing the incidence of musculoskeletal problems can be obtained from milk, cereals, meat, soy, and eggs.

Proper, balanced nutrition should be taken to maintain a normal body mass index. Excess intake of food may increase body mass index and can cause chronic diseases. Exercise is an important activity that, together with a balanced diet, can help us maintain body weight and at the same time build muscle strength. With increasing age our body requirements change, calling for changes in our food plan. Those who suffer from chronic diseases should consult a dietician. Resources are available on the Internet that may help us plan a healthy diet. One should take care each day in observing the content of food consumed, because the choices we make affect our long-term health and there is no cure for most chronic diseases.

SOME OF THE CHRONIC DISEASES

Cystic Fibrosis

Cystic fibrosis is caused by a mutation in the cystic fibrosis transmembrane conductance regulator gene and is inherited from either parent. Each year 1,000 new cases of cystic fibrosis are detected in the United States (Grosse et al., 2004). The incidence of this disease is higher in Whites as compared with African Americans and Asian Americans. In cystic fibrosis patients, mucus that is secreted in different organs of the body is thicker than normal. Thick mucus in the bronchi obstructs airways and ducts in glands such as the pancreas, causing pancreatitis. Frequent infections, infertility, and indigestion are other symptoms. Treatment involves support, medications to liquefy mucus, and intake of nutritious food.

Cardiovascular Disease

Cardiovascular diseases are usually preventable. Risk factors such as physical inactivity, smoking, diabetes, high cholesterol, and high blood pressure can be effectively managed and controlled. Twenty-nine percent of deaths that occur worldwide are a result of cardiovascular diseases (**Figure 7-8**) (WHO/Cardiovascular diseases, 2010). In the United States, 26% of deaths (more than 1 in 4) are attributable to cardiac causes (CDC/ Heart disease, 2010). No racial or gender prevalence differences have

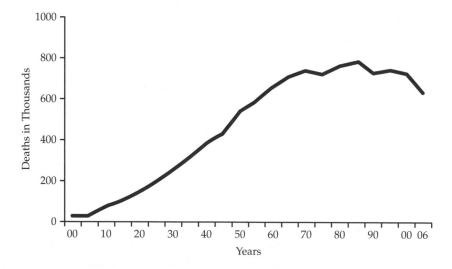

FIGURE 7-8   Deaths from heart disease in the United States from 1900 to 2006. *Source:* CDC, NCHS.

been observed (although mortality rates are higher in postmenopausal women). Healthcare costs, the costs of medication, loss of productivity, and emergency medical bills are higher for those with cardiovascular disease, whether for acute or chronic episodes. Salt consumption should be decreased. Restaurants should be discouraged to use salt in excess (in some restaurants we could not find salt bottles on tables—a good sign of behavioral change). These cost-effective, preventive, affordable measures can save millions of dollars and the lives of those for whom we care.

Diabetes Mellitus

Lack of or decrease in insulin levels and insulin resistance cause diabetes mellitus. Insulin regulates glucose levels in the blood, and increased levels of glucose affect almost all organs in the body. The progression of organ diseases caused by diabetes mellitus depends on the blood glucose control. The prevalence of diabetes increases with age. The prevalence of diabetes mellitus has increased in all age groups from 1990 to 2007 (**Figure 7-9**). Overweight and obesity lead to insulin resistance; as

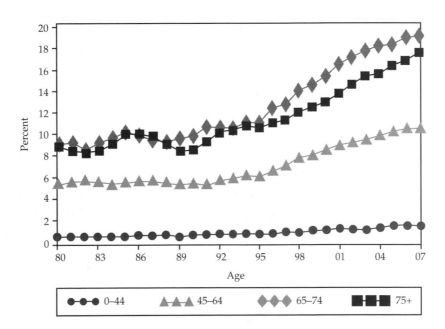

FIGURE 7-9 Percentage of the civilian, noninstitutionalized population with diagnosed diabetes by age, United States, 1980–2007.
Source: From CDC. Diabetes mellitus. Retrieved September 21, 2010, from http://www.cdc.gov/diabetes/statistics/prev/national/figbyage.htm

obesity prevalence increases, the risk of diabetes mellitus also increases. Pregnant women are at increased risk of developing diabetes. Some 24 million people suffer from diabetes, and 57 million more are prediabetic (CDC, Diabetes, 2010). The incidence of diabetes mellitus is higher in Native Americans and Alaskans. Good nutrition, better blood glucose control, use of insulin or antidiabetic drugs (patient compliance), and regular medical check-ups are advised.

Chronic Disease Surveillance

Morbidity data provide information about persons who have a disease. These data may be collected by federal or state programs who fund services, managed care companies, hospitals, or disease control programs, to name a few. These sources are restricted, however, to the populations they serve. Surveillance, conducted across the country under the guidance of CDC and its partners, can document the burden of chronic diseases and identify health risk behaviors among various population groups in different locations. Results from these surveys and registries are used to monitor disease trends, develop prevention programs, and monitor prevention efforts. **Table 7-3** provides a brief description of selected surveillance systems identified by CDC.

Disability-Adjusted Life Year

The disability-adjusted life year is an indicator of health outcomes that measures the time lived with disability and time lost due to premature death (United Nations Educational Scientific and Cultural Organization; http://www.unesco.org/water/wwap/wwdr/indicators/pdf/F1_Disability_adjusted_life_year.pdf). See WHO/global burden of disease http://www.who.int/healthinfo/global_burden_disease/metrics_daly/en/index.html.

Quality Adjusted Life Year

The quality-adjusted life year is a frequently used outcome measure in cost utility analysis that incorporates the quality or desirability of a health state with the duration of survival. See CDC, http://www.cdc.gov/dhdsp/library/pdfs/Economic_Evaluation_Glossary.pdf.

Table 7-3   Major Chronic Disease Surveillance Systems of the Centers for Disease Control and Prevention

Surveillance System	Description (Year of Earliest Data)
Behavioral Risk Factor Surveillance System (BRFSS)	Ongoing state-based telephone survey monitoring behaviors such as physical activity, diet, and tobacco and alcohol use and conditions such as asthma, diabetes, and participation in health screening among adults (1984).
Chronic Disease Indicators	97 indicators developed by consensus allowing states to uniformly define, collect, and report disease data. Categories include physical activity & nutrition; tobacco & alcohol use; cancer; cardiovascular disease; diabetes, & arthritis (1999).
Health-Related Quality of Life (HRQOL)	Identify unmet population physical and mental health needs; recognize trends, disparities, and determinants of health; and inform decision making and program evaluation (1993).
National Assisted Reproductive Technology Surveillance System (NASS)	Assistive reproductive technology treatment outcomes from all infertility clinics in the United States, including patient profile, treatment reasons, procedure type, outcomes, and clinic contact information (1992).
National Diabetes Surveillance System	Documents the public health burden of diabetes and its complications in the United States (1994).
National Health Interview Survey (NHIS)	Large-scale household population interview survey tracking health status, healthcare access, and progress toward achieving national health objectives (1957).
National Health and Nutrition Examination Survey (NHANES)	Assesses the health and nutritional status of adults and children in the United States combining interviews and physical examinations (1960).
National Oral Health Surveillance System (NOHSS)	Data pooled from state-based and national surveys to monitor trends in key indicators of oral health status, oral healthcare utilization, receipt of preventive interventions such as water fluoridation and dental sealants, and state oral health program infrastructure (1998).

(continues)

Table 7-3   Major Chronic Disease Surveillance Systems of the Centers for Disease Control and Prevention *(continued)*

Surveillance System	Description (Year of Earliest Data)
National Program of Cancer Registries	Funds population-based cancer registries in 45 states, the District of Columbia, Puerto Rico, and the U.S. Pacific Island jurisdictions to collect data on the occurrence of cancer; the type, extent, and location of the cancer; and the type of initial treatment (1992).
National Youth Tobacco Survey	School-based survey of public school students enrolled in grades 6–12 monitoring tobacco-related beliefs, attitudes, behaviors, and exposure to pro and anti tobacco influences to inform the development, implementation, and evaluation of prevention programs (1999).
Pediatric (PedNSS) and Pregnancy (PNSS) Nutrition Surveillance·System	Nutritional status and behavioral indicators of low-income infants, children, and pregnant and postpartum women in federally funded maternal and child health programs (1973).
Pregnancy Risk Assessment Monitoring System	State-specific, population-based data on maternal attitudes and experiences before, during, and shortly after pregnancy (1987).
State Tobacco Activities Tracking and Evaluation (STATE) System	Electronic data warehouse, integrating data from multiple sources, behaviors, demographics, economics, environment, funding, health consequences, costs, and legislation related to tobacco use (1984).
United States Cancer Statistics (USCS)	Federal statistics on cancer incidence from registries with high quality data and mortality statistics (1999).
Youth Risk Behavior Surveillance System	Monitors health risk behaviors, including obesity, and asthma and related indicators among youth and adults (1991).

Source: CDC. Chronic disease prevention & promotion. Retrieved September 21, 2010, from http://www.cdc.gov/chronicdisease/stats/index.htm

IMPLICATIONS FOR CLINICAL PRACTICE _____

Surveillance of Own Practice

Surveillance has become easy with softwares that are used to document patient information in clinical settings. Clinicians should document patient risk factors for chronic diseases. Data can be analyzed and the area of need (most prevalent risk factor) can be assessed within a short period of time. Conclusions drawn from these data help us formulate strategies and, when looking at population-wide risk factors, help bolster collaboration with community partners. Clinicians can reduce risk both by treating the patients and by offering education on risk factors to those who visit clinical settings. For example, each patient should be asked whether he or she smokes tobacco; the clinician can then encourage the patient to quit smoking and introduce helpful and supportive resources.

Knowledge of Risk Factors, Populations at Risk

Because we know that most pregnant women need folic acid and iron, a wise strategy is to prescribe these for all pregnant women to preclude fetal neurological growth problems. Seafood is rich in iodine, but if an individual does not eat seafood because of reasons of culture or geographic location, it can be difficult to get sufficient amounts of iodine. Although iodine-deficient foods are consumed in many parts of the world, the availability of iodized salt in the community has greatly reduced the incidence of stillbirths and goiter from lack of iodine. Iodine prophylaxis (related to iodine supplementation) may induce hyperthyroidism (Stanbury et al., 1998). However, the incidence of iodine deficiency is higher and the number of people who will benefit from iodized salt is great, as compared with the low incidence of hyperthyroidism that occurs in few parts of the world.

Risk factors are unearthed as the prevalence of diseases gain public health importance. WHO community programs are changing the picture of the incidences of global diseases. Nevertheless, local public health problems are often best managed by local government. For example, in Nalgonda, a district in India, the fluoride content in the water (at 10 to 12 ppm) is 10 times greater than maximum permitted levels (1.5 ppm). For years this problem was ignored because of local politics, and thousands were affected with fluorosis. In this condition, fluoride accumulates to detrimental levels in bones, teeth, and other organs of the body. After years of drinking water with high fluoride levels, one develops dental, skeletal, ophthalmic, and gastrointestinal disorders. In the United States controlled safe water fluoridation is encouraged in many states to prevent tooth decay. Deformities caused by fluoride excess can be misdiagnosed as rheumatoid arthritis.

Interdisciplinary Care Teams

The concept of interdisciplinary teamwork on public health issues is successfully growing in the community. Most public health problems are multidimensional in nature, requiring experts from different specialties to formulate strategies. For example, tobacco smoking is a risk factor for many diseases; the immense chronic disease burden on the healthcare system associated with smoking makes this a major public health issue. It is difficult to quit smoking, and it is the individual's responsibility to direct efforts in the right direction. At the same time we have a collective responsibility to help those who want to quit because secondhand smoke affects others. The clinician's role is to prescribe alternative forms of tobacco to taper dependence, treat diseases, and educate individuals about the long-term effects of related chronic diseases. Public health policy needs to be designed and public health laws need to be effectively implemented. Information on harmful effects of tobacco should be disseminated. For all these efforts, funding for programs and expertise is needed.

Chronic Care Model

The chronic care model was developed to address concerns related to the increasing prevalence of chronic diseases in the world. The model components include community resources, self-management support, delivery system design, decision support, and a clinical information system. Community resources should be assessed, and collaboration with community partners should be nurtured to plan and implement strategies targeting the needs of a target population. Patients are educated on a number of issues related to a chronic disease, including medications and diet. The services are evaluated, and identified shortcomings in the delivery system are rectified. Adherence to standards of care and disease management guidelines should be audited in the clinical setting. Technology should also be effectively used in the clinical setting to track details related to patient care. Providers should continue medical education to keep abreast of updated disease management practices. Effective communication, provider and patient education, and assessment of needs to strengthen provider and delivery systems for optimal care are important to reduce suffering for those with chronic diseases. Studies evaluating use of the chronic care model have found improved clinical outcomes for patients, increased patient knowledge on chronic disease, and enhanced provider compliance with disease management guidelines (Piatt et al., 2006).

Ecological and Social Determinants of Health

Disparities in health care exist in relation to improper management of the healthcare delivery system, lack of education, poverty, inadequate access to health care, politics, socioeconomic and racial discrimination, and even corruption. Health, an individual right, is often lost in the battle. The impact of these factors on the long-term support of individuals suffering from chronic diseases is far-reaching and often unimaginable. The constant presence of and exposure to environmental risks is also challenging. For example, people living around nuclear reactors are constantly exposed to nuclear radiation. People living in basements are exposed to radon gas (without radon detectors) in some parts of the United States. Shipyard workers are exposed to asbestos and may develop mesothelioma. Coal mine workers inhale coal dust and suffer with severe lung problems. Even though we are aware of the risk and results of such exposure, and although worker safety strategies are usually in place, cases are still reported.

Risk Factor Versus Population Approaches

Many public health practitioners, policymakers, and epidemiologists worldwide have embraced Geoffrey Rose's population-based prevention concept: a strategy of disease prevention that aims to shift the population distribution of a risk factor in a favorable direction by applying interventions to an entire population. Strategies that have traditionally used epidemiological methods to study disease causation in the search for risk factors and their quantification within individuals are shifting focus to population-based perspectives. Rose (1992) compares the traditional high-risk approach of individual case-centered prevention with the population strategy of controlling the determinants of disease and shifting of the whole distribution of exposure in a favorable direction. He argues that the factors that explain the distribution of disease within a population do not necessarily explain the differences in disease rates between populations. The population, not individual behavior, is the main determinant of absolute level of risk.

Some disagree with Rose and like to target interventions to the individuals in whom the risk factor is detected (Malik, 2006). Treatment directed toward risk factors may not treat the disease but may decrease exposure to risk. The risk factor is not eliminated from the environment we live in by treating an individual. The number of interventions on an individual increases with the increase in number of risk factors. Clinicians treat individuals, understanding the global picture of an individual considering the comorbid conditions. Population strategies are important to decrease the risk of transmission and the likelihood that others will also share the burden of chronic disease. Education plays an important role in implementing population strategies.

KEY POINTS

- Chronic disease is defined as a prolonged suffering of a disease because a cure is not available or not possible. The patient's episodic exacerbations are treated, and follow-up is essential.
- Chronic diseases consume both individual and community resources. Educating patients is key to effective long-term planning and strategies.
- Risk factors and protective factors should be identified for every chronic disease. Our objective of care should be to decrease the influence of risk factors and increase the influence of protective factors.
- Social determinants of health impact the quality of health care received by an individual in the community.
- For chronic diseases it is important to treat risk factors and also to implement population-based strategies.
- Interdisciplinary care is usually better than one individual's expert decisions or perceptions.
- Chronic disease surveillance helps us measure the effect of our efforts on community health.

CRITICAL QUESTIONS

1. How can we decrease prevalence of chronic diseases?
2. What models of care are effectively implemented in healthcare systems to help those suffering from chronic diseases?
3. What is the most prevalent risk factor in your patients, and how do you plan to address it?
4. How should one suffering with a chronic disease plan his or her long-term management of resources?

RESOURCES

National Physical Activity Plan
http://www.physicalactivityplan.org/
WIN Weight-control Information Network
http://www.win.niddk.nih.gov/statistics/index.htm

The WHO Global Burden of Disease Project
   http://www.who.int/healthinfo/global_burden_disease/en/
   http://www.who.int/healthinfo/global_burden_disease/GBD_
   report_2004update_full.pdf
National Highway Traffic Safety Administration
   http://www-fars.nhtsa.dot.gov/Crashes/CrashesAlcohol.aspx
U.S. Department of Agriculture—Food Pyramid
   http://www.mypyramid.gov/
Chronic Care Model
   http://www.improvingchroniccare.org/index.php?p=The_Chronic_Care_
   Model&s=2
UNESCO/ DALY
   http://www.unesco.org/water/wwap/wwdr/indicators/pdf/F1_Disability_
   adjusted_life_year.pdf
National Vital Statistics Report/Mortality Data
   http://www.cdc.gov/NCHS/data/nvsr/nvsr58/nvsr58_19.pdf

REFERENCES

Centers for Disease Control and Prevention. (2010). Cholesterol Facts and Statistics. Retrieved from http://www.cdc.gov/cholesterol/facts.htm
Centers for Disease Control and Prevention. (2010). Smoking and Tobacco use. Retrieved from http://www.cdc.gov/tobacco
Centers for Disease Control and Prevention. (2010). Physical Activity. Retrieved from http://www.cdc.gov/physicalactivity
Centers for Disease Control and Prevention. (2010). Heart Disease. Retrieved from http://www.cdc.gov/heartdisease
Centers for Disease Control and Prevention. (2010). Diabetes data and trends. Retrieved from http://apps.nccd.cdc.gov/DDTSTRS/default.aspx
Flegal, K. K. M. (2010). Prevalence and trends in obesity among US adults, 1999-2008. *Journal of the American Medical Association, 303*(3), 235–241.
Grosse, S., Boyle, A. G., Botkin, R. J., Comeau, M. A., Kharrazi, M., Rosenfeld, M., et al. (2004). Newborn Screening for Cystic Fibrosis. Retrieved from http://www.cdc.gov/mmwr/preview/mmwrhtml/rr5313a1.htm
Helmrich, S. P., Ragland, D. R., Leung, R. W., & Paffenbarger, R. S., Jr. (1991). Physical activity and reduced occurrence of non-insulin-dependent diabetes mellitus. *New England Journal of Medicine, 325*(3), 147–152.
Malik, P. (2006). The axiom of Rose. *Canadian Journal of Cardiology, 22*(9), 735.
McGinnis, J. M., & Foege, W. H. (1993). Actual causes of death in the United States. *Journal of the American Medical Association, 270*(18), 2207–2212.

McKenna, M., & Collins, J. (2010). Current issues and challenges in chronic disease control. In P. L. Remington, R. C. Brownson, & M. V. Wegner (Eds.), *Chronic disease epidemiology and control* (3rd ed., pp. 1–26). Washington, DC: American Public Health Association.

National Highway Traffic Safety Administration. (2010). Impaired Driving. Retrieved from http://www.nhtsa.com/Impaired

National Institute of Mental Health. (2010). Mental Health, Statistics. Retrieved from http://www.nimh.nih.gov/health/topics/statistics/index.shtml

Piatt, G. A., Orchard, T. J., Emerson, S., Simmons, D., Songer, T. J., Brooks, M. M., et al. (2006). Translating the chronic care model into the community: Results from a randomized controlled trial of a multifaceted diabetes care intervention. *Diabetes Care, 29*(4), 811–817.

Rose, G. (1992). *The strategy of preventive medicine.* Oxford, UK: Oxford University Press.

Sobieszczanska, M., Kalka, D., Pilecki, W., & Adamus, J. (2009). Physical activity in basic and primary prevention of cardiovascular disease. [Aktywnosc fizyczna w podstawowej i pierwotnej prewencji choroby sercowo-naczyniowej.] *Polski Merkuriusz Lekarski: Organ Polskiego Towarzystwa Lekarskiego, 26*(156), 659–664.

Stanbury, J. B., Ermans, A. E., Bourdoux, P., Todd, C., Oken, E., Tonglet, R., et al. (1998). Iodine-induced hyperthyroidism: Occurrence and epidemiology. *Thyroid: Official Journal of the American Thyroid Association, 8*(1), 83–100.

World Health Organization. (2010). Physical Activity. Retrieved from http://www.who.int/topics/physical_activity/en

World Health Organization. (2010). Cardiovascular Diseases. Retrieved from http://www.who.int/cardiovascular_diseases/en

Yasmin, S., Afroz, B., Hyat, B., & D'Souza, D. (2010). Occupational health hazards in women beedi rollers in Bihar, India. *Bulletin of Environmental Contamination and Toxicology, 85*(1), 87–91.

Xu, J. Q., Kochanek, K. D., Murphy, S. L., & Tejada-Vera, B. (2010). Deaths: Final data for 2007. National Vital Statistics Reports (Vol. 58, No. 19). Hyattsville, MD: National Center for Health Statistics. Released May 2010. Retrieved from http://www.cdc.gov/nchs/data/nvsr/nvsr58/nvsr58_19.pdf

CHAPTER 8

Genetic Epidemiology

"We wish to suggest a structure for the salt of deoxyribose nucleic acid (D.N.A). This structure has novel features which are of considerable biological interest."

—J. D. Watson & F. H. C. Crick, 1953

Kiran Macha
John P. McDonough

OBJECTIVES

- Explain the inheritance of diseases based on Mendel's laws of inheritance.
- Discuss outcomes of the Human Genome Project.
- Describe the mechanisms that influence gene expression.
- List the ways the environment can influence gene expression.

INTRODUCTION

Observations have led to theories, and theories have led to scientific advancements. Mendel's laws of inheritance, the observations of Charles Darwin, and the discovery of the structure of deoxyribonucleic acid (DNA) by Watson and Crick have all contributed to the acceleration of genetic research. The developments of microscopy, laboratory techniques and equipment, and testing methods have assisted scientists in their yearning for understanding. The findings of the Human Genome Project have begun to unearth the secrets of life. As we continue to learn more about genes, the responsibility for us to direct the use of genetic knowledge for human benefit becomes greater.

Genetic epidemiology has been defined as "... a science which deals with the etiology, distribution, and control of disease in groups of relatives and with inherited causes of disease in populations" (Morton, 1993, p. 523).

GENETICS IN A NUTSHELL

The basic unit of life is the cell. Trillions of cells in the human body coexist; they may differ in structure and function, and the internal milieu is adapted to perform a specific function. The nucleus where chromosomes are contained is known to control the functions of a cell. In each human cell (except gametes), 46 chromosomes are present, of which 44 are known to be autosomes and two are sex chromosomes. Females have two X sex chromosomes (XX) and males have X and Y sex chromosomes in the nucleus of a cell. Chromosomes are made up of DNA and proteins called histones (**Figure 8-1**). From DNA, ribonucleic acid (RNA) is produced and from RNA, functional proteins are produced. Proteins are made up of small subunits called amino acids, which are the building blocks of a cell.

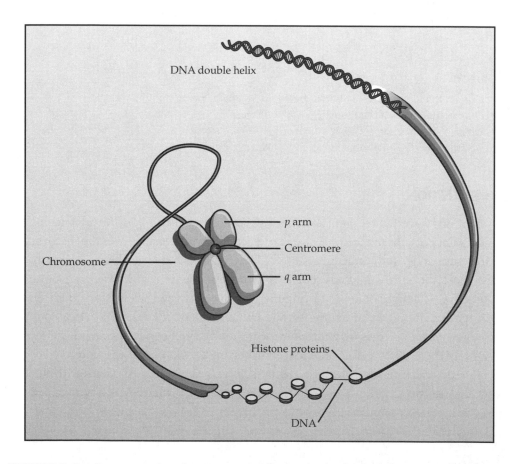

FIGURE 8-1   Structure of a chromosome. The *p* arm is short and *q* arm is longer; the ends of the chromosome are called telomeres. The *p* and *q* arms meet at the centromere. *Source:* National Library of Medicine. Accessed July 10, 2010.

DNA and RNA are made up of nucleotides, with each nucleotide composed of three components:

1. A nitrogenous base, classified in one of two groups:
   a. Purines: adenine and guanine
   b. Pyrimidines: thymine, uracil, and cytosine
2. A sugar molecule
3. A phosphate group

A nitrogenous base attached to a sugar molecule is known as a nucleoside. A nucleoside attached to a phosphate group forms a nucleotide. **Table 8-1** summarizes the differences between DNA and RNA.

DNA has two strands that are arranged in the form of a double helix (**Figure 8-2**). These two strands are held together by hydrogen bonds between the nitrogenous bases. Two hydrogen bonds exist between adenine and thymine, and three hydrogen bonds exist between guanine and cytosine. Covalent bonds exist between the sugar molecule and nitrogenous base. A phosphodiester bond exists between the sugar and phosphate group. Sugar molecules and phosphate groups form the backbone of the DNA structure. The double-helical structure of DNA is maintained by the attractive and repulsive forces between the molecules (**Figure 8-3**).

Public Health Applications

Ionizing radiation can break any of the bonds within the makeup of our cells and can cause disease. Exposure to x-ray, magnetic resonance imaging, and computed tomography is common in the medical field. Professionals who work in nuclear facilities and live near them are especially vulnerable to radiation exposure. The nuclear bombing of Hiroshima and Nagasaki resulted in a higher incidence of leukemia for those living

Table 8-1 Differences Between DNA and RNA	
DNA	**RNA**
Double stranded	Single stranded
Deoxyribose is the sugar molecule	Ribose is the sugar molecule
Thymine (T), adenine (A), cytosine (C), and guanine (G) are the nitrogenous bases	Uracil (U), adenine (A), cytosine (C), and guanine (G) are the nitrogenous bases
Longer than RNA	Smaller than DNA

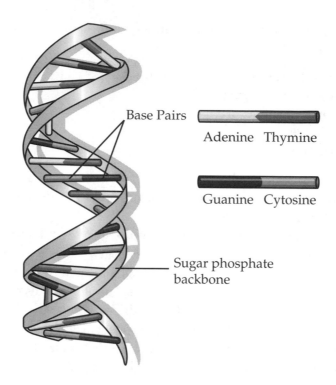

FIGURE 8-2   DNA is a double-stranded helix.
Source: National Library of Medicine. http://ghr.nlm.nih.gov/handbook/basics/dna. Accessed July 10, 2010.

nearby. Conversely, ionizing radiation can be used beneficially in the treatment of cancers. Radiation levels and health status in the community should be monitored. Any abnormal rise in the incidence of disease caused by radiation effects should be investigated.

Ribonucliec Acid and Protein Synthesis

RNA is of three different types: *rRNA (ribosomal RNA)* is present in the nucleolus, produced from DNA, and participates in the formation of *mRNA (messenger RNA)*. mRNA is transported from nucleus to cytoplasm and carries coded information for protein synthesis. mRNA in association with the ribosome and with the help of *tRNA (transporter RNA)* produces proteins. tRNA brings amino acids to the protein synthesis site. The process of formation of RNA from DNA is known as transcription. The process of formation of proteins from RNA is known as translation and occurs in the cytoplasm.

S - SUGAR
P - Phosphate

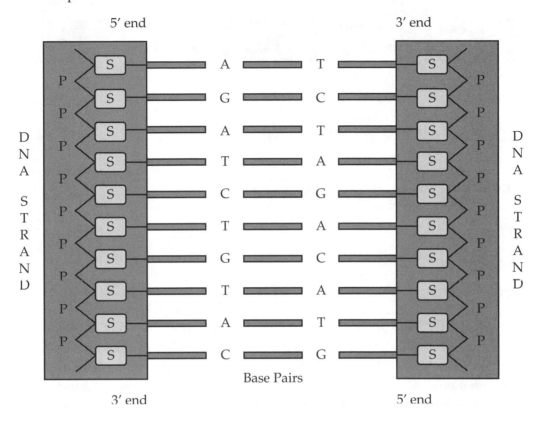

FIGURE 8-3   A DNA segment showing nitrogenous bases, with the sugar molecule and phosphate group positions.
Source: Picture courtesy of Dr. Kiran Macha.

The part of the DNA that codes for a specific protein is called a gene, and the complete set of genes that code for all proteins in the body is known as the genome. Several genes exist in the DNA, and each one codes for a specific protein; these proteins, in turn, are the building blocks of a specific structure or organ in the body (**Figure 8-4**). For example, hair (keratin) is made of proteins that are different from those making up muscle (actin and myosin). Both DNA and RNA carry genetic information for making proteins, because the genetic code exists in both of them.

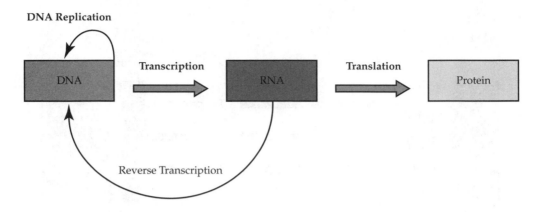

FIGURE 8-4   Proteins cannot produce nucleic acid.
Source: Picture courtesy of Dr. Kiran Macha.

Genetic Code

Three nucleotides (nitrogenous bases) form a codon (genetic code), and each codon is specific for an amino acid. Each amino acid can have one or more codes. For example, UUU and UUC both are specific codes for phenylalanine. The ATG code in DNA and the AUG code in RNA are known as "start codons" (they signal the start of protein synthesis). UAA, UAG, and UGA are known as "stop codons" (they end the RNA translation process). The genetic code is the information that is required for the synthesis of all proteins in the body, which are essential to human life.

Important Enzymes and Their Function

One or both strands of DNA can be replicated, and complementary strands can be produced. To separate the two strands of DNA, enzymes called topoisomerases are needed. The DNA polymerase enzyme brings the nucleotides to the replication site that are complementary to the DNA strand, allowing the production of a complementary DNA strand. This process is known as DNA replication. In the transcription process (DNA to RNA), DNA-dependent RNA polymerase enzyme is involved.

In bacteria, restriction endonuclease enzymes were discovered; these are highly specialized enzymes capable of cutting the DNA at specific sites. The DNA fragments can then be joined together by an enzyme called DNA ligase, with rDNA as the result. The DNA methylation process is known to protect DNA from restriction enzymes. RNA can produce DNA with the help of reverse transcriptase (RNA-dependent DNA polymerase) enzyme (in retroviruses).

Public Health Applications

Antibiotics such as norfloxacin, ofloxacin, and ciprofloxacin inhibit DNA topoisomerases or DNA gyrases in bacteria, but they have no effect on DNA topoisomerases within the human cell (Rose, 1988). With the help of rDNA technology, insulin and growth hormones are produced for human use.

Genetic Information Transmission

The genetic information is transferred through sperm and ovum. Sperm is produced as a result of meiotic divisions containing either one X chromosome or Y chromosome. Ova carry only the X chromosome. If sperm with an X chromosome enter the ovum, the zygote will have two XX chromosomes and the result is a female. If sperm with a Y chromosome enter the ovum (X chromosome), the result is a male (with XY chromosomes). So, the zygote carries genetic information from both parents. During the DNA replication process in the zygote, an important event known as "crossing over" may occur. During crossing over, a part of the paternal chromosome may be exchanged with the maternal chromosome and vice versa. This exchange of genetic information further increases the complexity of the features in the resultant end product—the human being.

Because genes are inherited from the DNA of both the mother and father, the two strands of DNA are not similar. So, each human has two genes for any given trait. The sequence of nucleotides may be similar or different on these genes located at same locus in the chromosomes. The variants of a gene are known as alleles. Some alleles are dominant, and some may be recessive. If a similar sequence of nucleotides is found in the genes of a trait on both strands of DNA, then the genotype (genetic makeup) is considered to be homozygous. If the sequence of nucleotides is different in the genes of a given trait on both DNA strands, then the genotype is considered to be heterozygous. These minor differences at the microscopic (genotype) level manifest at the macroscopic (phenotype) level (or, in the way physical characteristics for traits present themselves).

Sometimes nucleotides may be deleted from or inserted into the DNA sequence. When the insertion or deletion occurs in pairs of three (genetic code), the result of translation is the generation of a whole new protein (with more amino acids) or a protein with less amino acids. These mutations occur frequently, and point mutations that can cause the replacement of a single nucleotide with another can also greatly affect gene expression.

Epigenes

The word "epigenes" comes from "epi," which means "upon/on top of," and "genes," representing the nucleotide sequence in DNA. Epigenes influence genetic expression without altering the nucleotide sequence in the genes. The study of epigenes is known as epigenetics. Histones in the chromatin keep the DNA tightly coiled, and in this state it is not available to participate in transcription. The acetyl groups attached to the histones play an important role in keeping the DNA in this offline state. In contrast, methyl groups when attached to cytosine bases in DNA result in the deacetylation of the histones, making DNA available for the transcription process (**Figure 8-5**). DNA transcription can also be affected by phosphorylation and ubiquitylation of histones. These mechanisms do not alter the nucleotide sequence of DNA. Epigenes, like DNA, are inherited. For example, the color of the iris may be different between twins. This variation in color for individuals with the same genetic makeup (genotype) is explained by the influence of epigenes on gene expression (phenotype).

Genetic imprinting is a mechanism by which the suppression of a gene on a DNA strand because of the methylation process may result in the expression of the gene sequence located on another DNA strand. Through this process the parent-specific allele for a trait received from either the mother or father will be expressed.

Public Health Applications

Food is designed with the addition of colors, additives, and preservatives. Human exposure to chemicals in foods, teratogenic drugs, and toxic environmental contaminants may cause epigenetic changes that can negatively impact our health.

Single-Nucleotide Polymorphisms

Replacement of a single nucleotide in the genetic sequence results in the insertion of a different amino acid in the protein, for example, UUU codes for phenylalanine and UUA codes for leucine. So, if uracil is replaced by adenine in the genetic code, instead of phenylalanine, leucine will occupy the position in the protein. Single-nucleotide polymorphisms result in changes in the amino acid sequence in a protein in such a way that the functional structure of a protein may not be formed. As well, the solubility and the stability of the protein may be lost (Sunyaev et al., 2001).

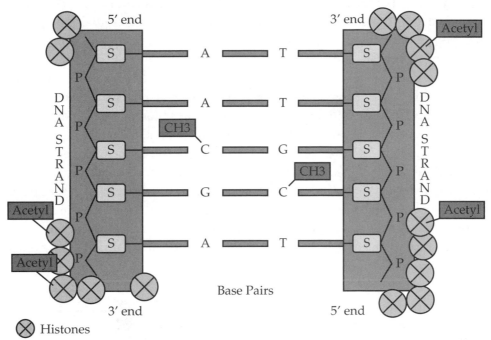

FIGURE 8-5   Epigenetic changes occur as a result of methylation of the cytosine bases and deacetylation of the histones.
Source: Picture courtesy of Dr. Kiran Macha.

Haplotypes

Reproduction and the exchange of genetic material between paternal and maternal chromosomes (crossing over) enable the progression of genetic complexity. This evolutionary process did not affect all segments of chromosomes. These unchanged inherited segments of chromosomes, known as haplotypes, are found in many people in the population (Gabriel, 2002).

Public Health Applications

The study of haplotypes led to the understanding of diseases that may arise because of changes that occur in the nucleotide sequence in these chromosome segments. The International HapMap Project is gathering information about haplotypes from researchers around the world.

GREGOR JOHANN MENDEL'S LAWS OF INHERITANCE _____

Gregor Mendel, an Austrian monk, is well known as the "Father of Genetics." He conducted pioneering experiments on inheritance in peas in the mid-19th century, with his conclusions having a far-reaching impact in the field of genetics. Mendel proposed the existence of a dominant and recessive "factor" (later referred to as genes). His Law of Segregation states that each allele is inherited from a parent and separates during the production of gametes (**Figure 8-6**). His Law of Independent Assortment states that the inheritance of an allele (dominant or recessive) is a random phenomenon.

The abnormal gene can be inherited either through autosomal or sex chromosomes. If a child inherits an abnormal gene, this may result in the outright manifestation of a disease, mild disease symptoms, or no disease symptoms at all. Sometimes even though the abnormal gene is present, the individual may not suffer from disease because of the absence of triggers. But these individuals are at risk of developing the disease.

Two copies of the same gene (one allele inherited from each parent) are present in an individual. If one of the alleles is abnormal, the protein produced by that allele is

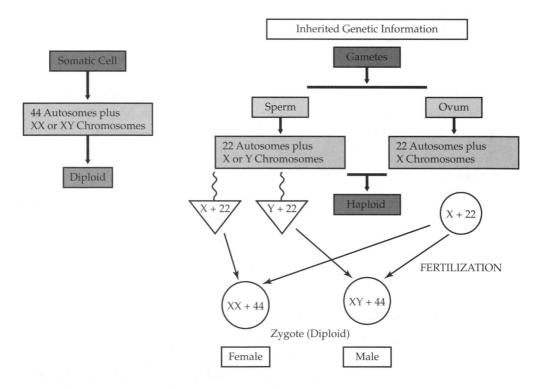

FIGURE 8-6 Genetic information is inherited through gametes.
Source: Picture courtesy of Dr. Kiran Macha.

abnormal. The other normal allele may produce enough protein to overcome the deficiency. Sometimes the abnormal protein is produced in greater quantity than the normal protein and can thus cause disease. In dominant disorders one abnormal gene is enough to inherit disease, and in recessive disorders two abnormal genes need to be inherited to suffer from disease.

Public Health Applications

According to Mendelian principles, the inheritance of disorders is predictable. Genetic disorders are classified into the following categories.

Autosomal Dominant Disorders

In Case 8-1 the female parent has a dominant gene. There is a 50% chance that children suffer from the disease. In diagram **Case 8-1** the "r" is the abnormal dominant gene and "R" is the normal gene.

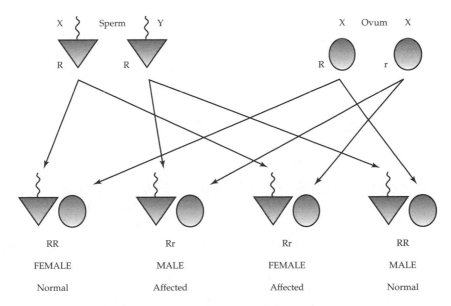

CASE 8-1
Source: Picture courtesy of Dr. Kiran Macha.

In Case 8-2 both parents have a dominant gene that is inherited by the children. There is a 75% chance that children may suffer from the disease. The child with two abnormal genes may suffer from severe disease because there is no normal gene to compensate for the abnormal gene, resulting in abnormal protein production. In diagram **Case 8-2** "r" is the abnormal dominant gene and "R" is the normal gene.

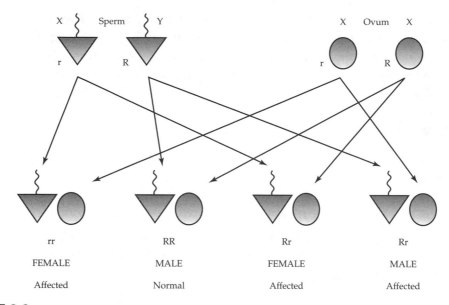

CASE 8-2
Source: Picture courtesy of Dr. Kiran Macha.

Examples of autosomal dominant disorders are shown in **Table 8-2**.

Table 8-2	Autosomal Dominant Diseases	
Autosomal Dominant Disorder	**Genes Affected**	**Abnormal Protein**
Huntington's disorder	CAG trinucleotide repeats are found on the short arm of chromosome 4	Huntington protein accumulations cause disease CNS affected
Neurofibromatosis	Mutation involving *NF-1* and *NF-2* genes	Abnormal neurofibromin and merlin proteins are produced, respectively CNS affected
Myotonic dystrophy	Type 1: *DMPK* gene Type 2: *ZNF9* gene	Type 1: Deficiency of dystrophy myotonic protein kinase Type 2: Abnormal zinc finger protein
Tuberous sclerosis	*TSC1* gene is located on chromosome 9 *TSC2* gene is located on chromosome 16	*TSC1* mutation produces abnormal hamartin protein *TS2* mutation produces abnormal tuberin protein CNS affected

Table 8-2   Autosomal Dominant Diseases *(continued)*

Autosomal Dominant Disorder	Genes Affected	Abnormal Protein
Polycystic kidney disease	*PKD1* gene *PKD2* gene *PKHD1* gene	*PKD1:* Abnormal polycystin protein *PKD2:* Abnormal polycystin protein *PKHD1:* Abnormal fibrocystin protein Kidney, pancreas, liver, CNS affected
Familial polyposis coli	*APC* gene	Abnormal APC protein (APC protein is a tumor suppressor protein). GIT affected
Hereditary spherocytosis	Spectrin alpha and beta genes are located on chromosomes 1 and 14, respectively	Spectrin deficiency Red blood cells affected
Von Willebrand	*VWF* gene	Von Willebrand factor deficiency disease Blood clotting affected
Marfan syndrome	*FBN-1* gene located on chromosome 15	Deficiency of fibrillin-1 protein Bones, lungs, eyes, heart, and blood vessels affected
Ehlers-Danlos syndrome	Mutations in *ADAMTS2, COL1A1, COL1A2, COL3A1, COLL5A2, PLOD1,* and *TNXB* genes	Deficiency in collagen protein Skin and bones affected
Osteogenesis imperfecta	Mutations in *COL1A1* (chromosome 17), *COL1A2* genes	Collagen protein deficiency Bones affected
Achondroplasia	Mutations in *FGFR3* gene	Fibroblast growth factor receptor 3 protein deficiency Bones affected
Familial hypercholesterolemia	Mutations in *APOB, LDLR, LDLRAP1,* and *PCSK9* genes	*APOB:* Apolipoprotein B-100 *LDLR:* Low-density lipoprotein receptor *LDLRAP1:* Low-density lipoprotein receptor adaptor protein 1

(continues)

Table 8-2 Autosomal Dominant Diseases *(continued)*		
Autosomal Dominant Disorder	**Genes Affected**	**Abnormal Protein**
		PCKSK9: Proprotein convertase subtilisin/kexin type 9 Above proteins involved in lipid metabolism and abnormal production of these proteins affects lipid metabolism
Acute intermittent porphyria	*PBGD* gene mutation	Porphobilinogen deaminase deficiency
Notes: CNS, central nervous system; GIT, Gastrointestinal tract.		

Autosomal Recessive Disorders

In Case 8-3 the female parent carries a recessive gene. There is a 50% chance the children will inherit the abnormal gene. The symptoms in carriers of an abnormal recessive gene are often mild, and the individual may not be affected. In diagram **Case 8-3** "R" is the normal gene and "r" is the abnormal recessive gene.

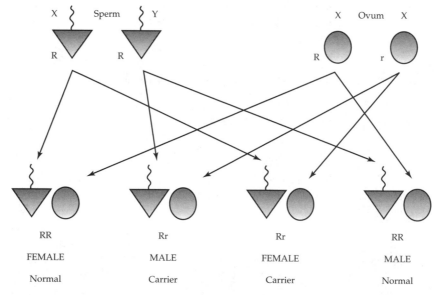

CASE 8-3

Source: Picture courtesy of Dr. Kiran Macha.

In Case 8-4 both parents carry a recessive gene. There is a 25% chance the children will suffer from disease and a 50% chance they will carry the abnormal gene. The symptoms in carriers of abnormal genes are often mild, and the individuals may not be affected. In diagram **Case 8-4** "R" is the normal gene and "r" is the abnormal recessive gene.

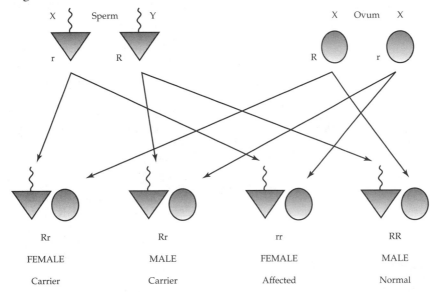

CASE 8-4
Source: Picture courtesy of Dr. Kiran Macha.

Examples of autosomal recessive disorders are show in **Table 8-3**.

Table 8-3 Autosomal Recessive Disorders		
Autosomal Recessive Disorder	**Genes Affected**	**Abnormal Protein**
Cystic fibrosis	Mutation in *CFTR* gene	Deficiency of CFTR protein (chloride channels)
Phenylketonuria	Mutations in *PAH* gene	Deficiency of an enzyme, phenylalanine hydroxylase
Galactosemia	Mutations in *GALE*, *GALK1*, and *GALT*	Deficiency of enzymes UDP-galactose-4-epimerase, galactokinase 1, and galactose-1-phosphate uridylyltransferase, respectively.
		(continues)

Table 8-3   Autosomal Recessive Disorders *(continued)*

Autosomal Recessive Disorder	Genes Affected	Abnormal Protein
Homocystinuria	Mutations in *CBS, MTHFR, MTR,* and *MTRR* genes	Deficiency of cystathionine beta-synthase, 5, 10-methylenetetrahydrofolate reductase enzyme
Examples of lysosomal storage disorder		
Gaucher disease	*GBA* gene mutation	Beta-glucocerebrosidase
Niemann-Pick disease	*NPC1, NPC2,* and *SMPD1* gene mutation	Sphingomyelinase
Tay-Sachs disease	*HEXA* gene mutation	Hexosaminidase A enzyme deficient
Alpha-1-antitrypsin deficiency	*SERPINA1* gene mutation	Deficiency of alpha-1-antitrypsin enzyme
Wilson disease	*ATP7B* gene mutation	Deficiency of ATPase, CU++ transporting, beta-polypeptide
Hemochromatosis	*HAMP, HFE, HFE2, SLC40A1,* and *TFR2* gene mutations	Deficiency of hepcidin antimicrobial peptide, HFE protein, hemojuvelin, ferroportin 1, and transferring receptor 2
Examples of glycogen storage disorder		
Von Gierke disease	*G6PC* gene	Glucose 6-phosphatase
Pompe disease	*GAA* gene	Lysosonal acid alpha-glucosidase
Forbes disease	*AGL* gene	Amylo-1,6 glucosidase
Andersen disease	*GBE1* gene	Branching enzyme
McArdle disease	*PYGM* gene	Myophosphorylase
Hers disease	*PYGL* gene	Liver phosphorylase enzyme deficiency
Sickle cell disease	*HBB* gene mutations	Beta-globin deficiency
Thalassemia	*HBB* and *HBA1* and *HBA2* gene mutations	Beta-globin deficiency and alpha-globin deficiency
Congenital adrenal hyperplasia	*CYP21A2* gene mutation	21-Hydroxylase deficiency
Alkaptonuria	*HGD* gene mutation	Deficiency of homogentisate oxidase enzyme

Table 8-4 Autosomal Trisomy Disorders		
Autosomal Trisomies	**Trisomy of the Chromosome**	**Abnormalities**
Down syndrome	Trisomy 21	Mental retardation, prominent epicanthal fold, simian crease, duodenal atresia, septum primum, and increased risk of Alzheimer disease
Edwards syndrome	Trisomy 18	Mental retardation, rocker bottom feet, micrognathia, congenital heart disease, clenched hands, and prominent occiput
Patau's syndrome	Trisomy 13	Mental retardation, microcephaly, cleft lip, cleft palate, polydactyly, and congenital heart disease

Autosomal Trisomy

In this genetic disorder, instead of two copies of chromosomes, there are three copies of chromosomes seen together. Examples of autosomal trisomy disorders are shown in **Table 8-4**.

X-Linked Dominant Disorders

In Case 8-5 the dominant gene is present on the X chromosome of the male parent, with 50% of the children suffering from disease. In diagram **Case 8-5** "R" is an abnormal dominant gene present on X chromosome and "r" is a normal gene.

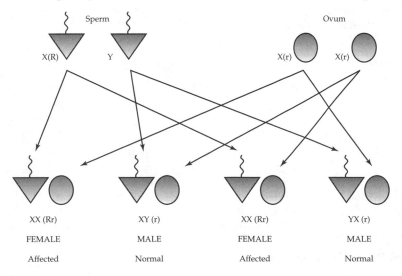

CASE 8-5
Source: Picture courtesy of Dr. Kiran Macha.

In Case 8-6 the dominant abnormal gene is present on X chromosomes of both parents, with 75% of the children affected with the disease. In diagram **Case 8-6** "R" is the abnormal dominant gene present on X- chromosomes and "r" is a normal gene.

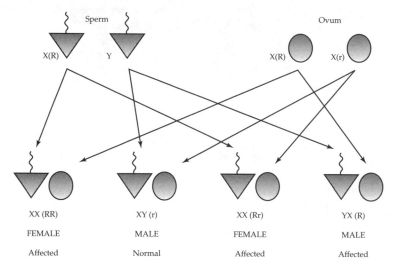

CASE 8-6
Source: Picture courtesy of Dr. Kiran Macha.

Examples of X-linked dominant disorders are shown in **Table 8-5**.

Table 8-5 X-Linked Dominant Disorders		
X- Linked Dominant Disorder	**Gene Affected**	**Abnormal Protein**
Coffin-Lowry syndrome	*RPS6KA3* gene mutations	Ribosomal S6 kinase protein deficiency
Incontinentia pigmenti	*IKBKG* gene mutations	Nuclear factor kappa B
Familial vitamin D-resistant rickets	Phosphate-regulating gene (*PHEX*) gene mutation	Abnormal PHEX protein produced
Hereditary nephritis/ Alports syndrome	*COL4A3, COL4A4,* and *COL4A5* gene mutations	Abnormal collagen synthesis

X-Linked Recessive Disorders

In Case 8-7 an abnormal recessive gene is present on the X chromosomes (female parent): 25% of children suffer from disease, 50% are not affected, and 25% carry the abnormal gene. In diagram **Case 8-7** "R" is the normal gene and "r" is the abnormal gene present on the X chromosome.

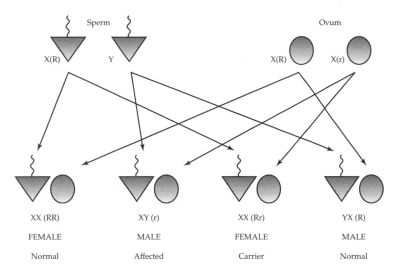

CASE 8-7

Source: Picture courtesy of Dr. Kiran Macha.

In Case 8-8 the abnormal recessive genes are present on the X chromosomes of both parents: 50% of children are affected, 25% are carriers, and 25% are not affected. In diagram **Case 8-8** "R" is the normal gene and "r" is the abnormal gene present on the X chromosome.

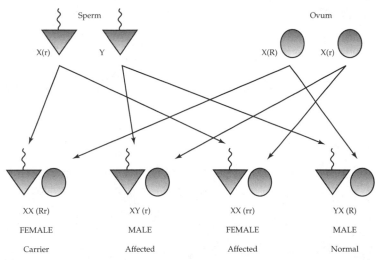

CASE 8-8

Source: Picture courtesy of Dr. Kiran Macha.

In Case 8-9 the abnormal recessive gene is present on the X chromosome of the male parent, with 50% of children not affected and 50% carrying the recessive gene. In diagram **Case 8-9** "R" is a normal gene and "r" is the abnormal gene on the X chromosome.

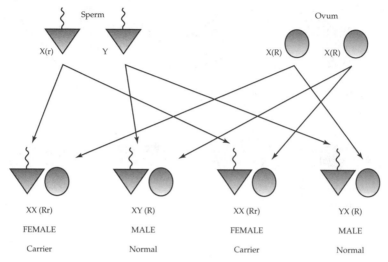

CASE 8-9
Source: Picture courtesy of Dr. Kiran Macha.

Examples of X-linked recessive disorders are shown in **Table 8-6**.

Table 8-6 X-Linked Recessive Disorders		
X- Linked Recessive Disorder	**Gene Affected**	**Abnormal Protein**
Hemophilia	*F8* (hemophilia A) and *F9* (hemophilia B) gene mutations	Coagulation factor VIII and coagulation factor IX deficiency, respectively
Duchenne and Becker muscular dystrophy	Mutations in *DMD* gene	Deficiency in dystrophin protein
Lesch-Nyhan syndrome	Mutations in *HPRT1* genes	Deficiency of hypoxanthine phosphoribosyltransferase 1
Hunter disease	*IDS* gene mutation	Deficiency of iduronate 2-sulfatase deficiency
Menkes disease	*ATP7A* gene mutations	Deficiency of ATPase, CU++ transporting, beta-polypeptide

Table 8-6   X-Linked Recessive Disorders *(continued)*

X- Linked Recessive Disorder	Gene Affected	Abnormal Protein
Glucose-6-phosphate dehydrogenase deficiency	*G6PD* gene mutations	Deficiency of enzyme glucose 6-phosphate dehydrogenase
Fabry disease	Mutations in *GLA* gene	Deficiency of enzyme alpha-galactosidase A
Wiskott-Aldrich syndrome	Mutations in *WAS* genes	Deficiency of WASP protein
Bruton agammaglobulinemia	*BTK* gene mutations	Bruton tyrosine kinase deficiency
Color vision deficiency	*CNGA3, CNGB3, GNAT2, OPN1LW, OPN1MW,* and *OPN1SW* gene mutations	Deficiency of CNG channel proteins, transducin, and photopigment

Y-Chromosome Linked Disorders

If an abnormal gene is present on the Y chromosome, only the males inherit and suffer from the disease. "R" is the abnormal gene present on Y chromosome, shown in diagram **Case 8-10**. Examples of Y-chromosome linked disorders are shown in **Table 8-7**.

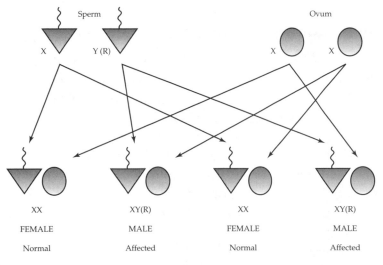

CASE 8-10

Source: Picture courtesy of Dr. Kiran Macha.

Table 8-7 Y-Chromosome Linked Disorders		
Y-Chromosome Linked Disorders	Gene Affected	Abnormal Protein
Y chromosome infertility	Mutations in *USP9Y* gene	Deficiency of ubiquitin-specific protease 9
46, XX testicular disorder	Mutations in *SRY* gene	Deficiency of sex-determining region Y protein
Swyer syndrome	Mutations in *SRY* gene	Deficiency of sex-determining region Y protein

CHARLES DARWIN'S THEORY OF NATURAL SELECTION

Application of the "Theory of Natural Selection" proposed by Charles Darwin in modern genetics explains some of the phenomena we have witnessed. Darwin's theory is based on the observation of phenotypic variations in animals and the influence of the environment on the selection of the species. Genetic variations over time lead to phenotypic variations by producing individuals of the same species but with different physical features. Those features that allowed the individual to best adapt to a changing environment also allowed that individual to survive, thus contributing to evolution of the species.

GENE MAPPING AND THE HUMAN GENOME PROJECT

Genetics has had its own growing pains. The idea of exploring the human gene and gathering all known information about it developed into the Human Genome Project. This global collaborative project was conducted from 1990 to 2003 to map and sequence the entire human genome. The National Institutes of Health and Department of Energy in the United States in association with several international organizations conducted this study. The outcomes of this research were not only related to learning about human genetics but also led to many innovations and technological developments. Genes that are responsible for many forms of cancer, for diseases such as diabetes, for cardiovascular events, and for diseases with limited knowledge (causation) are now being explained.

More than 1,800 genes linked to disease have been identified. Some 1,000 genetic tests that diagnose genetic diseases and risk for disease have been developed. Gene therapy is the subject of ongoing research. We now also better understand the effects of therapeutic drugs at the genetic level. We have data to prove health risks of toxic chemicals. The discovery of epigenes is another major breakthrough. The Human Genome Project has not only helped us explore new avenues but has also raised many questions that need to be answered in the future.

DNA BIOBANKING

The knowledge of genes (Human Genome Project), evidence of gene–environment interactions, and the identification of the genetic markers for diseases propelled the concept of DNA biobanking. Biobanks in European and North American countries are collecting human tissue, blood, and buccal smears from patients suffering from well-documented diseases. The biobanks allow geneticists to research and strengthen evidence of linkages between specific genes and disease. Other uses of these resources include the development of pharmacogenetics. Global ethical, legal, and confidentiality issues continue to challenge biobanking, because the idea of usage of this genetic material for future unknown purposes is a general public concern (Melas, Sjoholm, & Forsner, 2010). Biobanking is a complex and expensive undertaking demanding technology-equipped laboratories and needs to be closely monitored by government agencies.

GENETIC TESTING

Efforts toward the identification of the "ideal genetic composition" in a human to overcome the pain of life seem to be never-ending. (As Buddhists say, "to live is to suffer.") The natural genetic phenomenon that humans are trying hard to understand is complex, with many factors playing a role in unraveling its mysteries. The discovery of certain events may lead, or even mislead, us to do further research. With the discovery of biomarkers, the race persists to identify a genetic link for every disease with the idea of finding ways to treat disease at the genetic level. Genetic testing identifies and confirms the presence of a disease and provides us time to formulate a plan of action to counter the effects of the disease. To obtain embryo tissue material for the prenatal diagnosis of diseases through genetic testing, amniocentesis and chorionic villous biopsy are invasive procedures performed. Genetic testing is also widely used in forensic medicine. (Issues that challenge genetic testing are discussed in Chapter 12, "Ethical and Legal Issues in Epidemiology.") Health insurance companies may or may not cover genetic testing.

Newborn Screening

The screening of newborn infants is a great boon for the current generation. A few drops of blood can screen children for hundreds of infectious, endocrine, hematological, metabolic, and genetic diseases. Diseases that are known to cause harm or disability or to be life-threatening are identified and diagnosed, and treatment can be initiated even before the symptoms manifest. Blood samples from the newborn can be collected by hospital personnel if the facilities are capable of performing genetic tests in their laboratories and they are allowed to do screening. Most newborn blood samples are sent to state public health laboratories for screening purposes. Guidelines for the collection of blood and other instructions for infant screening programs are listed on the Centers for Disease Control and Prevention website and also on state health department websites. State laws mandate that information gathered in association with genetic testing be kept confidential.

Importance of Early Identification of Diseases

Phenylketonuria is a genetic metabolic condition that occurs as a result of a lack of phenylalanine hydroxylase enzyme. Phenylalanine and tyrosine are essential amino acids required for the formation of a protein. Tyrosine is produced from phenylalanine and is also an essential amino acid. Without the enzyme essential to catalyze this reaction, phenylalanine amino acid levels are elevated in the blood. The results of such elevation are mental retardation and seizures. To prevent the progression of this disease to such extreme levels, dietary modification is an option to keep the levels of phenylalanine low. Early identification and elimination of phenylalanine from the diet slows progression of the disease.

Sickle cell anemia is an abnormal condition that causes red blood cells to change shape. Hemoglobin is abnormal in this condition and occurs because of the presence of valine instead of glutamine amino acid at the sixth position in the beta globin. Patients suffer from severe respiratory infections and are susceptible to deadly bacteria, like pseudomonas. *Salmonella* may cause bone infections in those who suffer from sickle cell disease. The sickle cells can block the arteries and cause damage to the spleen. Prophylactic administration of penicillin to these children is known to protect them from severe bacterial infections and prevent deaths. The silent human immunodeficiency virus infectious epidemic that can be transmitted from mother to infants is a growing burden to the community. Early detection of the antibodies helps us to monitor the status of the disease and administer antiretrovirals when necessary.

The following chemicals, enzymes, drugs, hormones, and infectious disease agents that cause diseases are screened as part of the infant screening program:

Acarboxyprothrombin
Acylcarnitine
Adenine phosphoribosyl
    transferase
Adenosine deaminase
Albumin
Alpha-fetoprotein
Amino acid profiles
Arginine (Krebs cycle)
Histidine/urocanic acid
Homocysteine
Phenylalanine/tyrosine
Tryptophan
Andrenostenedione
Antipyrine
Arabinitol enantiomers
Arginase
Benzoylecgonine (cocaine)
Biotinidase
Biopterin
C-reactive protein
Carnitine
Carnosinase
CD4
Ceruloplasmin
Chenodeoxycholic acid
Chloroquine
Cholesterol
Cholinesterase
Conjugated 1-ß hydroxy-
    cholic acid
Cortisol
Creatine kinase
Creatine kinase MM
    isoenzyme

Cyclosporin A
D-penicillamine
De-ethylchloroquine
Dehydroepiandrosterone
    sulfate
DNA (PCR)
    acetylator polymorphism
    Alcohol dehydrogenase
    Alpha-1-antitrypsin
    Cystic fibrosis
    Duchenne/Becker
        muscular dystrophy
    Glucose-6-phosphate
        dehydrogenase
    hemoglobinopathies
    A,S,C,E
    D-Punjab
    Beta-thalassemia
    Hepatitis B virus
    HCMV
    HIV-1
    HTLV-1
    Leber hereditary optic
        neuropathy
    MCAD
    RNA
    PKU
    Plasmodium vivax
    Sexual differentiation
    21-Deoxycortisol
Desbutylhalofantrine
Dihydropteridine
    reductase
Diptheria/tetanus
    antitoxin

Erythrocyte arginase
Erythrocyte
    protoporphyrin
Esterase D
Fatty acids/acylglycines
Free ß-human chorionic
    gonadotropin
Free erythrocyte
    porphyrin
Free thyroxine (FT4)
Free tri-iodothyronine
    (FT3)
Fumarylacetoacetase
Galactose/gal-1-
    phosphate
Galactose-1-phosphate
    uridyltransferase
Gentamicin
Glucose
Glucose-6-phosphate
    dehydrogenase
Glutathione
Glutathione perioxidase
Glycocholic acid
Glycosylated hemoglobin
Halofantrine
Hemoglobin variants
Hexosaminidase A
Human erythrocyte
    carbonic anhydrase I
17-Alpha-
    hydroxyprogesterone
Hypoxanthine
    phosphoribosyl
    transferase

Immunoreactive trypsin
Lactate
Lead
Lipoproteins
  (a)
  B/A-1
  ß
Lysozyme
Mefloquine
Netilmicin
Phenobarbitone
Phenytoin
Phytanic/pristanic acid
Progesterone
Prolactin
Prolidase
Purine nucleoside
    phosphorylase
Quinine
Reverse tri-iodothyronine
    (rT3)
Selenium
Serum pancreatic lipase
Sissomicin
Somatomedin C
Specific antibodies
  Adenovirus

Antinuclear antibody
Anti-zeta antibody
arbovirus
Aujeszky disease virus
Dengue virus
Dracunculus medinensis
Echinococcus granulosus
Entamoeba histolytica
enterovirus
Giardia duodenalisa
Helicobacter pylori
Hepatitis B virus
IgE (atopic disease)
Influenza virus
Leishmania donovani
leptospira
Measles/mumps/rubella
Mycobacterium leprae
Mycoplasma pneumoniae
Onchocerca volvulus
parainfluenza virus
Plasmodium falciparum
Poliovirus
Pseudomonas aeruginosa
Respiratory syncytial
    virus
Rickettsia (scrub typhus)

Schistosoma mansoni
Toxoplasma gondii
Trepenoma pallidium
Trypanosoma cruzi/rangeli
Vesicular stomatis virus
Wuchereria bancrofti
Yellow fever virus
Specific antigens
Succinylacetone
Sulfadoxine
Theophylline
Thyrotropin (TSH)
Thyroxine (T4)
Thyroxine-binding
    globulin
Trace elements
Transferrin
UDP-galactose-4-
    epimerase
Urea
Uroporphyrinogen I
    synthase
Vitamin A
White blood cells
Zinc protoporphyrin

Source: Centers for Disease Control and Prevention. Retrieved June 10, 2010, from http://www.cdc.gov/labstandards/nsqap_bloodspots.html

Normal DNA Repair Mechanisms and Gene Therapy

DNA glycosylases recognize damaged portions of bases in DNA and are responsible for their removal (base excision repair). Where there is a mismatch of DNA base pairs (for example, adenine pairs with cytosine rather than with thymine), inappropriate bases are removed through the mismatch repair mechanism. Nucleotides are also removed from damaged portions of DNA, with new nucleotides generated and integrated (nucleotide excision repair). Phosphatidylinositol-3-kinases recognize damaged portions of DNA and signal genetics repair (Christmann, 2003). When one or all mechanisms of DNA repair fail, one may suffer from a disease because the protein needed to maintain a specific bodily function is not produced.

Interestingly, it is not only the failure of the gene repair mechanisms; other factors also play a role in sustaining DNA damage. The environment, the foods we eat, and the adaptation of the body to its own physiological needs can alter gene expression. These complex interactions pose a challenge because it is difficult to distinguish causes for changes in gene expression caused by one factor alone.

Public Health Applications

Failures of the above mechanisms that protect genetic structures can lead to diseases. Some diseases such as cancer are irreversible. Advanced techniques and research have been progressing in the direction of gene therapy even though the U.S. Food and Drug Administration has not permitted the treatment of the general population with such therapy.

Learning about the behavior of viruses and genomics has helped us to use them in gene therapy (**Figure 8-7**). Viruses have either DNA or RNA (capable of generating DNA). Viruses such as adenoviruses, herpes simplex, and retroviruses can be used as

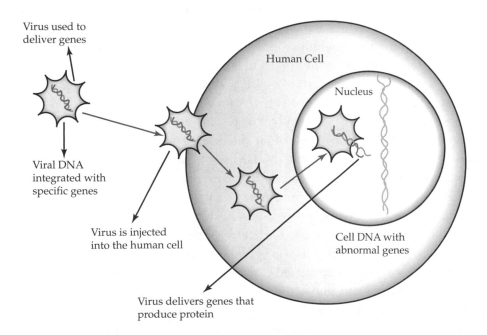

FIGURE 8-7   Genetic therapy and steps involved in using a virus.
Source: Picture courtesy of Dr. Kiran Macha.

vectors to deliver genes into cancer cells or cells with abnormal DNA. Challenges associated with this form of gene therapy include the body's immune response to viruses, skills in targeted cell approaches, and how responses are measured after interventions.

Nanotechnology has opened up another avenue for therapy, because genetic material can be attached to micromolecules and delivered to target cells. Research on gene therapy has been conducted in association with Huntington disease, blood disorders, melanoma, and lung cancer. Gene therapy raises several issues: Instead of curing one disease, therapy may generate another disease because we have yet to master this important science.

GENETIC COUNSELING

The story of genetics is not yet over because the complexities in details seem to create more enthusiasm. Healthcare professionals, geneticists, and genetic counselors study genetics and can then offer their understanding through public education and genetic counseling. It is clear from the research that gene–environment interactions may have an impact on the expression of genes. Diseases such as obesity, heart disease, diabetes, and cancers are prevalent in the community. New risk factors such as childhood obesity are growing in incidence and will likely impact the prevalence of chronic diseases such as diabetes and cardiovascular disease. The changing dynamics of the genetic pool cannot be monitored because this is not a cost-effective strategy. The identification of new genetic diseases will help us to develop screening tests. However, disease risk factors are increasing healthcare costs. Education and lifestyle changes are the most cost-effective methods to decrease risk for a number of prevalent diseases.

Those who are already affected by diseases linked to their genetics need support and should be educated properly about the disease and its cause. Community resources that can help one cope with disease need to be introduced. The impacted individual should be informed as to likely future events in the disease process as well as measures that offer protection from environmental triggers, if any. The need for genetic testing of family members should also be determined, and the family should be educated about the disease process. The effects of genetic disease on marriage and the potential for inheritance of the disease by children should be carefully communicated. One should also research any related ethical, legal, and discrimination ramifications associated with the disease, and appropriate agencies should be notified if such issues are encountered. Healthcare professionals such as physicians and nurses can be trained as genetic counselors. Genetic counselors are trained to do this job, and the role of advanced practice nurses is more important than the role of counselors.

PHARMACOGENETICS AND PHARMACOGENOMICS

Drugs administered to treat disease pass through a series of events. The drugs may interact with enzymes in the liver or elsewhere and may be transported attached to proteins. The action of the drug may be based on its attachment to receptors or ion channels on cell membranes. Drugs are eventually metabolized by enzymes in the liver. These enzymes, receptors, ion channels, and transporters are all proteins, with their production also dependent on genes. Mutations in genes may alter protein structures and in turn affect physiology. A drug may produce an effect in some but may not produce the same effect in others because of receptor differences. (For example, salbutamol works well for many in treating asthma but may not work for everyone because of receptor differences.) When a drug is administered to a group of people, the effects observed in each individual may be different. Some drugs may significantly decrease the risk of a disease for a particular ethnic group, such as diuretics for African Americans, but have a lesser impact for others.

Pharmacogenetics and pharmacogenomics involve the study of the interaction between genetics and therapeutic drugs. Pharmacogenetics looks for the genetic cause when an unusual response is detected in an individual after the administration of a drug. Pharmacogenomics is based on linking the identified genetic differences in populations to drug responses. Because genetic makeup controls both metabolic and physiological factors, its understanding allows the determination of risk of suffering from a disease. Targeting the treatment of disease for each individual is not cost-effective, and ethical issues must always be addressed. Current research in pharmacogenetics is focused on cardiac, respiratory, and psychiatric conditions.

IMPROVING PUBLIC HEALTH THROUGH GENETIC STUDIES

Breast Cancer Genes

The discovery of the *BRCA1* and *BRCA2* genes that are related to breast cancer was well received. However, the fact that only 3% to 8% of breast cancers appear to be caused by mutations in these genes is challenging (Rosman, Kaklamani, & Pasche, 2007). Further exploration and understanding of the genes linked to breast cancer is essential, with efforts also directed to understanding the complex interaction of environmental factors in the development of breast cancer. Genetic testing screens individuals and can predict the chances of evolution of normal breast cells into cancerous tissue. Prevention measures such as changes in lifestyle, avoiding estrogen or progesterone hormone intake based on the hormonal receptors present on cancer cells, and surgical options may decrease suffering from this form of cancer.

Mental Health

Depression, bipolar disorder, and schizophrenia are some common psychiatric disorders. Most of those who suffer from psychiatric illness are known to have a history of similar suffering in the family. This correlation explains the heritable nature of the disease. Exploration for genetic linkages was successful in locating the genes that cause these diseases. For example, *DRNBP1* and *NRG1* have been linked to schizophrenia.

Accumulations of amyloid beta protein in the brain cells are known to cause Alzheimer disease. The amyloid precursor protein, or *APP*, gene is present on chromosome 21. Family history plays an important role in predicting this disease. Identification of the possibilities of the expression of Alzheimer disease can help healthcare providers formulate a health plan in anticipation of this event. Regular physical, neurological, and mental status examinations coupled with laboratory tests can track progression of the disease, and early countermeasures may slow down the disability.

The incidence of autism, a neurological disorder with social interaction and communication problems, is growing in children. The LRRN3 and LRRTM3 brain proteins have been found to be linked to autism. The theory that autism is linked to vaccines (as an environmental trigger) is yet to be proved. Early interventions can positively impact autism, as we understand the cause and pathophysiological process of the disease.

Exploration for Predictors

The idea to correlate race with the incidence of a particular genetic disease may not be of great help, because humans have been migrating and reproducing since time immemorial. Examining subgroups may, however, helps us predict some genetic diseases. For example, Tay-Sachs disease is an autosomal recessive, lysosomal storage disorder known to be common in Ashkenazi Jews. Tay-Sachs disease in children causes blindness, seizures, mental retardation, and death at an early age. The Amish community is known to suffer from many genetic disorders caused by the common practice of marriage of closely related individuals in the community.

Epidemiological studies conducted to identify minor differences in incidence statistics of a disease based on race may help us to explore the socioeconomic causes and genetic factors that potentiate the disease expression. For example, the incidence of coronary artery disease is higher in African Americans than in Whites and Hispanics. African Americans are genetically more susceptible to high blood pressure. Culture, economy, education, and lifestyle are some of the socioeconomic factors that may increase the disease risk.

Advance practice nurses should understand the role of genetics in the web of disease causation. The pointers to a genetic disease are available in health communications with a patient. Factors such as a broad genetic knowledge base, communication skills, and the availability and affordability of genetic testing matter to our clinical practice. Tentative health plans should be designed for patients based on specific predictable events of a genetic disease. Encouragement of prevention measures such as lifestyle modifications, exercise, smoking cessation, dietary modifications, and avoidance of teratogens during pregnancy may all decrease disease incidence.

KEY POINTS

- DNA and RNA carry genetic information in the form of a triplet code. DNA produces RNA, and RNA produces proteins.
- Proteins are essential components of the human body. Changes in genes as a result of reproduction, mutations, or recombinations may produce abnormal proteins that cause disease.
- The interaction of genes and the environment is known to affect genetic expression. The food we eat and the fluids we drink can affect our genes.
- Family history is a key predictor of the possibility of inheritance of genetic disease.
- The Human Genome Project unearthed the secrets of DNA, improved our techniques, and generated questions for the future.
- Our life expectancy has been increased with medical technology and public health measures. Longer lives with minimum disability associated with aging may be achieved with genetic solutions.
- Legal and ethical issues associated with genetic testing are complex.
- Pharmacogenetics may revolutionize the way we treat people in the future.

CRITICAL QUESTIONS

1. How do you believe we can better our health through an understanding of genetics?
2. What measures do you suggest to minimize gene changes?
3. Why should we invest in expensive genetic research?
4. The genetic code is not all there is to know but is a starting point in our understanding of genetics. How can we focus genetic research for the benefit of humankind?

RESOURCES

Human Genome Epidemiology Network, Centers for Disease Control and Prevention
  http://www.cdc.gov/genomics/hugenet/default.htm
National Human Genome Research Institute
  http://www.genome.gov/
American Society of Human Genetics
  http://www.ashg.org/
National Society of Genetic Counselors
  http://www.nsgc.org/
National Center for Biotechnology Information
  http://www.ncbi.nlm.nih.gov/gene
Human Genome Project Information
  http://www.ornl.gov/sci/techresources/Human_Genome/medicine/genetherapy.shtml

REFERENCES

Christmann, M. (2003). Mechanisms of human DNA repair: An update. *Toxicology, 193*(1-2), 3.

Gabriel, S. S. B. (2002). The structure of haplotype blocks in the human genome. *Science, 296*(5576), 2225–2229.

Melas, P. A., Sjoholm, L. K., & Forsner, T. (2010). Examining the public refusal to consent to DNA biobanking: Empirical data from a Swedish population-based study. *Journal of Medical Ethics, 36*(2), 93–98.

Morton, N. E. (1993). Genetic epidemiology. *Annual Review of Genetics, 27*, 523–538.

Rose, K. M. (1988). DNA topoisomerases as targets for chemotherapy. *FASEB Journal, 2*(9), 2474.

Rosman, D. S., Kaklamani, V., & Pasche, B. (2007). New insights into breast cancer genetics and impact on patient management. *Current Treatment Options in Oncology, 8*(1), 61–73.

Sunyaev, S., Ramensky, V., Koch, I., Lathe, W., Kondrashov, A. S., & Bork, P. (2001). Prediction of deleterious human alleles. *Human Molecular Genetics, 10*(6), 591–597.

Watson, J. D., & Crick, F. H. (1953). Molecular structure of nucleic acids; a structure for deoxyribose nucleic acid. *Nature, 171*(4356), 737–738.

CHAPTER 9

Environmental Epidemiology

"The more we exploit nature, the more our options are reduced, until we have only one: to fight for survival."

—Morris K. Udall

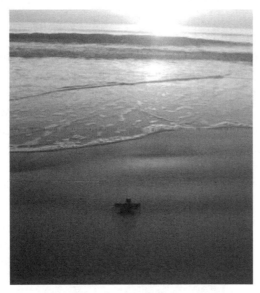

Source: Courtesy of Nonie Sullivan.

Michele S. Bednarzyk
Lillia M. Loriz

OBJECTIVES

- Identify ways environmental epidemiology contributes to public health.
- Describe how to assess environmental problems.
- Identify the role of the clinician in environmental epidemiology.
- Describe how human activity has interfered with and has affected the environment and human health.

HISTORY OF ENVIRONMENTAL EPIDEMIOLOGY

There has been a relationship between the environment and human health for centuries. Hippocrates (460–377 BC), author of *Epidemic I, Epidemic III*, and *On Airs, Waters and Places*, made a connection between disease and environmental conditions, especially in relation to water and seasons (Jones, 1923). He observed that different diseases occurred in different places and that malaria and yellow fever were common in swampy areas. Some 2,000 years later, Bernardino Ramazzini (1633–1714) authored the first notable book on occupational health and industrial hygiene, *De morbis artificum diatribe (The Diseases of Workers)*, published in 1700. In his work he identified several adverse health outcomes associated with chemicals, dust, metals, and other abrasive agents encountered by workers in various occupations (Cumston, 1926).

Environmental epidemiology is a subdivision of epidemiology, deriving historically from chronic disease epidemiology. Environmental epidemiology is the study of health-related events in specified populations that are influenced by physical, chemical, biological, and psychosocial factors in the environment. How to prevent and control health problems is also part of this line of study. The focus on population and emphasis on identifying causal relations distinguishes it from environmental health, which is more comprehensive (Goldsmith, 1967). Environmental epidemiology seeks to clarify the relationship between environmental factors and human health by focusing on specified populations or communities. This knowledge is based on the observation that most diseases are not random occurrences but rather are related to environmental factors that vary according to population subgroups, place, and time. Environmental epidemiological studies are concerned not only with those who get a disease but also with those who do not and in identifying why the two groups differ.

TYPES OF HEALTH EFFECTS AND ENVIRONMENTAL EXPOSURES

Health Effects

Environmental epidemiology deals with a broad array of disease and health states. Heading that array, of course, in terms of gravity, is mortality, including case fatality rates. The next concept is morbidity, which is estimated in a variety of ways, such as reported new cases of illness, aggravation of preexisting illness, the occurrence of episodes of hospitalization or demands for medical service, the occurrence of accidents, the impairment of function, or the production of symptoms (Goldsmith, 1969). Other less obvious effects are also of importance, such as biochemical and physiological reactions, which may not be easily understood in relation to long-term implications; the occurrence of annoyance reactions; and the storage of potentially harmful material such as lead and pesticides in the human body.

Environmental Exposures

Exposures to chemical or biological agents can occur through inhalation, oral ingestion, or occasionally absorption through the skin. Toxicity of the substance may vary considerably depending on the exposure mode. The location of exposures and the manner in which the given pollutant is introduced are also quite varied. In the case of radiation, exposures occur as a result of natural background levels, which vary to some extent. There are occupational exposures, such as medical diagnostic and therapeutic radiation, and the possible community exposures in association with nuclear power development. Similarly, regarding pesticides, exposure can be found incidentally in people who live adjacent to areas being sprayed, as residue in food, and occasionally as a food chain gradient; there is the possibility of absorption through handling and occupational exposures of workers. Thus, the types of environmental exposures are quite varied, and they have a tendency to interact (**Figure 9-1**).

Complex diseases have both genetic and environmental components. Understanding the contribution of environmental factors to disease susceptibility requires a more comprehensive view of exposure and biological response than has traditionally been applied. Exposure is defined as the "contact between an agent and a target" (World Health Organization, 2004). For risk assessment this definition of exposure has been applied primarily to the individual or human population as a target of exposure and to a chemical as an agent of exposure; however, the target of exposure can be an organ, tissue, or cell, and the agent of exposure can be a biological, physical, or psychosocial stressor or the byproduct of a given exposure agent. Exposure science is required to incorporate consideration of life stage, genetic susceptibility, and interaction of nonchemical stressors for holistic assessment of risk factors associated with complex environmental disease. Achieving this goal requires the establishment of new capabilities to identify biologically relevant exposure metrics that can be directly associated with key events in a disease process and with an individual's exposure profile.

Wild (2005) proposed the need for a "step change" in exposure assessment and articulated a vision for exposure measurement calling for an "exposome," or measurement of the life course of environmental exposures, to provide the evidence base for public health decisions to address environmental health. Wild discussed the potential of emerging technologies to provide this new generation of exposure information. In their guest editorial in *Environmental Health Perspectives*, Smith and Rappaport (2009, p. A334) argued that if we expect to have any success at identifying the contribution

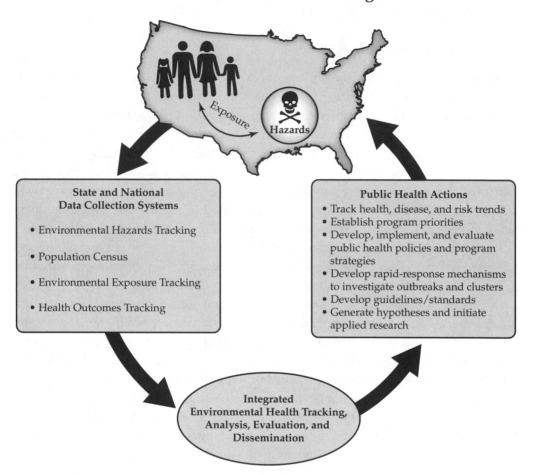

Environmental Public Health Tracking Network

FIGURE 9-1   The Centers for Disease Control and Prevention and Agency for Toxic Substances and Disease Registry developed a model in their proposed plan for an environmental public health tracking network.
Source: Picture courtesy of the Centers for Disease Control and Prevention, Agency for Toxic Substances and Disease Registry: http://www.atsdr.cdc.gov/ Accessed August 20, 2010.

of environmental factors on chronic diseases, "we must develop 21st-century tools to measure exposure levels in human populations" and quantify the exposome. The National Academy of Sciences Committee on Emerging Science for Environmental Health Decisions, sponsored by the National Institute of Environmental Health Sciences, organized a workshop in February 2010 that launched a discussion on resources needed to make the exposome a reality.

The Exposure Biology Program of the National Institutes of Health Genes, Environment and Health Initiative, led by the National Institute of Environmental Health Sciences, invests in innovative new technologies to determine how environmental exposures—including diet, physical activity, stress, and drug use—contribute to human disease. These technologies include sensors for chemicals in the environment and new ways to characterize dietary intake, levels of physical activity, responses to psychosocial stress, and measures of the biological response to these factors at the physiological and molecular levels. These new tests will provide the improved accuracy and precision needed to determine how environmental and lifestyle factors interact with genetic factors to determine the risk of developing disease. One critical aspect of this program is the idea of integrating these measures of the environment together with the expected result that we will be able to determine, with a level of confidence never before possible, who was exposed, to how much of what, where, what they were doing at the time, and how their bodies are responding to that stress. Although the Exposure Biology Program is still in a developmental stage, many early successes are starting to emerge and beginning the initial transition into environmental epidemiology studies (Birnbaum, 2010).

ENVIRONMENTAL DISASTER EXAMPLES

Hurricane Katrina

Hurricane Katrina made landfall on Monday, August 29, 2005, as a category 4 hurricane and passed within 10 to 15 miles of New Orleans, Louisiana. The storm brought heavy winds and rain to the city, and the damage breached several levees protecting New Orleans from the water of Lake Pontchartrain. The levee breaches flooded up to 80% of the city with water, reaching a depth of 25 feet in some places. Among the widescale impacts of Hurricane Katrina, the storm caused significant loss of life and disrupted power, natural gas, water, sewage treatment, road safety, and other essential services to the city. Early in the disaster response and recovery, federal, state, and local elected officials and public health and environmental leaders recognized the significant role of environmental health in the post-hurricane rebuilding of New Orleans.

At the request of Secretary Michael Leavitt of the Department of Health and Human Services and Administrator Steve Johnson of the U.S. Environmental Protection Agency, the Director of the Centers for Disease Control and Prevention, Dr. Julie Louise Gerberding, created the Environmental Health Needs Assessment and Habitability Taskforce (EH-NAHT). The taskforce was charged with identifying the overarching environmental health issues faced by New Orleans to reinhabit the city.

The EH-NAHT collaborated extensively with a diverse group of federal, state, and local partners, including the New Orleans City Public Health Department, the Louisiana Department of Health and Hospitals, and Louisiana Department of Environmental Quality, Federal Emergency Management Agency, and U.S. Army Corps of Engineers. The team was guided by the following questions:

1. What are the core fundamental environmental health issues to be addressed?
2. Which agencies and organizations at the federal, state, or local level are responsible for, or involved in, the various environmental health issues?
3. What progress has been made and what challenges exist?
4. What is the timetable to address these environmental health issues?
5. What resources exist or need to be brought to bear to address these environmental health issues?
6. What are the key milestones and endpoints that define success?

The team identified 13 environmental health issues and supporting infrastructure to address. This initial assessment included drinking water, wastewater, solid waste/debris, sediments/soil contamination (toxic chemicals), power, natural gas, housing, unwatering/flood water, occupational safety and health/public security, vector/rodent/animal control, road conditions, underground storage tanks (e.g., gasoline), and food safety. After the initial assessment, the EH-NAHT categorized these issues by increasing time and complexity to full restoration of services. Occupational safety and health as well as public security was identified as cross-cutting all other areas. Long-term solutions to these many issues are critical to allow resumption of normal life in New Orleans and to prevent reoccurrence of such an event in this area (for more information, go to http://www.bt.cdc.gov).

Union Carbide: Disaster at Bhopal

In the early hours of Monday, December 3, 1984, a toxic cloud of methyl isocyanate gas enveloped the hundreds of shanties and huts surrounding a pesticide plant in Bhopal, India. Later, as the deadly cloud slowly drifted in the cool night air through streets in surrounding sections, sleeping residents awoke, coughing, choking, and rubbing painfully stinging eyes. By the time the gas cleared at dawn, many were dead or injured. Four months after the tragedy, the Indian government reported to its Parliament that 1,430 people had died. In 1991 the official Indian government panel charged with tabulating deaths and injuries updated the count to more than 3,800 dead and approximately 11,000 with disabilities. Although it was not known at the time, the gas was formed when a disgruntled plant employee, apparently bent on spoiling a batch of methyl isocyanate, added water to a storage tank. The water caused a reaction that built up heat and pressure in the tank, quickly transforming the chemical compound into a lethal gas that escaped into the cool night air.

The plant was operated by Union Carbide India Limited, just over 50% of which was owned by Union Carbide Corporation. The first report of the disaster reached Union Carbide executives in the United States more than 12 hours after the incident. By 6:00 AM in the United States, executives were gathering with technical, legal, and communications staff at the company's Danbury, Connecticut, headquarters. Information was sparse, but as casualty estimates quickly climbed, the matter was soon recognized as a massive industrial disaster (by Jackson B. Browning, Retired Vice President, Health, Safety, and Environmental Programs; Union Carbide Corporation).

REQUIREMENTS OF AN ENVIRONMENTAL STUDY

There are four essential requirements for the conduct of effective work in environmental epidemiology: (1) an appropriate study design and suitable set of statistical strategies; (2) the capacity to design, carry out, and report the necessary procedures for dependable research; (3) access to populations of sufficient size and appropriate characteristics for study; and (4) an adequate support base in resources and in personnel for carrying out the necessary work. It cannot be assumed that good study design is sufficient to ensure good epidemiological studies because there are always factors of population accessibility and unestimated variables that influence results of work in the field.

Compared with experimental research on related problems, the epidemiological studies of environmental effects tend to be expensive; hence there is greater importance given to the planning and design of studies. Most epidemiological research deals with tests of association. Almost never can a single epidemiological study be interpreted with respect to causation. Thus, it is of great importance that precise language be used to make it clear that, for an identified problem, a statistical association is being sought and evaluated and a necessary and sufficient cause is usually not approachable solely by a single epidemiological study (Cetta, Benoni, Zangari, Guercio, & Monti, 2010).

FACTORS AFFECTING ENVIRONMENTAL EPIDEMIOLOGY

Epidemiological studies, even well-planned ones, often suggest but do not prove causation. Because of the long lead time necessary for determining such effects as genetic and chronic disease associations, studies can hardly be justified if they lead to delaying the adoption of policies to minimize the risk. Yet if it happens that experimental and epidemiological data converge on even an approximate dose–response relationship, policies to avoid a given "response" are scientifically supportable. Some examples of how environmental epidemiological information influenced public health decisions and policy are provided here.

Example 1: Air Quality and Coronary Artery Disease

The National Academy of Science and National Research Council Committee on Effects of Atmospheric Contaminants on Human Health and Welfare includes as one of eight tentative conclusions "a possible effect of increased ambient levels of carbon monoxide in coronary vascular disease." The Federal Air Quality Criteria for Carbon Monoxide treat both epidemiological and toxicological results separately. It is doubtful if either toxicological or epidemiological results alone would have been of comparable importance for these policy considerations. By contrast, Federal Air Quality Criteria for Oxides of Nitrogen are based primarily on epidemiological studies. They are currently being contested by representatives of the motor vehicle industry. This relationship has been used by the California State Department of Health and the Air Resources Board of California as one basis for air quality standards (Bahadori & Barr, 2010).

Example 2: Detecting Medication Metabolites in Sewage Discharge and River Water

Both public water supplies and private wells can be a source of toxic exposure, especially for industrial solvents, heavy metals, pesticides, and fertilizers. For example, an Environmental Protection Agency groundwater survey detected trichloroethylene in approximately 10% of the wells tested. It is estimated to be in 34% of the nation's drinking water supplies. Up to 25% of the water supplies have detectable levels of tetrachloroethylene. Methylene chloride may remain in groundwater for years. Some solvents can volatilize from showers and during laundering of clothes, thereby creating a risk of toxicity via inhalation. Nitrates, a common contaminant of rural shallow wells, pose a risk of methemoglobinemia, especially to infants.

Some medications are known to withstand activated sludge treatment at sewage treatment plants, but less is known about how much of the drug metabolites may make their way into waterways that receive sewage treatment plant discharge. After the sewage treatment process, the excreted active metabolite remains in sewage treatment plant effluent and travels to waterways where the effluent is discharged. According to CA.gov, the U.S. Geological Survey in 2002 sampled streams in 30 states. Of the 139 streams tested, 80% had measurable concentrations of prescription and non-prescription drugs, steroids, and reproductive hormones. Exposure to even low levels of drugs has negative effects on fish and other aquatic species and also may negatively affect human health. CA.gov offers guidance to help the public dispose of pharmaceutical waste in a safe, efficient, and environmentally sound manner, using methods that are convenient, cost-effective, sustainable, and environmentally sound. There is no question that the disposal of personal care products and drugs is a huge environmental issue, not only in the United States but all over the world (Eisenstadt, 2005).

Example 3: Soil Contamination

In January 2010 the Maine Department of Environmental Protection (DEP) measured the concentrations of drugs in samples collected at three landfills, selected because they were receiving only household waste and not biosolids that might contain human-excreted drugs. DEP scientists were surprised to find what could amount to yearly emissions of hundreds of pounds of active pharmaceutical ingredients from over-the-counter and prescription drugs. Researchers were not surprised to find active pharmaceutical ingredients but were surprised at the high levels. The pain reliever acetaminophen, for example, was present in samples from one landfill at the highest level of any drug measured in the study. The prescription antibiotic ciprofloxacin was present at moderate concentrations, and lab tests even found cocaine in one landfill, according to the DEP's unpublished findings. Other drugs found in all three landfills included low concentrations of estrone (from hormone replacement therapy), albuterol (an asthma drug), and the antibiotic penicillin in the range of tens to hundreds parts per billion (Lubick, 2010).

Pharmaceuticals are not the only toxins that can have an effect on our environment. Manufacturing 1 pound of methamphetamine creates 5 pounds of toxic waste. Chemical byproducts from methamphetamine are found in parks and forests and can linger in soil and groundwater for years, posing immediate and long-term environmental health risks. The number of methamphetamine labs has been decreasing since 2005, but methamphetamine cooks are finding new ways to produce this dangerous drug in smaller mobile labs. The chemicals are highly toxic, and waste dumped into streams, rivers, fields, backyards, and sewage systems can contaminate water resources for humans and animals.

Coca plants, the source of cocaine, are grown in the rainforests of Colombia. Nearly 500,000 acres of Colombian natural forest are destroyed every year, mainly because of the planting of coca plants, and the primary cause of air pollution in the Colombian jungle is the burning of forest to make way for coca plants. The production of 2 pounds of coca paste generates 1,300 pounds of trash and contaminates 200 gallons of water. Consequently, for every 1 gram of cocaine consumed, 43 square feet of Columbian rain forest is destroyed.

Approximately 60% of outdoor marijuana cultivation in the United States takes place on America's public lands where growers are less likely to be discovered because of their remote location. This comes at a high cost to the environment: For every acre of forest where marijuana is grown, 10 acres are damaged by fertilizers and other toxic chemicals. Between 2007 and 2008, 700 marijuana growing sites were found in California's national forests and parks.

Table 9-1 Environmental Toxins and Related Diseases		
Toxin	**Location**	**Disease and/or Symptoms**
Heavy metals Metals like arsenic, mercury, lead, aluminum, and cadmium, which are prevalent in many areas of our environment, can accumulate in soft tissues of the body.	Found in drinking water, fish, vaccines, pesticides, preserved wood, antiperspirant, building materials, dental amalgams, and chlorine plants.	Can cause cancer, neurological disorders, Alzheimer disease, fatigue, nausea, abnormal heart rhythm, and damage to blood vessels
Polychlorinated biphenyls (PCBs) This industrial chemical has been banned in the United States for decades yet is a persistent organic pollutant that's still present in our environment.	Found in farm-raised salmon. Most farm-raised salmon, which accounts for most of the supply in the United States, are fed meals of ground-up fish that have absorbed PCBs in the environment.	Can cause cancer and impaired fetal brain development
Dioxins Chemical compounds formed as a result of combustion processes such as commercial or municipal waste incineration and from burning fuels (like wood, coal, or oil).	Found in animal fats. Over 95% of exposure comes from eating commercial animal fats.	Can cause cancer, reproductive disorders, chloracne, skin rashes, and skin discoloration

Table 9-1 Environmental Toxins and Related Diseases *(continued)*

Toxin	Location	Disease and/or Symptoms
Pesticides Pesticide residues have been detected in 50–95% of U.S. foods.	Found in bug sprays, commercially raised meats, and other foods	Can cause cancer, Parkinson's disease, miscarriage, nerve damage, and birth defects
Phthalates These chemicals are used to lengthen the life of fragrances and soften plastics.	Found in plastic wrap, plastic bottles, and other plastic food containers. All these can leach phthalates into our food.	Can cause endocrine system damage (phthalates chemically mimic hormones and are particularly dangerous to children)
Volatile organic compounds (VOCs)	Found in drinking water, paint, deodorants, cosmetics, and dry-cleaned clothing.	Can cause cancer, eye irritation, headaches, and memory impairment
Asbestos This insulating material was widely used from the 1950s to 1970s. Problems arise when the material becomes old and crumbly, releasing fibers into the air.	Found in flooring insulation, ceilings, water pipes, and heating ducts from the 1950s to 1970s.	Can cause cancer, scarring of the lung tissue, and mesothelioma
Chlorine This highly toxic, yellow-green gas is one of the most heavily used chemical agents.	Found in household cleaners and drinking water.	Can cause sore throat, coughing, eye irritation, rapid breathing, narrowing of the bronchi, wheezing, blue coloring of the skin, pain in the lung region, and lung collapse
Chloroform This colorless liquid has a pleasant, nonirritating odor and a slightly sweet taste and is used to make other chemicals. It's also formed when chlorine is added to water.	Air, drinking water, and food can contain chloroform.	Cancer, potential reproductive damage, birth defects, dizziness, fatigue, headache, and liver and kidney damage

What Can We Do?

Daughton (2009) made a "call to stakeholders" to integrate a variety of professional disciplines involving analytic chemists, environmental engineers, social psychologists, physicians, pharmacologists, pharmacists, drug designers, and health insurers to provide a framework for this issue. The "call" was given to formulate an interdisciplinary action group to steer this mass of data and information into a more logical and standardized focus. An informal proposal was made to capitalize on the readily "available, published literature containing a wealth of data not yet examined and certainly never thoroughly mined, compiled, summarized, evaluated, and distilled into useful insights and knowledge" (Daughton, 2009, p. 2493).

Daughton further revealed that within the first 2 months of 2009, more literature was published on this topic than in all of 1999. However, in reality, rapid inflation of published literature does not necessarily promote an expanded scope of this problem. Rather, it serves to increase the volume of unknown data and continues to impede maximum focus on select interventions to promote optimum solutions for our planet and its inhabitants. The lack of sufficient synoptic review greatly increases the risk of duplication of prior work and thwarts streamlined strategies to remedy this seemingly insurmountable pandemic (Daughton, 2009).

CLINICIANS ROLE

What Is the Purpose of Taking an Exposure History?

Most environmental and occupational diseases either manifest as common medical problems or have nonspecific symptoms. Yet environmental factors rarely enter into the clinician's differential diagnosis. As a result, clinicians miss the opportunity to make correct diagnoses that might influence the course of disease in some afflicted individuals. Most environmental and occupational diseases either manifest as common medical problems or have nonspecific symptoms (e.g., headache, difficulty concentrating, behavioral problems, rashes, asthma, angina, myalgia, difficulty conceiving, spontaneous abortion) (Marshall, Weir, Abelsohn, & Margaret, 2002). Unless an exposure history is pursued by the clinician (**Figure 9-2**), the etiological diagnosis might be missed, treatment may be inappropriate, and exposure can continue.

Most people with illness caused or exacerbated by exposure to hazardous substances obtain their medical care from clinicians who are not specialists in either environmental or occupational medicine. Consideration of environmental factors rarely enters into the clinician's history taking or diagnosis (Marshall et al., 2002). In a study of a primary care practice in an academic setting, only 24% of 625 charts reviewed included any mention of the patient's occupation; only 2% included infor-

Exposure History Form

Part 1. Exposure Survey   Name _____   Date _____

Please circle the appropriate answer. Birth date _____   Sex (circle one): Male   Female

1. Are you currently exposed to any of the following?

   metals   no   yes

   dust or fibers   no   yes

   chemicals   no   yes

   fumes   no   yes

   radiation   no   yes

   biologic agents   no   yes

   loud noise, vibration, extreme heat or cold

2. Have you been exposed to any of the above in the past?   no   yes

3. Do any household members have contact with metals,
   dust, fibers, chemicals, fumes, radiation, or biologic agents?   no   yes

If you answered *yes* to any of the items above, describe your exposure in detail—how you were exposed, to what you were exposed. If you need more space, please use a separate sheet of paper.

4. Do you know the names of the metals,
   dusts, fibers, chemicals, fumes, or radiation
   that you are/were exposed to?   no   yes ⟶ | If *yes*, list them below

5. Do you get the material on your skin or
   clothing?   no   yes

6. Are your work clothes laundered at home?   no   yes

7. Do you shower at work?   no   yes

8. Can you smell the chemical or material you are
   working with?   no   yes

9. Do you use protective equipment such as
   gloves, masks, respirator, or hearing protectors?   no   yes ⟶ | If *yes*, list the protective equipment used

FIGURE 9-2   Taking an exposure history.

Source: CDC, Agency for Toxic Substances & Disease Registry. website: http://www.atsdr.cdc.gov/csem/exphistory/ehcover_page.html; Accessed September 1, 2010.

10. Have you been advised to use protective equipment?   no   yes

11. Have you been instructed in the use of protective
    equipment?   no   yes

12. Do you wash your hands with solvents?   no   yes

13. Do you smoke at the workplace?   no   yes   At home? no   yes

14. Are you exposed to secondhand tobacco smoke at the
    workplace?   no   yes   At home? no   yes

15. Do you eat at the workplace?   no   yes

16. Do you know of any co-workers experiencing similar or
    unusual symptoms?   no   yes

17. Are family members experiencing similar or unusual
    symptoms?   no   yes

18. Has there been a change in the health or behavior of
    family pets?   no   yes

19. Do your symptoms seem to be aggravated by a specific
    activity?   no   yes

20. Do your symptoms get either worse or better at work?   no   yes
                                              at home?   no   yes
                                        on weekends?   no   yes
                                        on vacation?   no   yes

21. Has anything about your job changed in recent months
    (such as duties, procedures, overtime)?   no   yes

22. Do you use any traditional or alternative medicines?   no   yes

---

If you answered *yes* to any of the questions, please explain.

FIGURE 9-2   Taking an exposure history. *(continued)*

Part 2. Work History   Name _____
A. Occupational Profile   Birth date _____ Sex: Male   Female

The following questions refer to your current or most recent job:

Job title: _____   Describe this job: _____

Type of industry: _____   _____

Name of employer: _____   _____

Date job began: _____   _____

Are you still working in this job? yes   no   _____

If *no*, when did this job end?_____   _____

Fill in the table below listing all jobs you have worked including short-term, seasonal, part-time employment, and military service. Begin with your most rcent job. Use additional paper if necessary.

Dates of Employment	Job Title and Description of Work	Exposures*	Protective Equipment

*List the chemicals, dusts, fibers, fumes, radiation, biologic agents (i.e., molds or viruses) and physical agents (i.e., extreme heat, cold, vibration, or noise) that you were exposed to at this job

FIGURE 9-2   Taking an exposure history. *(continued)*

Have you ever worked at a job or hobby in which you came in contact with any of the following by breathing, touching, or ingesting (swallowing)? If *yes*, please check the box beside the name.

☐ Acids	☐ Ethylene dibromide	☐ Radiation
☐ Alcohols (industrial)	☐ Ethylenen dichloride	☐ Rock dust
☐ Alkalies	☐ Fiberglass	☐ Silica powder
☐ Ammonia	☐ Halothane	☐ Solvents
☐ Arsenic	☐ Isocyanates	☐ Styrene
☐ Asbestos	☐ Ketones	☐ Talc
☐ Benzene	☐ Lead	☐ Toluene
☐ Beryllium	☐ Mercury	☐ TDI or MDI
☐ Cadmium	☐ Methylene chloride	☐ Trichloroethylene
☐ Carbon tetrachloride	☐ Nickel	☐ Trinitrotoluene
☐ Chlorinated naphthalenes	☐ PBBs	☐ Vinyl chloride
☐ Chloroform	☐ PCBs	☐ Welding fumes
☐ Chloroprene	☐ Perchloroethylene	☐ X-rays
☐ Chromates	☐ Pesticides	☐ Other (specify)
☐ Coal dust	☐ Phenol	
☐ Dichlorobenzene	☐ Phosgene	

B. Occupational Exposure Inventory   *Please circle the appropriate answer.*

1. Have you ever been off work for more than 1 day because of an illness related to work?		no yes
2. Have you ever been adivsed to change jobs or work assignments because of any health problems or injuries?		no yes
3. Has your work routine changed recently?		no yes
4. Is there poor ventilation in your workplace?		no yes

Part 3. Environmental History   *Please circle the appropriate answer.*

1. Do you live next to or near an industrial plant, commercial business, dump site, or nonresidential property?	no yes
2. Which of the following do you have in your home? *Please circle those that apply.* Air conditioner Air purifier Central heating (gas or oil?) Gas stove Electric stove Fireplace Wood stove Humidifier	
3. Have you recently acquired new furniture or carpet, refinished furniture, or remodeled your home?	no yes

FIGURE 9-2   Taking an exposure history. *(continued)*

4. Have you weatherized your home recently?   no   yes

5. Are pesticides or herbicides (bug or weed killers; flea and tick sprays, collars, powders, or shampoos) used in your home or garden, or on pets?   no   yes

6. Do you (or any household member) have a hobby or craft?   no   yes

7. Do you work on your car?   no   yes

8. Have you ever changed your residence because of a health problem?   no   yes

9. Does your drinking water come from a private well, city water supply, or grocery store?   no   yes

10. Approximately what year was your home built? _____

If you answered *yes* to any of the questions, please explain.

FIGURE 9-2   Taking an exposure history. *(continued)*

mation about toxic exposure, duration of present employment, and former occupations (ATSDR, 2008). A chart review of 2,922 histories taken by 137 third-year medical students showed that smoking status was documented in 91% of cases, occupation in 70%, and specific occupational exposures in 8.4%. Patients younger than 40 years of age and women were significantly less likely than older patients or men to have their occupation and industry noted. Findings from another recent study showed that work-related issues might not be adequately addressed or documented in the provider's clinical notes, and opportunities for preventive care relating to work-related injuries and illnesses may not be realized in the primary care setting (Thompson, Brodkin, Kyes, Neighbor, & Evanoff, 2000).

CONCLUSIONS

Understanding the connection between our health and our environment, with its mixture of chemicals, diet, and lifestyle stressors, is no less important than understanding the intricacies of the human genome. The advances we have made are a beginning, but they also point to the continuing limitations of our capabilities and our understanding. We as a community need to increase our efforts to address these gaps in, for instance, the integration of environmental measures to identify the source of exposure, the use of biomonitoring to determine the dose of toxicants an individual receives, and the integration of this knowledge into the development of interventions to improve public health. As clinicians, we need to remain committed to working with the National Institutes of Health and other federal agencies, including the U.S. Environmental Protection Agency, National Institute for Occupational Safety and Health, and other parts of the Centers for Disease Control and Prevention, to help the field of exposure science evolve to meet emerging public health challenges. We must look forward to the increased contributions of exposure scientists as we work to understand the role of environment in the etiology of disease.

KEY POINTS

- Environmental epidemiology is the study of the distribution and determinants of health-related states or events in specified populations that are influenced by physical, chemical, biological, and psychosocial factors in the environment. It also involves the application of this study to prevent and control health problems.
- The population focus of environmental epidemiology and emphasis on identifying causal relationships distinguishes it from environmental health, which is more comprehensive.
- Environmental epidemiology should consider a full range of existing environments: the inner versus outer environment; the personal versus ambient environment; the solid, liquid, and gaseous environments; the chemical, biological, physical, and socioeconomic environments.
- The systems approach in environmental epidemiology considers the fact that environmental exposures may derive from multiple sources, they may enter the body through multiple routes, and elements in the environment can change over time because of constant interaction, altering the degree to which they are harmful. Viewing a health problem in its entirety through a systems approach involves (1) determining the source and nature of each environmental contaminant or stress, (2) assessing how and in what form it comes into contact with people, (3) measuring the health effect, and (4) applying controls when and where appropriate.
- Changes in the environment caused by human interference in matter cycles (hydrological cycle, the nitrogen cycle, the phosphorous cycle, the sulfur cycle,

and the carbon cycle) have resulted in environmental problems and adverse affects to human health.

- Epidemiological findings contribute to preventing and controlling health-related states or events by providing useful information for directing public health policy and planning as well as informing individuals about adverse health behaviors.

CRITICAL QUESTIONS

1. List the most prevalent environmental hazards in the United States and the diseases associated with them.
2. What effects depend on the patient's characteristics such as age, gender, and underlying disease in identifying the outcomes of environmental exposures?
3. To what extent is mortality and morbidity accelerated by short- and long-term exposure to air and water pollution?
4. What would the advanced practice nurse look for in an environmental exposure history? What specifically would you be addressing?

RESOURCES

- Department of Health and Human Services
- Agency for Toxic Substances and Disease Registry
- Health Resources and Services Administration
- Office of Public Health and Science
- Centers for Disease Control and Prevention
  - National Institute for Occupational Safety and Health
- U.S. Food and Drug Administration
- National Institutes of Health
  - National Cancer Institute
  - National Institute of Biomedical Imaging and Bioengineering
  - National Institute of Environmental Health Sciences
  - National Library of Medicine
  - National Center for Complementary and Alternative Medicine

Other websites:

http://www.healthandenvironment.org/

http://www.epa.gov/iris/

http://www.who.int/quantifying_ehimpacts/publications/preventingdisease/en/

REFERENCES

Agency for Toxic Substances & Disease Registry. (2008). Case studies in environmental medicine. Retrieved from http://www.atsdr.cdc.gov/csem/exphistory/ehprimary_care.html

Bahadori, T., & Barr, D. (2010). Close encounters: Reflections on the successes and near misses of exposure science. *Journal of Exposure Science and Environmental Epidemiology, 20*, 1.

Birnbaum, L. (2010). Applying research to public health questions: Biologically relevant exposures. *Environmental Health Perspectives, 118*(4), A152.

Cetta, F., Benoni, S., Zangari, R., Guercio, V., & Monti, M. (2010). Epidemiology, public health, and false-positive results: The role of the clinicians and pathologists. *Environmental Health Perspectives, 118*(6), A240.

Cumston, C. (1926). *An introduction to the history of medicine.* New York: Alfred A. Knopf.

Daughton, C. G. (2009). Chemicals from the practice of healthcare: Challenges and unknowns posed by residues in the environment. *Environmental Toxicology and Chemistry, 28*, 2490–2494. Retrieved from http://www3interscience.wiley.com/journal/123234094/issue

Eisenstadt, L. (2005). *Drugs in the water.* Retrieved from http://www.bu.edu/sjmag/scimag2005/features/drugsinwater.htm

Goldsmith, J. (1967). Environmental epidemiology and the metamorphosis of the human habitat. *American Journal of Public Health, 57*, 1532–1549.

Goldsmith, J. (1969). Non-disease effects of air pollution. *Environmental Research, 2*, 93–101.

Jones, W. (1923). *Hippocrates* (vol. I, pp. 71–137). London: William Heinemann.

Lubick, N. (2010). Drugs in the environment: Do pharmaceutical take-back programs make a difference? *Environmental Health Perspectives, 118*, 210–214.

Marshall, L., Weir, E., Abelsohn, A., & Margaret, S. D. (2002). Occupational and environmental exposure. *Canadian Medical Association Journal. 167*(7), 744.

Smith, M., & Rappaport, S. (2009). Building exposure biology centers to put the E into "G × E" interaction studies. *Environmental Health Perspectives, 117*, A334–A335.

Thompson, J. N., Brodkin, C. A., Kyes, K., Neighbor, W., & Evanoff, B. (2000). Use of a questionnaire to improve occupational and environmental history taking in primary care physicians. *Journal of Occupational and Environmental Medicine / American College of Occupational and Environmental Medicine, 42*(12), 1188–1194.

Wild, C. (2005). Complementing the genome with an "exposome": The outstanding challenge of environmental exposure measurement in molecular epidemiology. *Cancer Epidemiology, Biomarkers & Prevention, 14*, 1847–1850.

World Health Organization. (2004). Protection of the human environment. Retrieved from http://www.who.int/phe/en

CHAPTER 10

Role of Culture in Epidemiology

"Culture is the process by which a person becomes all that they were created capable of being."
—Thomas Carlyle

Kiran Macha
John P. McDonough
Juergen Osterbrink

OBJECTIVES

- Describe the role played by culture in the field of epidemiology.
- Explain the beliefs that support traditional cultural practices that may affect health.
- Describe the relationship between food and health status.

INTRODUCTION

Culture has played an important role in the growth of the United States. After World War II the United States saw a surge in immigration numbers. Cultural diversity caused by immigration and the intermixing of races has led to an exchange of cultural beliefs. The United States is now a melting pot of different cultures. Knowledge and understanding of traditional health beliefs, medical and healing practices, and foods that are specific to a culture contribute to more effective advanced nursing practice. The term "cultural epidemiology" is becoming popular in recent years because some of the epidemiological studies are more focused on health issues related to culture.

Advanced practice nurses must be able to identify cultural values, beliefs, and practices and proactively modify treatment methods accordingly to affect more positive patient outcomes. Using a cross-cultural interview when taking a patient's history can promote establishment of a positive, supportive, and trusting relationship with the patient. As a healthcare provider, one should also remember to elicit information about use of nontraditional therapies, because these healing practices may contribute to restoring the health of the patient. Transcultural training helps us to become competent practitioners toward reducing health disparities in the community. Advance practice nurses who are culturally aware are likely to provide more compassionate care. Understanding and respecting the cultural beliefs of a patient can also help us establish a relationship with the patient's family. Healthcare providers without transcultural training may unknowingly inflict cultural pain in their patients. Transculturally prepared advanced practice nurses are more likely to provide culturally sensitive care that is better accepted by the patient and likely to result in better health outcomes.

Culture has its own inherent effect on wellness and the likelihood of incidence of disease. The biases and stereotypical attitudes of healthcare providers in the community toward a culture can be reduced through understanding. In this chapter we will learn more about the health beliefs, traditional medical practices, and dietary preferences specific to a few cultures. Learning these facts can allow us to better prepare our approach to working with a patient and to improve our diagnosis, may help us better trace the source of an incident, and may even change the direction of global epidemiology issues.

CULTURAL BELIEFS AND ISSUES MAY IMPACT HEALTH

Native Americans living in the United States are often secluded from the modern American society. The U.S. Department of Health and Human Services established the Indian Health Service to improve the health of Native Americans. Given the isolation and wide dispersal geographically of Native Americans, their different views on life, and their dependency on herbal medicine and traditional healing practices, practitioners are challenged to educate and offer proper care to these Americans. Native Americans generally consider health to be a balance of mind, body, spirit, and nature. According to their belief systems, nature is respected, everything is interconnected (**Figure 10-1** is an example), and silence is encouraged. Socioeconomic barriers impacting Native American tribal members include poverty, lack of knowledge of disease, inadequate transportation, communication difficulties, and access to health care. The incidence of diabetes is growing in this population, calling for a change in dietary habits. Advanced practice nurses can work more readily with Native Americans if they can learn and respect their beliefs.

Religious customs can seclude one or more individuals from the society at large, with advantages and disadvantages. For example, the Amish community rejects worldly possessions and lives in complete modesty. These Americans do not drive cars or use modern machinery, do not use electricity, and do not purchase health insurance. Folk medicine in the community relies heavily on herbal medicines, and prayer is encouraged. Marriages between close relations in the community may explain the higher incidence of genetic disorders. Healthcare decisions are made in the

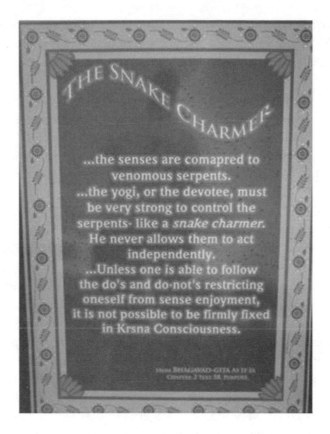

FIGURE 10-1 Many cultures believe that everything in nature is connected.
Source: Picture courtesy of Dr. Kiran Macha. From Bhagavad-Gita As It Is. Chapter 2 Text 58, Purport.

best interest of the community. Amish pregnant women do not receive prenatal care, and Amish midwives deliver babies at home. They believe in using Barouche doctors who use hands-on techniques for healing.

In this century the United States is facing a new cultural issue once perceived as an illness in the field of psychiatry. The concept of marriage only between a man and a woman, a holy relationship according to many religions (and explained for many in relation to the creation of two sexes by God), is now being reframed and challenged in the community. Even though most religions do not support the concept of the co-existence of same-sex partners, it is difficult for gays and lesbians to follow religious doctrines and live in rejection. European countries are generally more relaxed with the gay and lesbian concept than the Western world. Recently, in the United States

President Barack Obama signed an Executive Order directing hospitals receiving Medicare and Medicaid funding to give gay and lesbian patients the ability to choose who can make healthcare decisions for them. With greater acceptance, gay and lesbian couples are increasingly adopting children, although some believe this may create confusion for children who often must explain the parenting concept to others. The incidence of suicides in the gay and lesbian community is higher compared with the general population. Advanced practice nurses are encouraged to learn more about the gay and lesbian community, to avoid discrimination based on sexual orientation, and to comfort patients to enhance the process of communication toward better health care.

With a population of 1 billion, India has seen less than 1 million of its numbers immigrate to the United States in the past decade. Most Indian Americans are working in the fields of medicine and technology. Hinduism is the most common religion, with Indians often worshipping multiple gods (**Figure 10-2**). They believe in amulets and herbal medicines. Hindus avoid meat and may restrict themselves to a vegetarian diet. Spices are used in the preparation of foods with the belief that they help in digestion and also prevent disease. Hindu followers believe in Karma, that is, what we do, either good or bad, comes back to us. Marriage, festivals, and traditional customs are very important to the Hindus. Most Indian Americans are well educated, speak English, and adapt to Western culture easily. A high percentage of Indians work in the United States as software developers, often suffering from syndromes associated with the computer technology industry. Vegetarian diet is deficient of vitamin B12 and protein, and spices interact with allopathic medications.

Some traditional Hispanic women avoid viewing an eclipse during certain times, such as pregnancy. They believe this astronomical event may cause congenital disorders in the infants exposed to it, so they wear metal keys to deflect the eclipse (Poma, 1987). A traditional Chinese health belief is based on "yin and yang" (cold and hot), the two opposite conditions. Yin is considered a negative force, and yang a positive force. The practices that restore health based on these holistic beliefs are common in China. Use of opposite force is encouraged to treat the conditions that follow because of yin or yang, and thus the balance of forces is restored in the body. For example, excess "hot" energy can be counterbalanced by cooling herbal teas and vice versa.

A strange but common belief exists with Chinese women during the postpartum period. After giving birth, for a period of one month (called *Zuo yuezi*, "doing the month") women live in partial seclusion. They consume more overall, avoid cold food, and eat hot food, believing it is protein rich. They do not wash their hair or bathe during this period, believing this activity may cause headaches. This concept is believed by the Chinese to restore women's health (Raven, Chen, Tolhurst, & Garner, 2007).

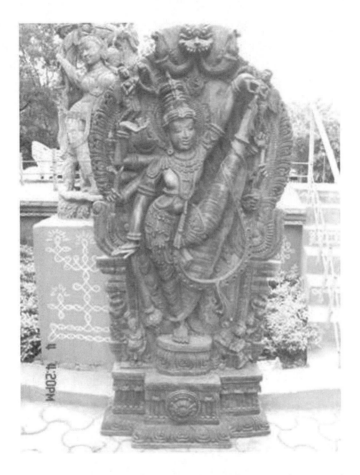

FIGURE 10-2   God, prayer, and meditation are part of many cultures such as Hinduism.
Source: Picture courtesy of Dr. Kiran Macha.

Vietnamese believe in traditional holistic treatments for the restoration of health. "Coining," "steaming," and "cupping" are often used. In cupping, a small heated glass is placed on certain points on the body. Steaming includes boiling a mixture of medical herbs with steam, which is then inhaled. Coining includes rubbing a coin on the spine to relieve illness. The belief behind these holistic treatment methods is that the illness is caused by bad spirits, and these actions expel them and cleanse the body (Wright, Jolly, Cassandra, & Rankin, 2002). Traditional Vietnamese healers also believe mental illness can be treated by contacting the bad spirit and seeking the reason for torment (Malarney, 2010). Benefits associated with a belief in contacting spirits are prevalent in many cultures in the world.

Eggs have healing powers, according to beliefs held by Peruvians. When a person is suffering from any illness, an egg is rubbed all over the body for a specified period of time and is then placed in a glass of warm water. If the cup is soon filled with a frothy white material, this is interpreted to mean the illness has left the body. Even though "second generation" immigrants generally undergo acculturation and assimilation in the United States, some customary generational health beliefs are deeply rooted. Filipinos believe illness is associated with spiritual causes or the result of wrongdoings. They also believe that casting of evil eye can cause illness. *Mang-ga-gas* are spiritual healers who Filipinos believe can protect you from evil eye. *Hilot* is the traditional art of healing that uses massage, body manipulation, and herbal medicines to cure illness. Filipinos also believe in amulets that give protection from bad spirits (Moran, 1999).

Traditional healers in rural Turkey recommend the eating of raw gallbladder and/or bile of carp to improve visual acuity. Cases of acute renal failure and acute hepatitis have been reported after ingesting these, but no improvements in visual acuity have been reported.

Brazilians use a 28-bead necklace to help women remember events (representing the fertilization period) associated with the menstrual cycle. The first bead is red in color and indicates the first day of menses. The next seven beads are brown in color and represent a time of infertility. Next, 11 white beads designate the fertile window, followed with fluorescent beads indicating a woman's peak days of ovulation. A black rubber band is moved from bead to bead to indicate the day of the menstrual cycle. The fluorescent beads glow in the dark to indicate the ovulation or fertility period (Institute for Reproductive Health, 1995).

Haitians living in poverty cannot afford a modern healthcare system. They believe that illness is a form of punishment from God for not obeying his rules and that the connection between man and God is weak during periods of illness or disease (Colin & Paperwalla, 1996). *Pedisyon* (perdition), also known as "arrested pregnancy syndrome," is representative of a common cultural belief among Haitians. It is thought that the reason behind arrest of pregnancy is that the blood flow to the uterus has been diverted to menstrual blood. Haitians believe the state characterized as menstruation may last for years until a "cure" is obtained and the pregnancy can then resume (Thomas & DeSantis, 1995).

Health is the greatest gift that is bestowed by God or Allah for Muslims. Muslims pray five times a day to maintain purity of thought. Before offering prayers, their face and extremities are washed. Alcohol and pork are considered as *haram* and are prohibited. The incidence of beef tapeworm infection is higher in underdeveloped countries. Women do not show their face and body to men and are covered with fabric *purdah* or scarf. Muslim women do not like to be seen by a male healthcare provider. *Halal* meat is preferred because it is prepared by observing certain religious guidelines. The preservation of cultural beliefs and practices is very important for those with this belief system. By permitting followers of the Muslim religion to pray five times a day, respecting women's needs in a healthcare setting, and by not offering food considered as *haram*, a healthcare provider can promote trust and establish good communication with Muslim patients.

Italians as well as Asian Indians attribute the cause of illness to the evil eye (*malocchio*) and curses (*castiga*). Italians believe there are two types of evil eye: (1) Malevolent evil eye is an intentional look meant to cause harm to an individual, and (2) involuntary evil eye is caused by someone gazing at another for too long in an admiring or envious way. Amulets and spells are believed to prevent and cure misfortune from evil eye (Stefco, 2007).

Female circumcision is an act of cruelty. The law prohibits such acts in the United States. In other parts of the world such as some African nations, female circumcision is encouraged, with female genital organs removed partially or completely (Kouba, 1985). The removal of female genitalia is known to cause serious emotional disturbances in women, and the pain can be traumatic.

Black and white beads (*Konta d'odju*) are used to keep evil spirits away from patients and children in the Cape Verde culture. Neighbors in this society are considered as immediate family and are often consulted in times of need. These people prefer to eat red meat, fried food, and dairy products, making it difficult to meet these cultural dietary preferences in a hospital setting (Carvalho, Robinson, & Rundle, 1999)

TRADITIONAL HEALTHCARE SYSTEMS

Practices within healthcare systems differ based on the culture, access to modern health care, and economic status. Each culture through years of practice has developed its own system and methods to cure illness. Researchers are now comparing the benefits of many complementary and alternative practices and medicines with allopathic approaches. Some cultural methods have been proven to have a placebo effect on individuals, whereas others have produced an extraordinary outcome that cannot be explained with scientific knowledge. Advanced practice nurses should remember to ask patients during history taking about their experiences involving the practices of other health systems and about the use of herbal medicines. Herbal medicines can interact with allopathic medicines and cause adverse reactions. Knowledge of many traditional practices may help you appreciate different views of the healing process, and you may wish to refer patients for the benefits they offer.

Tibetans living in Tibet (and most of them currently living in India) practice a method called Healing Chö, which means "cutting through." This healing practice does not involve any massages, coining, cupping, or physical exertion to relax the body. Rather, anyone can bring a pillow and blanket and lie down, relax, and hear traditional chants and music. The belief is that the vibrations from mantras and music create harmony in our system.

Germans developed a homeopathic medical system in the late 1800s by gathering information from various other medical systems. The principle of treating "like with like" is followed in this approach to healing. A person suffering from illness is exposed to small doses or therapeutic amounts of chemicals that are intended to stimulate or potentiate our body's immune system. Chemicals derived from herbs taken in excess amounts may cause adverse reactions. These practices are widely used in India, Canada, and the United States.

The origins of naturopathy can be traced to ancient Greece. To be with nature, to use substances available in nature, and to hold the belief that your body should be allowed to recover by itself is common in this medicine. This system of practice focuses primarily on the prevention of disease, and some specific diseases are also treated. Naturopathic practitioners are known as naturopaths. By avoiding the risk factors, one can stop suffering from the recurrence of disease.

The Chinese developed a system involving manipulation of the meridian flow of energy in the body by inserting needles at specific points for specific diseases. One of the oldest medical practices, acupuncture is widely practiced in the United States with often positive results if one meets with a good practitioner. The insertion of needles at certain points seems to release opioids in the brain that decrease sympathetic stimulation in the body. The opioid effects can relax muscles, lower blood pressure, and promote sleep. Cupping is another Chinese technique developed to create a vacuum at certain points by using glass and bamboo cups in such a way that the vacuum formed applies pressure on these points. The cupping may produce red marks on the body, resulting in increased chances that healthcare providers may believe these are signs of abuse (Pearson, 1997).

Kunz and Krieger developed therapeutic touch in the 1970s in the United States. It is believed that the energy that surrounds the human body extends beyond its physical contours and is unseen. During a period of stress or illness, positive energy can be produced through certain techniques of hand movements around the body without touching the human body, restoring the normal energy field. Because therapeutic touch is believed to relieve stress and to promote relaxation and recovery, the results of its use are being researched in many hospitals in the United States.

Healing touch also involves gentle hand techniques. The Japanese believe that by touching the patient and correcting the positions of the body, one can correct energy fields around the body and restore health. Reiki is a Japanese holistic hand technique developed to promote healing with the belief that the life force flows through us and is responsible for our well-being.

Ayurvedic medicine originated about 2,000 years ago in India (**Figure 10-3**). Many textbooks were written about the properties of herbs and the systems they affect. *Caraka Samhita* is a textbook of internal medicine, and *Sushruta Samhita* is a textbook of surgery involving Ayurvedic medicine. Sushruta (author of *Sushruta Samhita*), known as the father of surgery, has practiced and described more than 100 surgical techniques and has designed a number of surgical instruments. Ayurvedic

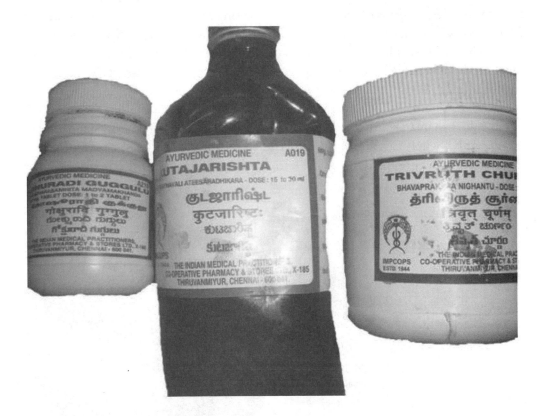

FIGURE 10-3   Ayurvedic medicine is prepared from herbs, minerals, and oils. The preparations of these medicines are described in detail in the ancient textbooks of Ayurvedic medicine.
Source: Picture courtesy of Dr. Suvarna Vemula.

medicine is widely practiced in India, where it is believed that many conditions treated with allopathic surgical practices may not need surgery but can be treated with herbal medicines or other Ayurvedic techniques. According to a National Health Survey conducted in 2000, around 200,000 people in the United States have used and benefited from complimentary and alternative medicine.

Unani medical practices are based on the teachings of the great Greek physician, Hippocrates. Unani is widely practiced and researched in India, and one can earn a medical degree in this medical system specialty. Unani supports the promotion of health and prevention and treatment of a disease. According to this system of beliefs, the body has the capacity to maintain blood, phlegm, yellow bile, and black bile, and the physician (known as *Hakim*) should aid in the restoration of balance of natural forces in the body. Proponents of this system believe illness can be cured in four different ways: *Elajbil Tadbeer* is an approach to treating disease using regimental therapy, *Elajbil Ghiza* is an approach to treating illness using diet therapy, *Elajbil Dawa* is an approach to restoring health using drugs (pharmacotherapy), and, *Elajbil Yad* uses surgical methods when all the above approaches fail to cure the disease (Rafatullah & Algasoumi, 2008).

Native Americans' belief in spirits, good and bad, led to the development of a ritual called shamanism that is believed to heal people from sickness. Shamanism is based on the belief that illness is caused by bad spirits and that the healing powers of good spirits can cure the illness. The entire community gathers at one place to con-

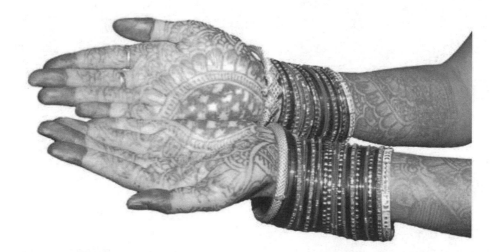

FIGURE 10-4   Hindus, Arabs, and Muslims use Mehndi or Henna for temporary tattooing.
Source: Picture courtesy of Dr. Suvarna Vemula.

duct this healing ritual, which can include dancing and chanting (American Cancer Society, 2010). In contrast to practices of tribes within the contiguous states, Alaskan natives more frequently access Western medicine, while also using traditional herbal medicines. They commonly use stinkweed to prevent infections.

Ancient Roman medicine involved both physical techniques, spiritual and religious rituals, and what we might call magical treatments. Valetudinarias are believed to be hospitals built by the Romans in the ancient days to treat people. Different specialties of medicine existed to treat different kinds of diseases. Romans boiled their surgical tools before use, pointing to their possible awareness of modes of transmission of bacteria and other agents that cause diseases. Physicians were held accountable for their mistakes, and laws such as "an eye for an eye" were established. The Aztecs developed a regimen for wound care by using urine to sterilize the area, applying herbs to stop bleeding, and using agave sap, a complex fructose, to reduce pain.

Appalachian folk medicine is based on faith and the use of herbal medicines. The widespread dispersal of Native Americans and other residents throughout this geographical region makes it difficult and expensive for physicians to reach and serve all Appalachians, many of whom cannot afford medical services. Appalachians are known to depend on herbs such as yellow root and snakeroot for the treatment of diseases. Magic and spiritual healing beliefs are also prevalent in this community.

Hawaiians believe they are connected with nature and that balance in health can be maintained through exercise and proper diet. For many decades, isolation from the mainland protected Hawaiian islanders from many diseases. Aggressive economic development in recent years has made them vulnerable to all diseases.

Western medicine and traditional medicine are equally preferred in Chile. The traditional ways of treating diseases is known as *Mapuche*. Proponents of Mapuche, like other traditional healing practices, believe in the body–spirit balance, and herbs play an important role in the treatment of diseases (Estomba, 2006).

Yoga sutras of Patanjali, forming the basis of Rajayoga, are designed to transform a human to a divine state, with meditation a major component. Hatha yoga is practiced for the purification of the physical body and to prepare one for meditation. Viapassna meditation was practiced by Lord Gautama Buddha to achieve nirvana (salvation). In the current world, yoga is practiced for the benefits that one derives such as relaxation, peace, and the reduction of anxiety. Meditation under the guidance of a spiritual master is recommended, because this practice can cause severe emotional disturbance if not undertaken in a proper way. Some of the saints teach kundalini yoga. Kundalini is believed to be a coiled energy that exists in the lower lumbar spine; the awakening of this serpent (coiled energy) is believed useful.

Some believe this energy can be awakened easily through certain yogic practices and rituals, but this has not been proven. It is often said that this energy is uncontrollable when awakened, and some believe the will of nature bestows the energy in only the few who are destined to bring change in this world. (One should not be misled by such beliefs that can, in and of themselves, cause severe emotional disorders.) Advance practice nurses can educate themselves on these issues and caution their patients on such practices.

The Greeks, Romans, Egyptians, and ancient Indians have practiced aromatherapy. Indians use attar (oil extracted from the petals of flowers such as the rose) to affect the mental state. Aromatic oils are used for massage and bathing to affect mood, decrease stress, and promote relaxation in the body. The olfactory nervous system is involved in this process of comfort healing.

TRADITIONAL METHODS OF HEALTH RESTORATION

Cultural health beliefs may evolve into common health practices in a community. These practices sometimes may have positive outcomes and may contribute to the development of modern treatments. For example, Russian Jews used mud baths and mineral waters to remove impurities from the body. Austrians practiced saltwater gargling for a sore throat. French Canadian cultures believed that an oatmeal bath would restore skin with a rash back to normal. Canadian Catholics suggest that the treatment for a fever is blankets, with sweating thought to drive heat out of the body. Africans and Ethiopians used boiled milk with honey added to treat a cold. In India and the United States, fenugreek is used to promote lactation. Iranians use frankincense as a disinfectant and antibacterial agent. Laughing has been found to reduce blood pressure and stress.

FOOD CULTURE THAT AFFECTS WELL-BEING

Knowledge of the benefits of different foods is important because food nourishes and heals the body. Each culture has its own style of food preparation, and some have beliefs associated with benefits related to the techniques they use to prepare food. Food specific to a culture is based on the availability of resources and values in the community. As an example, Hindus avoid eating meat, preferring vegetarian food for spiritual reasons and because they worship nature and animals. The diet specific to a culture can also be deficient of minerals and vitamins, causing severe health problems.

Learning about patient diets can help advanced practice nurses modify treatment for better patient outcomes, because we now know that diseases can be caused not only by pathogens but also by diet choices. For example, those who eat only corn for long periods of time may develop signs and symptoms of niacin deficiency because trypto-phan, an essential amino acid, is absent in maize that has not been properly prepared. Food in certain cultures is strongly believed to improve health, promote healing, and cleanse the soul. In India some believe that what you eat is what you become: A subtle food lightens your soul, whereas a gross or heavy food is a barrier to evolution of your soul. Muslims eat foods that are classified as *halal* and avoid foods classified as *haram*. Ramadan is an Islamic religious period during which Muslims do not eat during the day and pray five times a day. Pork and alcohol considered as *haram* are prohibited, whereas Islamic law does allow one to eat seafood (Gulam, 2003). In Somalia, camel milk is used to feed infants in addition to human breast milk. In Europe people love to grow and eat organic food to avoid pesticides, fertilizers, and other chemicals. Jews do not eat pork, and the meats they do consume must be considered as kosher (Rich, 2007). The Chi-nese eat clams believing they will bring prosperity and wealth. Ancient Egyptians used garlic for strength and to prevent respiratory diseases.

Spices are believed to be precious (**Figure 10-5**). Clove oil is believed to reduce dental pain. Green chilies can help protect the stomach from gastritis. Turmeric is an

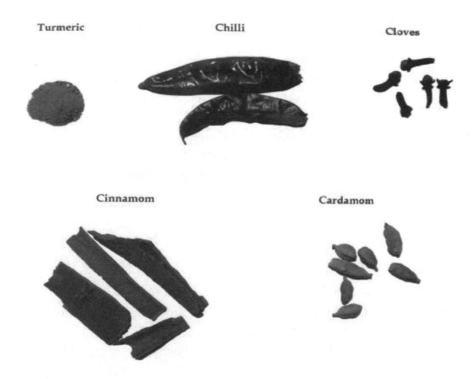

FIGURE 10-5 Spices contribute to the prevention of some diseases.
Source: Picture courtesy of Dr. Kiran Macha.

antibacterial agent and is applied on wounds. Turmeric is believed to protect us from intestinal cancers. Most Asian Indians use rich spices in their food preparation, many of which can promote positive health outcomes (Tapsell, 2006).

KEY POINTS

- Culture an integral part of a person's makeup. It may affect the well-being of an individual and may also influence health risks in a community.
- Traditional beliefs of many cultures are connected to nature, energy, and spirits.
- Objects such as amulets are believed by many to protect one from bad spirits and curses.
- Food is specific to a culture. By learning about a culture's diet, one can modify treatment.
- Prevention is a deep-rooted concept in all cultural practices.
- Herbal medicines are widely used. Practitioners should not fail to ask their patients about use of herbal medicines because they may interact with allopathic drugs.
- Alternative treatments are worth considering if the treatment is known to result in positive outcomes.
- Advanced practice nurses should learn about, respect, and educate patients on traditional medical practices.
- Spices are widely used by billions of people in the world and in many cases have been found to protect health and prevent disease.
- Ayurvedic medicine, homeopathic medicine, and Unani medicine are medical systems with proven health benefits.

CRITICAL QUESTIONS

1. How can culture influence statistics in epidemiology?
2. List disease conditions that cannot be treated with allopathic medicine but can be treated with alternative medicines.
3. How do you believe this chapter affected your perceptions and will affect your clinical nursing practice?
4. List the most common health beliefs of your culture.

ACKNOWLEDGMENT

We thank the graduate students who have taken the *Global Healthcare and Culture* course (2009, 2010) at the Brooks College of Health, University of North Florida, because their contributions as part of course assignments were used in writing this chapter.

RESOURCES TO DEVELOP CULTURE COMPETENCY

National Center for Culture Competence
   http://www11.georgetown.edu/research/gucchd/nccc/
University of Wisconsin, IME videos
   http://videos.med.wisc.edu/category.php?categoryid=18
U.S. Human Resources and Services Administration
   http://www.hrsa.gov/culturalcompetence/

REFERENCES

American Cancer Society. (2010). Native American healing. Retrieved from http://www.cancer.org/docroot/eto/content/eto_5_3x_native_american_healing.asp

Carvalho, M., Robinson, M., & Rundle, A. (1999). *Honoring patient preferences: A guide to complying with multicultural patient requirements.* San Francisco: Jossey-Bass.

Colin, J. M., & Paperwalla, G. (1996). Haitians. In J. G. Lipson, S. L. Dibble, & P. A. Minarik (Eds.), *Culture & nursing care: A pocket guide* (pp. 139–154). San Francisco: UCSF Nursing Press.

Estomba, D. (2006). Medicinal wild plant knowledge and gathering patterns in a mapuche community from north-western Patagonia. *Journal of Ethnopharmacology, 103*(1), 109.

Gulam, H. (2003). Care of the Muslim patient. *Australian Nursing Journal, 11*(2), 23–25.

Institute for Reproductive Health, Georgetown University, Center for Research on Maternal and Child Disease. (1995). Evaluation of the "collar" method of natural family planning. Washington, DC: Georgetown University Medical Center. Retrieved from http://www.fhi.org/en/rh/pubs/network/v17_1/nt1714.htm

Kouba, L. J. (1985). Female circumcision in Africa: An overview. *African Studies Review, 28*(1), 95.

Malarney, S. (2010). Vietnam. Retrieved from http://www.everyculture.com/To-Z/Vietnam.html

Moran, S. (1999). Filipino traditional healing practices. Retrieved from http://www.hawcc.hawaii.edu/nursing/filip1.htm

Pearson, B. (1997). Traditional Chinese medicine in the west. *Journal of the Australian Traditional Medicine Society, 3*(4), 127–128.

Poma, P. A. (1987). Pregnancy in Hispanic women. *Journal of the National Medicine Association, 79*(9), 929–935.

Rafatullah, S., & Algasoumi, S. (2008). Unani medicine: An integral part of health care system in India subcontinent. *European Journal of Integrative Medicine, 1*(1), 39–40.

Raven, J. H., Chen, Q., Tolhurst, R. J., & Garner, P. (2007). Traditional beliefs and practices in the postpartum period in Fujian Province, China: A qualitative study. Retrieved from http://www. ncbi.nlm.nih.gov/pmc/articles/PMC1913060/http://www.ncbi.nlm.nih.gov/pmc/articles/ PMC1913060/

Rich, T. R. (2007). Kashrut: Jewish dietary laws. Retrieved from http://www.jewfaq.org/kashrut. htm

Stefco, J. (2007). What is the evil eye? A brief history of the spell and possible cure. Retrieved from http://pagan-wiccan-practice.suite101.com/article.cfm/the_evil_eye

Tapsell, L. C. (2006). Health benefits of herbs and spices: The past, the present, the future. *Medical Journal of Australia, 185*(4), S4.

Thomas, J. T., & DeSantis, L. (1995). Feeding and weaning practices of Cuban and Haitian immigrant mothers. *Journal of Transcultural Nursing, 6*(2), 34–42. Retrieved from http://bearspace. baylor.edu/Charles_Kemp/www/haitian_refugees.htm

Wright, K., Jolly, K., Cassandra, R., & Rankin, V. (2002). Are you culturally aware? Retrieved from http://www.personal.uncc.edu/macurran/2002/webproject/asi.htm

CHAPTER 11

Nursing in Pandemics and Emergency Preparedness

The 1918–1919 influenza pandemic killed more people than any other outbreak of disease in human history. The lowest estimate of the death toll is 21 million, while recent scholarship estimates from 50 to 100 million dead [worldwide]. World population was then only 28% what is today, and most deaths occurred in a sixteen week period, from mid-September to mid-December of 1918 (Barry, 2004).

1918

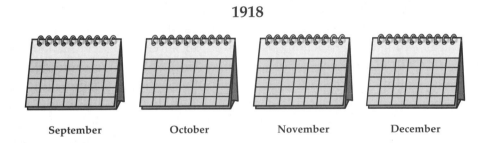

| September | October | November | December |

Carol A. Ledbetter
Margaret A. Holder

OBJECTIVES

- Analyze the characteristics of the 21st century pandemic, influenza A H_1N_1, and influenza A H_5N_1 epidemic of the late 20th century.
- Evaluate the principles of emergency preparedness related to both H_1N_1 and H_5N_1.

INTRODUCTION

There is ample evidence in the historical record that humanity has dealt with pandemics throughout the millennia (Martin, 2006; Moore, 2007). History is instructive and lets us know pandemics will occur again. Current history coupled with scientific information and emergency preparedness, however, will provide humanity with the tools needed to survive a pandemic.

PANDEMIC

According to the World Health Organization (WHO, 2005a), a pandemic is a global epidemic that spreads to more than one continent. The term "pandemic" is from the Greek word *pandemos*, *pan* meaning "all" and *demos* means "people." A more general definition suggests an outbreak of an illness that expands to different parts of the globe. History is replete with examples of pandemics throughout the centuries of recorded history (**Table 11-1**).

Avian Influenza Virus

In 1996 a strain of an avian influenza (bird flu), called H_5N_1, was isolated in a farm goose in Guangdong Province, China; the virus was highly pathogenic. Then, in 1997 H_5N_1 began killing chickens within 48 hours of exposure; there were few survivors. In February 2003 Hong Kong confirmed two cases of H_5N_1 in humans; the family had recently traveled to Fujian Province, China; there was one death. Hong Kong destroyed the entire population of poultry over 3 days. Experts believed that a pandemic had been averted by destroying the birds and eliminating human exposure. By December 2003 four large cats, two tigers and two leopards, fed with fresh chickens died in a Thailand zoo. By December 19, 2003, the Republic of Korea confirmed highly pathogenic H_5N_1 on three farms, killing poultry. By January 11, 2004, Vietnam identified H_5N_1 as the cause of a respiratory illness with high fatality in humans (WHO, 2005a).

The H_5N_1 virus continues to be of great concern for human health for three reasons: It has crossed the species barrier to infect humans (bird to human; cat to human), there is little preexisting natural immunity to H_5N_1 virus infection in the human population, and the severity and lethality of the disease is impressive. By August 2009, 440 people in 45 countries in Africa, Asia, and Europe had been infected with H_5N_1, and 262 had died; this is a 60% fatality rate. If H_5N_1 mutates and retains its lethality but becomes more easily transmitted from human to human, a devastating pandemic will occur. By comparison, the 1918 pandemic killed 2.5% of those infected (Pendergrast, 2010). H_5N_1 did not become a pandemic, but it remains a potential pandemic threat.

Table 11-1   Examples of Pandemics Throughout Recorded History

Antiquity
- Antonine Plague (possibly smallpox) 165–180 AD
- Plague of Cyprian 251–266 AD
- Plague of Justinian 541 AD
- Plague, also known as the Black Death 1300s AD
- Typhus 1501–1587 AD

18th Century
- Influenza 1732–1733 AD
- Influenza 1775–1776 AD

19th Century
- Cholera 1816–1826 AD
- Cholera 1829–1851 AD
- Influenza 1847–1848 AD
- Cholera 1852–1860 AD
- Bubonic Plague 1855 AD
- Influenza 1857–1859 AD
- Cholera 1863–1875 AD
- Influenza 1889–1892 AD
- Cholera 1899–1923 AD

20th Century
- The Great Influenza (avian flu) 1918–1920 AD
- El Tor (*Vibrio cholerae* [cholera]) 1960s AD
- HIV/AIDS 1980s to present

21st Century
- H_1N_1 (also known as the Swine Influenza) 2009

Source: Retrieved May 6, 2010, from www.medicalnewstoday.com

An Archetypal 21st Century Pandemic—H_1N_1 Influenza Virus

For the purpose of the discussion on pandemics, we focus on a novel avian influenza pandemic that began early in the 21st century. A viral pandemic occurs when a novel viral strain of an illness develops, the population has little or no immunity to the illness, and the virus moves easily from person to person. A novel virus pandemic is a virus that has never previously infected humans or has not infected humans for an extended period, and it is likely that only a very small number of the population, if any, have immunity or antibodies to protect them against the novel virus. The first 21st century novel pandemic virus is influenza A (H_1N_1), also known as the swine flu.

Influenza Viruses Transmission Dynamics

The natural home, or reservoirs, of the avian influenza virus, is in the gastrointestinal track of wild aquatic birds; their droppings contain millions of copies of the virus. Exposure to an avian influenza virus can cause disease in humans; however, the virus cannot be passed from one human to another. For an avian influenza virus to be infectious to humans and transmittable from human to human, the virus must first change. The change occurs in an intermediate host, most frequently pigs. Pigs serve as hosts and have receptors for both avian and human influenza viruses. In the pig the influenza virus undergoes genetic variation, developing new antigenic variants, or drift strains. Once the change occurs, a novel virus emerges (Ito et al., 1998; Novel Swine-Origin Influenza A (H_1N_1) Virus Investigation Team, 2009; Webster, 2002).

An influenza virus is usually spherical but can assume other shapes and is composed of eight genes. The surface has two types of glycoprotein protuberances, hemagglutinin and neuraminidase (e.g., H_1N_1), that supply the virus with the mechanism of attacking cells (**Figure 11-1**). The viral hemagglutinin binds with a cell-surface receptor called sialic acid that is specific for the influenza viruses (in humans); they both have shapes that fit tightly together. More viral hemagglutinin binds to more sialic acid receptors until the virus tightly adheres to the body of the target cell. Once attached to the cell, a pit forms beneath the virus and it slips into the cell. Inside the cell the host immune system cannot see the virus (Barry, 2004; National Institutes of Health, 2009).

Upon completing its cellular replication cycle, the final release of influenza virus from an infected cell surface relies on the action of the viral neuraminidase, which acts to remove sialic acid (the viral receptor) from the surface of the host cells. Without this step, the newly forming virus particles would immediately rebind to their receptor and not be efficiently released into the extracellular space, remaining attached to the cell in large clumps. Thus, the establishment of a productive influenza virus infection depends on both neuraminidase and hemagglutinin and a delicate balance between the functions of the two glycoproteins. It is also possible that the neuraminidase assists in evading host mucosal soluble mucin decoys during the process of infection. (Varki et al., 2009).

Influenza viruses are classified as type A, B, or C. Influenza A causes local epidemics and worldwide pandemics, influenza B does cause disease but does not cause

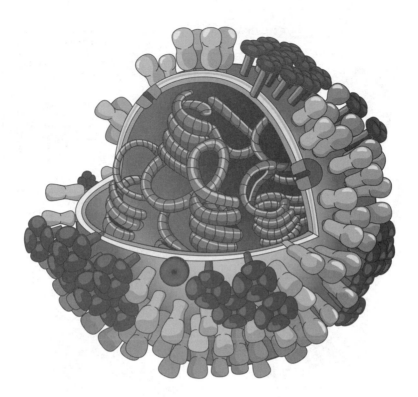

FIGURE 11-1   Graphical representation of a generic influenza virion's ultrastructure. The grey spikes are hemagglutinin and the black tree-like structures are neuraminidase. The green strands inside are ribonucleic acid (RNA).
Source: Picture courtesy of the Centers for Disease Control and Prevention, http://www.cdc.gov/media/subtopic/library/diseases.htm : Picture ID: 11822. Accessed July 9, 2010.

epidemics, and influenza C seldom causes disease in human beings (Novel Swine-Origin Influenza A (H₁N₁) Virus Investigation Team, 2009).

Antigenic Drift Versus Antigenic Shift

Antigenic drift (**Figure 11-2**) occurs in viral neuraminidase and hemagglutinin and is associated with seasonal epidemics. Influenza viruses change through antigenic drift, a process in which mutations occur in the virus genome and in turn cause changes in the viral neuraminidase and hemagglutinin. Antigenic drift is an unremitting process that results in the appearance of new viral strain variations. The

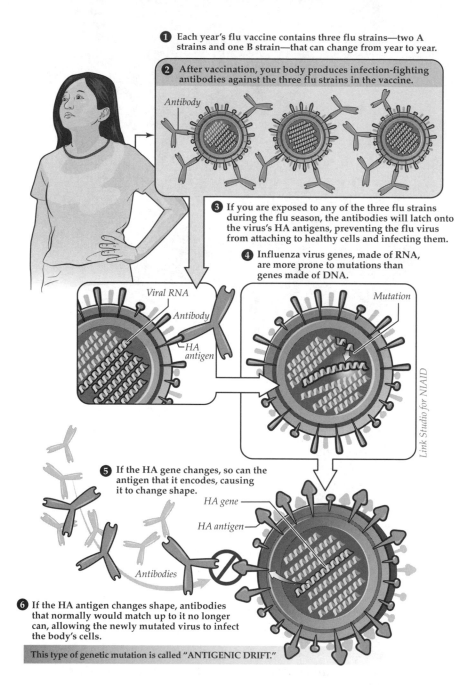

FIGURE 11-2   Antigenic drift.

Source: Picture courtesy of the National Institute of Allergy and Infectious Diseases (NIAID), http://www. niaid.nih.gov/topics/Flu/Research/basic/pages/antigenicdriftillustration.aspx; Accessed July 9, 2010.

amount of change can be slight or significant; over time, one of the new viral strains becomes dominant. The process of antigenic drift affects viruses that are in circulation worldwide. Antigenic drift is the reason vaccines must be updated annually and is also the reason influenza viruses can reinfect individuals repeatedly over the course of a lifetime.

Antigenic shift (**Figure 11-3**) is a process by which pandemic viruses arise. The genetic change enables an influenza strain to move from one animal species to another, including humans. During antigenic shift the viral neuraminidase and hemagglutinin are not changed but are replaced by different viral neuraminidase and hemagglutinin. As a result of antigenic shift, the human immune system sees the novel neuraminidase or neuraminidase–hemagglutinin combinations as something new and lacking antibody protection.

WHO Pandemic Phases

In 2009 the WHO revised the phase descriptions of pandemics. The grouping and description of pandemic phases were revised to make them easier to understand, more precise, and based on observable phenomena. Phases 1 to 3 correlate with preparedness, including capacity development and response planning activities, whereas phases 4 to 6 clearly signal the need for response and mitigation efforts. Furthermore, periods after the first pandemic wave are elaborated to facilitate postpandemic recovery activities (WHO, 2010a).

In nature, influenza viruses circulate continuously among animals, especially birds. Even though such viruses might theoretically develop into pandemic viruses, in phase 1 no viruses circulating among animals have been reported to cause infections in humans. In phase 2 an animal influenza virus circulating among domesticated or wild animals is known to have caused infection in humans and is therefore considered a potential pandemic threat. In phase 3 an animal or human–animal influenza reassortant virus has caused sporadic cases or small clusters of disease in people but has not resulted in human-to-human transmission sufficient to sustain community-level outbreaks. Limited human-to-human transmission may occur under some circumstances, for example, when there is close contact between an infected person and an unprotected caregiver. However, limited transmission under such restricted circumstances does not indicate that the virus has gained the level of transmissibility among humans necessary to cause a pandemic. Phase 4 is characterized by verified human-to-human transmission of an animal or human–animal influenza reassortant virus able to cause "community-level outbreaks."

The genetic change that enables a flu strain to jump from
one animal species to another, including humans, is called "ANTIGENIC SHIFT."
Antigenic shift can happen in three ways:

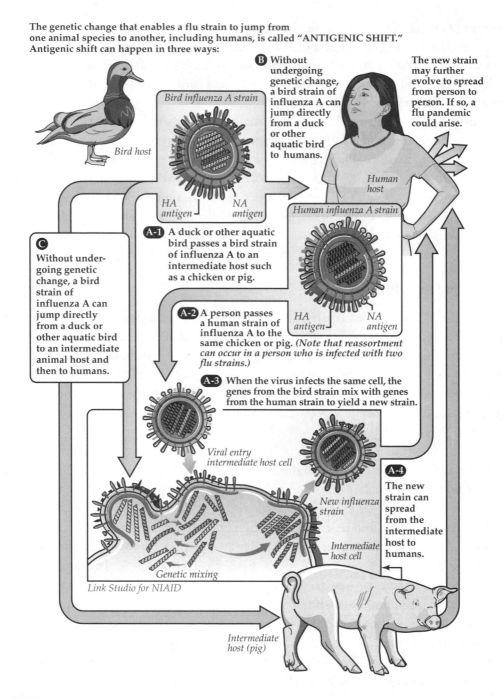

B Without undergoing genetic change, a bird strain of influenza A can jump directly from a duck or other aquatic bird to humans.

The new strain may further evolve to spread from person to person. If so, a flu pandemic could arise.

Bird influenza A strain

Bird host

HA antigen   *NA antigen*

Human host

Human influenza A strain

A-1 A duck or other aquatic bird passes a bird strain of influenza A to an intermediate host such as a chicken or pig.

C Without undergoing genetic change, a bird strain of influenza A can jump directly from a duck or other aquatic bird to an intermediate animal host and then to humans.

A-2 A person passes a human strain of influenza A to the same chicken or pig. *(Note that reassortment can occur in a person who is infected with two flu strains.)*

HA antigen   *NA antigen*

A-3 When the virus infects the same cell, the genes from the bird strain mix with genes from the human strain to yield a new strain.

Viral entry intermediate host cell

New influenza strain

A-4 The new strain can spread from the intermediate host to humans.

Intermediate host cell

Genetic mixing

Link Studio for NIAID

Intermediate host (pig)

FIGURE 11-3 Antigenic shift.

Source: Picture courtesy of the National Institute of Allergy and Infectious Diseases (NIAID), http://www.niaid.nih.gov/topics/Flu/Research/basic/pages/a AntigenicShiftIllustration.aspx; Accessed July 9, 2010.

The ability to cause sustained disease outbreaks in a community marks a significant upward shift in the risk for a pandemic. Any country that suspects or has verified such an event should urgently consult with WHO so that the situation can be jointly assessed and a decision made by the affected country if implementation of a rapid pandemic containment operation is warranted. Phase 4 indicates a significant increase in risk of a pandemic but does not necessarily mean that a pandemic is a foregone conclusion. Phase 5 is characterized by human-to-human spread of the virus into at least two countries in one WHO region. Although most countries will not be affected at this stage, the declaration of phase 5 is a strong signal that a pandemic is imminent and that the time to finalize the organization, communication, and implementation of the planned mitigation measures is short. Phase 6, the pandemic phase, is characterized by community-level outbreaks in at least one other country in a different WHO region in addition to the criteria defined in phase 5. Designation of this phase indicates that a global pandemic is under way (WHO, 2010a).

PANDEMIC EMERGENCY RESPONSE AND PREPARATION

An influenza pandemic is a catastrophic public health event. Given the significant growth in not only the human population but animal populations as well since the last major pandemic in 1968, the current environment may be even more conducive for the reassortment between animal and human influenza strains leading to a novel influenza virus that spreads between people and could cause a pandemic. It is expected that during a pandemic the virus spreads rapidly because of the interconnected nature of the world and the high level of global travel. The likelihood of tens of thousands of victims needing healthcare resources will overwhelm communities and existing healthcare services.

Whereas by definition a pandemic is a worldwide or national event, the greatest impact will be at the local level. During a pandemic event hospital and healthcare resources will be limited, and unlike a mass casualty, there will not be opportunities for replenishment from other communities. The hallmark of pandemics is a gradual increase in the number of people affected, rising to a catastrophic number of patients (Beach, 2010; http://www.osha.gov/Publications). The number of cases may at first decline as a result of treatment and prophylactic efforts only to increase because of reinfection with a different strain or as a result of an additional wave or waves of the disease. If a pandemic evolves to become severe and widespread over time, the following can also be expected:

- Vaccines, antiviral agents, and antibiotics to treat secondary infections will be in high demand and potentially in short supply;

- Medical facilities will be strained with demands to care for both influenza and noninfluenza patients.
- There will be potentially significant shortages of personnel to provide essential community services.

Healthcare facilities must consider how to maximize available care by estimating in advance staffing needed to care for patients and plan how to meet those needs when there is an increase in patients and/or a decrease in staff (Occupational Safety and Health Administration [OSHA], 2009). In all likelihood during a pandemic it will become necessary to allocate scarce resources in a manner that is different from normal circumstances but imperative if the system is to remain functioning and save as many lives as possible. Physicians and nurses with crucial knowledge of infectious and pulmonary diseases and critical care will need to be identified. Extensive advance planning is necessary to ensure adequate resources will be available. Preparedness planning efforts must be made to mitigate a pandemic's impact through prevention and public education (Beach, 2010; Columbia University School of Nursing, 2008; OSHA, 2009).

Pandemic Prepardness

The federal government bases its pandemic preparedness on assumptions from the Centers for Disease Control and Prevention (CDC) regarding the evolution and impacts of a pandemic. Defining the potential magnitude of a pandemic is difficult because of the large differences in severity for the three 20th century pandemics. Whereas the 1918 pandemic resulted in an estimated 500,000 deaths in the United States, the 1958 pandemic killed approximately 70,000 Americans and the 1968 pandemic caused an estimated 34,000 U.S. deaths. This difference largely relates to the severity of infections and the virulence of the influenza viruses that caused these pandemics (CDC, n.d.-a).

The 20th century pandemics also have shared similar characteristics. In each pandemic about 30% of the U.S. population developed illness, with about half of those Americans seeking medical care. Children under the age of 18 have tended to have the highest rates of illness, though not of severe disease and death. In each pandemic geographical spread was rapid and virtually all communities experienced outbreaks (DHHS, 2010). Based on these assumptions, the burgeoning throng of patients and "worried well" (otherwise healthy people who avoid the workplace for fear of exposure) may overwhelm local healthcare delivery systems. Many of our current systems are already operating at peak capacity, with scarce beds and overwhelmed emergency departments. During a pandemic an absenteeism rate of up to 40% coupled with an expected radically increased demand for services will place additional burden on local public health and direct care systems that have insufficient surge resources (GAO, 2008)

In the event of a pandemic, it is currently estimated that production of initial doses of a vaccine against a novel strain of influenza would take approximately 4 to 6 months (OSHA, 2009). Pandemic planning must include protocols and the stockpiling of supplies for administering pandemic influenza vaccine. Included in these protocols should be procedures to register, track, and contact individuals who have received immunizations. In contrast to the vaccine, antiviral medications for the treatment of influenza do not need to be "specific" to the circulating pandemic strain and therefore are more amenable to stockpiling (OSHA, 2009).

Role of the Advanced Practice Nurses

Given the potential scope of the pandemic's impact and the wide range of issues to be considered, communities and healthcare facilities must identify what resources will be needed, what processes and systems need to be put in place, and have contingency plans to mitigate the impact of a pandemic. The primary goal is to decrease the amount of infection and, by extension, reduce hospitalizations and deaths. Advanced practice nurses (APNs) are the frontline healthcare workers in direct contact with the public and are well positioned to assist local communities and healthcare facilities in addressing and defining essential staff and services. They are well suited and educationally prepared to take the lead in preparing for a pandemic disaster event.

Healthcare Facilities Planning

Each year, flu season can stress an emergency department's ability to maintain normal operations because of the increase in both outpatient volume and admissions. Although the precise effects on emergency department functions cannot be predicted with confidence, contingency plans should allow for a worse than normal flu season. At some critical point operations of hospitals will be affected, not only by the absence of the hospital's own workers but by slowdowns in transportation of supplies and support services, the impact of which is the inability to maintain normal operations, even for normal patient volumes. The DHHS (2005) has recommended that healthcare facilities consider developing institutional stockpiles of resources to counter supply shortages and transportation issues that may impact the ability to access federal and state supplies. As for supplies, many organizations have created a policy of keeping at least 30 days worth of supplies such as fuel, food, and water on hand. This provides a buffer in case there is a mismatch between what supplies can be delivered and what is truly needed in a crisis. However, a pandemic may affect a community and its resources for 6 to 8 weeks. The Joint Commission Disaster Guidance recommends that hospitals have a 48- to 72-hour stand-alone capability (DHHS, 2005; Joint Commission, 2006; MMCSR, 2010).

Alternate Care Sites

In the event of a pandemic, existing healthcare facilities and resources will be severely taxed. One big part of the solution is alternate care sites (ACS) that can relieve the pressure on hospitals (and the healthcare system in general) in times of high demand. ACS come in many shapes and sizes and can be used in a wide variety of ways, including direct care and screening sites. Call centers for advice lines can also be located at these sites.

There is a need to identify in advance the location of ACS and staffing to care for those not needing hospitalization and the "worried well." APNs are the ideal candidates for managing and staffing these sites, providing direct primary care for those not needing hospitalization. They also can take on the role of triage officer to redirect those needing more definitive care to hospitals. ACS are vital to prevent overwhelming traditional inpatient facilities and emergency departments in the event of a pandemic.

A major challenge for planners is that in contrast to hospitals and emergency medical systems, ACS do not currently exist as operating medical care systems. In fact, in many communities ACS have not even been carefully considered as an option for patient care. Therefore, it is imperative that the planning process for ACS begin early in the initial pandemic planning process (Cantrill, 2007).

Pandemic Severity Index

To better predict the impact of a pandemic and to provide local decision makers with recommendations that are matched to the severity of the pandemic, the CDC developed a pandemic severity index. This index (**Figure 11-4**) is modeled after the approach used to characterize hurricanes and has five different categories of pandemics, with category 1 representing moderate severity and category 5 representing the most severe. The severity of a pandemic is primarily determined by its death rate, or the percentage of infected people who die. A category 1 pandemic is as harmful as a severe seasonal influenza season; the outbreaks of 1958 and 1968 both fit into category

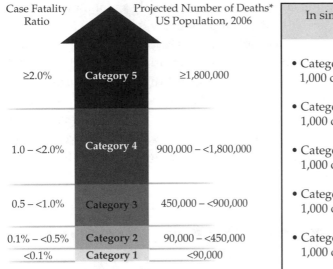

Case Fatality Ratio		Projected Number of Deaths* US Population, 2006
≥2.0%	Category 5	≥1,800,000
1.0 – <2.0%	Category 4	900,000 – <1,800,000
0.5 – <1.0%	Category 3	450,000 – <900,000
0.1% – <0.5%	Category 2	90,000 – <450,000
<0.1%	Category 1	<90,000

In simple terms the categories are as follows

- Category 1: less than 1 death per 1,000 cases

- Category 2: 1 to 5 deaths per 1,000 cases

- Category 3: 5 to 10 deaths per 1,000 cases

- Category 4: 10 to 20 deaths per 1,000 cases

- Category 5: More than 20 deaths per 1,000 cases

*Assumes 30% illness rate and unmitigated pandemic without interventions

FIGURE 11-4   Pandemic severity index.
Source: Picture courtesy of the Centers for Disease Control and Prevention, http://www.cdc.gov/media/pdf/MitigationSlides.pdf; Accessed July 13, 2010.

2, whereas a pandemic with the same intensity of the 1918 flu pandemic, or worse, is classified as category 5 (CDC, 2007).

Based on the severity of the pandemic, CDC may make recommendations designed to reduce contact between people to limit the spread of disease. Such recommendations may be as follows:

- Asking ill persons to remain at home or not go to work until they are no longer contagious (7 to 10 days). Ill persons will be treated with antiviral medication if drugs are available and effective against the pandemic strain.
- Asking household members of ill persons to stay at home for 7 days.
- Dismissing students from schools and closing child care programs for up to 3 months for the most severe pandemics and reducing contact among kids and teens in the community.
- Recommending social distancing of adults in the community and at work, which may include closing large public gatherings, changing workplace environments, and shifting work schedules without disrupting essential services.

Measures such as these are most effective if implemented early and uniformly across communities and can only be met with advanced planning and an aggressive community education program. The typical incubation period for influenza is approximately 2 days. Persons who become ill may shed virus and can transmit infection for one-half to 1 day before the onset of illness. Viral shedding and the risk of transmission is greatest during the first 2 days of illness. Children play a major role in transmission of infection and their illness rates are likely to be higher because they shed more virus over a longer period of time and they do not control their secretions as well (WHO, 2010b). **Table 11-2** outlines community mitigation strategies recommended for specific severity indexes.

Table 11-2   Community Mitigation Strategy by Pandemic Severity

Interventions* by Setting	Pandemic Severity Index		
	1	2 and 3	4 and 5
Home			
Voluntary isolation of ill at home (adults and children), combine with use of antiviral treatment as available and indicated	Recommend†§	Recommend†§	Recommend†§
Voluntary quarantine of household members in homes with ill persons¶ (adults and children), consider combining with antiviral prophylaxis if effective, feasible, and quantities sufficient	Generally not recommended	Consider**	Recommend**
School **Child social distancing**			
-dismissal of students from schools and school-based activities, and closure of child care programs	Generally not recommended	Consider; ≤4 weeks††	Recommend; ≤12 weeks§§
-reduce out-of-school social contacts and community mixing	Generally not recommended	Consider; ≤4 weeks††	Recommend; ≤12 weeks§§
Workplace/Community **Adult social distancing**			
-decrease number of social contacts (e.g., encourage teleconferences, alternatives to face-to-face meetings)	Generally not recommended	Consider	Recommend
-increase distance between persons (e.g., reduce density in public transit, workplace)	Generally not recommended	Consider	Recommend
-modify, postpone, or cancel selected public gatherings to promote social distance (e.g., stadium events, theater performances)	Generally not recommended	Consider	Recommend
-modify workplace schedules and practices (e.g., telework, staggered shifts)	Generally not recommended	Consider	Recommend

Generally not recommended = Unless there is a compelling rationale for specific populations or jurisdictions, measures are generally not recommended for entire populations because the consequences may outweigh the benefits.

Table 11-2   Community Mitigation Strategy by Pandemic Severity *(continued)*

Consider = Important to consider these alternatives as part of a prudent planning strategy, considering characteristics of the pandemic, such as age-specific illness rate, geographic distribution, and the magnitude of adverse consequences. These factors may vary globally, nationally, and locally.

Recommended = Generally recommended as an important component of the planning strategy.

*All these interventions should be used in combination with other infection control measures, including hand hygiene, cough etiquette, and personal protective equipment such as face masks. Additional information on infection control measures is available at www.pandemicflu.gov.
†This intervention may be combined with the treatment of sick individuals using antiviral medications and with vaccine campaigns, if supplies are available.
§Many sick individuals who are not critically ill may be managed safely at home.
¶The contribution made by contact with asymptomatically infected individuals to disease transmission is unclear. Household members in homes with ill persons may be at increased risk of contracting pandemic disease from an ill household member. These household members may have asymptomatic illness and may be able to shed influenza virus that promotes community disease transmission. Therefore, household members of homes with sick individuals would be advised to stay home.
**To facilitate compliance and decrease risk of household transmission, this intervention may be combined with provision of antiviral medications to household contacts, depending on drug availability, feasibility of distribution, and effectiveness; policy recommendations for antiviral prophylaxis are addressed in a separate guidance document.
††Consider short-term implementation of this measure—that is, less than 4 weeks.
§§Plan for prolonged implementation of this measure—that is, 1–3 months; actual duration may vary depending on transmission in the community as the pandemic wave is expected to last 6–8 weeks.
Source: From CDC. Retrieved July 13, 2010, from http://www.flu.gov/professional/community/commitigation. html#XIV (WHO, 2007).

Mitigation

The greatest potential for preventing the adverse effects of natural disasters exists during the preimpact phase. This involves delineating at-risk populations (vulnerability analysis), assessing the level of emergency preparedness and the flexibility of the existing surveillance systems, educating defined populations at risk, and training health and safety personnel. The critical component of any pandemic response is the early conduct of an assessment to identify urgent needs to determine relief priorities for an affected or potentially affected population. The primary goal of the mitigation phase is to lessen the impact of a pandemic before it strikes. Activities to focus on are those that reduce or eliminate a hazard including risk reduction (immunizations), treatment (including early antiviral administration), and prevention (public education).

An important community mitigation strategy is to keep people who are ill, even at the first sign, from entering the workplace and school. However, as the CDC observes, persons who become ill may shed virus and can transmit infection for one-half to one day before the onset of illness. Viral shedding and the risk for transmission will be greatest during the first two days of illness.

Children will play a major role in transmission of infection and their illness rates are likely to be higher because they shed more virus over a longer period of time and they do not control their secretions as well. Encouraging social distancing and frequent handwashing policies are important parts of any mitigation strategy (DHHS, 2005).

The combination of the effects of the disease and using these measures of social distancing and time off from work could adversely affect the business practices of all critical infrastructure operators, impeding their ability to maintain normal operations. The specific implications for the operations of each business from direct health impacts combined with the proposed disease containment strategies should be identified, assessed, and incorporated into their pandemic plan. Disruptions and failures at essential businesses will cause localized economic and social challenges and may affect other businesses in the sector, region, and, perhaps, the nation (U.S. Department of Homeland Security, 2006).

Pre-Event Planning

In considering how to meet the challenges of providing care under extreme circumstances, an organization must first identify those standards that should be maintained at all times, distinguishing them from those that may more readily be adapted when disastrous circumstances occur. The American Nurses Association has outlined specific guidance for professions during pandemics. The most critical standards for clinicians providing care (after triage has been performed and patients have been transferred for care) are:

- Maximizing worker and patient safety
- Maintaining airway and breathing, circulation, and control of blood loss
- Maintaining or establishing infection control (including continuity of medications for chronic conditions) (Columbia University School of Nursing, 2008)

Less important actions that could be delayed or eliminated for some period of time or assigned to family members, nonlicensed assistants, or volunteers include

- Routine care activities (e.g., blood pressure checks in nonacute patients, assisted ambulation, bathing, feeding)
- Administration of oral medications

- Extensive documentation of care
- Maintenance of complete privacy and confidentiality

Here again, APNs need to take the lead in identifying priorities and coordinating care.

Healthcare personal will be affected, either becoming ill themselves or having to care for ill family members or others. Identification of critical skills and essential personnel is an imperative. Plans need also to include stockpiling of supplies and equipment in the event of a breakdown of delivery services. Additionally, the identification of other facilities (ACS) to be used in the event of a shortage of hospital beds and treatment facilities, along with preplanning on their use, is needed. This planning involves a cooperative effort of leaders in the community, government, medical centers, public health officials, and local industry.

The Agency for Healthcare Research and Quality (AHRQ, 2005) expert panel recommended five principles to steer the development of mass casualty events (including pandemics) response plans:

1. In planning, the aim should be to keep the healthcare system functioning and to deliver acceptable quality of care to preserve as many lives as possible.
2. Planning a public health and medical response to a mass casualty event must be comprehensive, community based, and coordinated at the regional level.
3. There must be adequate legal framework for providing health and medical care in a mass casualty event.
4. The rights of individuals must be protected to the extent possible and reasonable under the circumstances.
5. Clear communication with the public is essential before, during, and after a mass casualty event.

Assessing the Need

In the confusion accompanying a pandemic event, managing a hospital can be challenging. Past events show patterns of hospital use. It is estimated that during a moderate to severe viral outbreak one-third of the population of the United States will become ill. Approximately 50% of those will require hospitalization. The strain on already overcrowded facilities will be immense. The DHHS (2010) estimates that during a moderate viral pandemic, 865,000 patients would be hospitalized, 128,750 in an intensive care unit (ICU) with 64,875 requiring ventilator assistance (**Table 11-3**). Potential shortages of ventilators will be particularly problematic. In the case of such

Table 11-3   Projected Number* of Episodes of Illness, Healthcare Utilization, and Death Associated With Moderate and Severe Pandemic Influenza Scenarios

Characteristic	Moderate (as in 1958/1968)	Severe (as in 1918)
Illness	90 million (30%)	90 million (30%)
Outpatient medical care	45 million (50%)	45 million (50%)
Hospitalization	865,000	9,900,000
ICU care	128,750[†]	1,485,000[†]
Mechanical ventilation	64,875[†]	742,500[†]
Deaths	209,000	1,903,000

*Estimates are based on extrapolation from past pandemics in the United States. Note that these estimates do not include the potential impact of interventions not available during the 20th century pandemics.
[†]At the present time, there are only 60,000 ICU beds in the United States, with an average utilization rate of around 85%, resulting in an available surplus of only 9,000 beds.
Source: From Flu.gov. Retrieved July 13, 2010, from http://www.hhs.gov/disasters/discussion/planners/playbook/panflu/index.html

a pandemic, hospitals may not have an adequate supply of reserve ventilators required to treat patients suffering from acute respiratory failure. Currently, the CDC has a reserve supply of thousands of mechanical ventilators under the Strategic National Stockpile.

The problem of over-reliance on hospitals was demonstrated in the spring of 2009, at the beginning of the H_1N_1 pandemic. Even though the outbreak was fairly mild, emergency departments in cities across the country saw huge increases in patient visits caused by actual illness and by the masses of concerned individuals who flocked to hospitals for care. In a pandemic, both the sick and concerned individuals must be served, whether with medical treatment or simply preventive care and information.

Software Modeling

CDC used FluSurge software (available at http://www.cdc.gov/flu/tools/flusurge/) using metro Atlanta as an example to illustrate the impact of an 8-week influenza pandemic with a 25% gross clinical attack rate. In this example, the demand on hospital resources peaked in week 5, with a maximum of 412 hospital admissions per day. Flu-

Surge estimated that during this week, 2,013 persons would be hospitalized, 583 would require use of the ICU, and 292 would need mechanical ventilation (these numbers, respectively, translate to 28% of all hospital beds, 77% of total ICU capacity, and 42% of all ventilators in metro Atlanta). Such an influenza pandemic would most likely result in 13,918 hospital admissions (ranging from 4,627 to 18,843) and 2,516 deaths (ranging from 1,173 to 4,530). These sample results illustrate how the next influenza pandemic may overwhelm existing hospital resources, given that hospitals increasingly operate at nearly full capacity. Public health officials and hospital administrators must plan for surges in demand for hospital services during the next pandemic.

Another tool for planning is the Hospital Surge Model. This software estimates the hospital resources needed to treat casualties arising from biological (anthrax, smallpox, pandemic flu), chemical (chlorine, sulfur mustard, or sarin), nuclear explosion, or radiological (dispersion device or point source) attacks. The Hospital Surge Model estimates

- The number of casualties arriving at the hospital, by arrival condition (e.g., mild or severe symptoms) and day
- The number of casualties in the hospital, by unit (emergency department, ICU, or floor) and day
- The cumulative number of dead or discharged casualties, by day
- The required hospital resources (personnel, equipment, and supplies) to treat casualties, by unit and day

This software can assist facilities for planning and resourcing materials and personnel during a pandemic (AHRQ, 2009).

Public Awareness

The general public will need detailed education concerning when to seek care, where to seek it, and how to protect themselves from the spread of disease. A mass immunization plan will need to be available. It is important to reinforce healthy habits (particularly hand washing and coughing protection). When pandemic planning became a major focused effort worldwide because of concerns regarding H_1N_1 in 2009, major social distancing actions (cancellation of school and public activities and events; 3- to 6-feet distances between people in work, school, and other public environments, etc.) were primary considerations.

The home will be particularly relevant in the case of a flu pandemic. Planners must emphasize the importance of the home as a "safe haven" and consider the use of primary care vans to go out into localities to provide services so that people may remain in their homes. In the case of a flu pandemic, primary care providers, including APNs, will in all likelihood be the first healthcare personnel contacted. They will have the responsibility to decide which patients will need hospitalization and who may be managed at home. The ambulatory care providers will be a critical element of a system to keep the hospitals from being overwhelmed during a pandemic (AHRQ, 2007).

It is imperative to establish a comprehensive public information strategy, such as the following (AHRQ, 2007):

- Use of mass media to provide the public information on preventive measures, home care management, and the appropriate time to seek healthcare services.
- Use of community healthcare call centers to reinforce mass messaging and to provide additional and more tailored information to individuals with questions and concerns. Review these issues for their value as potential mass media messages.
- Use of community call centers to assist with outpatient and home care monitoring and support, thereby helping to extend the reach of public health and healthcare systems into households.
- Use of information collected by the call centers for situational awareness and disease outbreak management and control.

INFLUENZA PANDEMIC PLANNING ISSUES

Because of the uncertainty of the nature of pandemics, pandemic plans must be flexible with built-in processes for obtaining "real-time" recommendations and updating plans accordingly. Some basic planning issues are as follows (OSHA, 2009):

- An influenza pandemic is not a contained or local event. It is widespread and therefore less federal, state, and local support is available at the individual facility level.
- An influenza pandemic is a sustained crisis. Expect the response to have a long duration (12–24 months).
- A pandemic may come and go in waves, each of which can last for 6 to 8 weeks.
- Prevention options (vaccine) and treatment options (medications) are fewer and more uncertain for pandemic influenza.
- It is likely that a vaccine will not be available early in the pandemic. Antiviral medication is in short supply, is highly susceptible to resistance, and may not be effective.

Reaction Phase

Phase 4 of the WHO pandemic preparedness plan involves rapid containment. Human to human transmission of an animal or human–animal influenza virus able to sustain community-level outbreaks has been verified. The estimated probability of pandemic is medium to high. In this phase efforts should center on containing the disease and reducing its spread through treatment and vaccination. The actions recommended in this phase include the following:

- Direct and coordinate rapid pandemic containment activities to limit or delay the spread of infection.
- Increase surveillance and monitor containment operations. Share findings with other organizations.
- Promote and communicate recommended interventions to prevent and reduce population and individual risk.
- Implement rapid pandemic containment operations and other activities.
- Activate contingency plans.

Communities and healthcare facilities must now be prepared to implement contingency plans. It is during this phase that previous cross-training and identification of essential personnel and their roles will come into play. Critical care nurses and respiratory care therapists may be in scarce supply. They may be needed to rove between patient care areas managing ventilator settings and care. APNs, particularly nurse anesthetists, will be in the unique position to coordinate ventilator care throughout the facility. Nurse practitioners and clinical nurse specialists may be called on to manage noncritical inpatient care as physician hospitalists become increasing more taxed managing critical care patients.

During this reaction phase all the preparations and contingencies in the preplanning and mitigation stages must now be activated. Patients will need to be treated, and opening of ACS previously planned should now occur to manage those not needing hospitalization but requiring care. These sites will need to be staffed and coordinated.

Many sick individuals will be managed safely at home. Voluntary quarantine of household members in homes with ill persons should now be encouraged, and the resultant impact on businesses (including healthcare organization) and schools must be determined and acted on. Public health departments must work closely with the media for information dissemination to prevent panic and misinformation. Activation of call centers and advice lines is now essential. Plans for mass immunizations must be activated once the vaccine is available. Antiviral therapy should be initiated according to specific recommendations and supplies. Decreasing social contacts (teleconferencing, telecommuniting, and canceling of large public events) may be necessary. Modification of school and work schedules will assist in social distancing. In a severe pandemic, a state of emergency may be declared.

Recovery Phase

No response to an extreme circumstance is complete until the participants have moved to the recovery phase, including reestablishing the medical and public health infrastructure, both physically and in human resources, disrupted by the disaster. This does not necessarily require fully returning to the preemergency status quo but simply achieving a level of staffing and supplies necessary to return to an ordinary level of care (Columbia University School of Nursing, 2008).

The main priority in the recovery phase is to restore minimum services and the return of a community to a stable state after a catastrophic event such as a pandemic. The goal of recovery is to ensure the economic sustainability of a community and the long-term physical and mental well-being of its citizens, to rebuild and repair the physical infrastructure, and to implement mitigation activities to reduce the impact of future disasters. At this stage influenza disease activity will have returned to levels normally seen for seasonal influenza. It is expected that the pandemic virus will behave as a seasonal influenza A virus. Even so, it is important to maintain constant surveillance and be ready to update pandemic preparedness and respond as needed to any change. Pandemic waves can be separated by months, and a critical task will be to balance information and activities with the possibility of another wave.

The post-peak period signifies that pandemic activity appears to be decreasing; however, it is uncertain if additional waves will occur, and communities need to be prepared for a second wave. Unlike nearly all other disasters, pandemic recovery duration and investments must be tempered by priorities for pandemic preparedness for follow-on waves. After a pandemic wave is over, it can be expected that many people will be affected in a variety of ways. Many may have lost loved ones, suffer from fatigue, or have financial losses as a result of the interruption of business. Governments or other authorities should ensure that these concerns can be addressed and support the rebuilding of the society (WHO, 2009).

Questions to be addressed in the recovery phase outlined by WHO (2009) are as follows:

- Is there a plan in place to ensure the quick revitalization of the community after a pandemic?
- Who should be responsible to provide social and psychological support to affected families and communities?

- How will support referrals be handled?
- Is there a mechanism in place to assess economic losses and to provide financial support to affected groups?

Essential services must develop and implement recovery plans for their service or organization:

- Define responsibilities for social, psychological, and practical support to affected families and communities. If needed, organize training and education for personnel involved.
- Assess how existing community groups (religious groups/churches, sports groups) can contribute to rebuilding the society. Identify contact persons within these groups.
- Consider whether recovery after a pandemic needs financial support from the government. If so, develop criteria for financial support and seek ways to ensure availability of funds.

Community and healthcare leaders should evaluate the following:

- Ensure evaluation of the response to the pandemic, once the first wave is over. Evaluation should focus on the response at all levels and should lead to recommendations for improvement.
- Ensure that results of research studies, both local and international, are made public to support improvement of response strategies and implementation of disaster plans.

The scope of emergency preparedness and recovery planning can be quite large, and as with the initial disaster response, it is important to think outside of the hospital when defining what essential nonhospital services can be restored quickly. OSHA (2009) recommends the following:

- Continue institutional surveillance of patients and facility/clinic staff for influenza-like illness.
- Return to normal facility operations as soon as possible.
- Review pandemic influenza plan based on experience during the first pandemic wave. Incorporate lessons learned into preparation for subsequent pandemic waves.
- Identify and anticipate resource and supply chain issues.
- Continue to emphasize communication within healthcare facilities and between healthcare facilities, state health departments, and the federal government.

Planning and preparedness for implementing pandemic strategies is complex and requires participation by all levels of government and all segments of society. Pandemic mitigation reaction and recovery strategies call for specific actions by individuals, families, businesses and employers, and organizations. Building a foundation of community and individual and family preparedness and developing and delivering effective risk communication for the public in advance of a pandemic is critical. If embraced earnestly, these efforts will result in enhanced ability to respond not only to pandemic influenza but also to multiple hazards and threats. Although the challenge is formidable, the consequences of facing a severe pandemic unprepared will be intolerable.

KEY POINTS

- When a pandemic influenza virus emerges, its global spread is considered inevitable.
- Preparedness activities should assume that the entire world population is susceptible.
- Countries might, through measures such as border closures and travel restrictions, delay arrival of the virus but cannot stop it.
- Most people have little or no immunity to a pandemic virus. Infection and illness rates soar. A substantial percentage of the world's population will require some form of medical care.
- Nations are unlikely to have the staff, facilities, equipment, and hospital beds needed to cope with large numbers of people who suddenly fall ill.
- Death rates are high, largely determined by four factors: the number of people who become infected, the virulence of the virus, the underlying characteristics and vulnerability of affected populations, and the effectiveness of preventive measures.
- Past pandemics have spread globally in two and sometimes three waves.
- The need for vaccine is likely to outstrip supply.
- A pandemic can create a shortage of hospital beds, ventilators, and other supplies. Surge capacity at nontraditional sites such as schools may be created to cope with demand.
- Difficult decisions will need to be made regarding who gets antiviral drugs and vaccines.
- Travel bans, closings of schools and businesses, and cancellations of events could have major impact on communities and citizens.
- Care for sick family members and fear of exposure can result in significant worker absenteeism.

- Communications and information are critical components of pandemic response. Education and outreach are critical to preparing for a pandemic. Understanding what a pandemic is, what needs to be done at all levels to prepare for pandemic influenza, and what could happen during a pandemic helps us make informed decisions both as individuals and as a nation.

CRITICAL QUESTIONS

1. Considering your local community, how would your organization implement the U.S. DHHS Pandemic Influenza Plan that provides guidance to national, state, and local policy makers and health departments?
2. How would your community prepare for a pandemic outbreak?
3. Identify the guidance, checklists, and information that will assist healthcare providers and service organizations in your local area in planning and responding to a pandemic flu outbreak?
4. What are the local, national, and global resources that provide healthcare workers and other public officials and communities with real-time pandemic information?

REFERENCES

Agency for Healthcare Research and Quality (AHRQ). (2005). Altered standards of care in mass casualty events: Bioterrorism and other public health emergencies. Retrieved from http://www.ahrq.gov/research/altstand/

Agency for Healthcare Research and Quality (AHRQ). (2007). Mass medical care with scarce resources: A community planning guide. Retrieved from http://www.ahrq.gov/research/mce/

Agency for Healthcare Research and Quality (AHRQ). (2009). Hospital surge model. Retrieved from http://hosptialsurgemodel.ahrq.gov

Barry, J. M. (2004). *The great influenza: The epic story of the deadliest plague in history*. New York: Viking.

Beach, M. (2010). *Disaster preparedness and management*. Philadelphia: F. A. Davis.

Cantrill, S. (2007). Alternative care sites. Retrieved from http://www.ahrq.gov/research/mce/mce6.htm

Centers for Disease Control and Prevention (CDC). (2007). *Community strategy for pandemic influenza mitigation in the United States*. Washington, DC: Department of Health and Human Services.

Centers for Disease Control and Prevention (CDC). (n.d.-a). History of flu pandemics. Retrieved from http://pandemicflu.gov/professional/community/commitigation.html

Centers for Disease Control and Prevention. (n.d.-b). Goals of community measures. Retrieved from http://www.cdc.gov/media/pdf/MitigationSlides.pdf

Columbia University School of Nursing. (2008). Adapting standards of care under extreme conditions: Guidance for professionals during disasters, pandemics, and extreme emergencies. Retrieved from http://www.nursingworld.org/MainMenuCategories/HealthcareandPolicyIssues/DPR/TheLawEthicsofDisasterResponse/AdaptingStandardsofCare.aspx

Ito, T., Couceiro, J. N., Kelm, S., Baum, L. G., Krauss, S., Castrucci, M. R., et al. (1998). Molecular basis for the generation in pigs of influenza A viruses with pandemic potential. *Journal of Virology, 72*(9), 7367–7373.

Joint Commission. (2006). *Surge hospitals: Providing safe care in emergencies.* Oakbrook Terrace, IL: Joint Commission Resources.

Martin, P. M.-G. (2006). 2,500-year evolution of the term epidemic. *Emerging Infectious Diseases, 12*(6), 976–980.

Mass Medical Care with Scarce Resources (MMCSR, 2010). Retrieved from http://www.ahrq.gov/research/

Moore, P. (2007). *The little book of pandemics: 50 of the world's most virulent plagues and infectious diseases.* London: Collins.

National Institute of Allergy and Infectious Diseases. (2009a). Flu (influenza) antigenic drift. Retrieved from http://www.niaid.nih.gov/topics/Flu/Research/basic/Pages/AntigenicDrift Illustration.aspx

National Institute of Allergy and Infectious Diseases. (2009b). Flu (influenza) antigenic shift. Retrieved from http://www.niaid.nih.gov/topics/Flu/Research/basic/Pages/AntigenicShift Illustration.aspx

National Institutes of Health. (2009). NCBI bookshelf. Retrieved from http://www.ncbi.nlm.nih.gov/bookshelf/br.fcgi?book=glyco2&part=ch39

Novel Swine-Origin Influenza A (H_1N_1) Virus Investigation Team. (2009). Emergence of a novel swine-origin influenza A (H_1N_1). *New England Journal of Medicine, 360,* 2605–2615.

Occupational Safety and Health Administration (OSHA). (2009). Pandemic influenza preparedness and response guidance for healthcare workers and healthcare employers. Retrieved from http://www.osha.gov/Publications/OSHA_pandemic_health.pdf

Pendergrast, M. (2010). *Inside the outbreaks: The elite medical detectives of the epidemic intelligence service.* Boston: Houghton.

U.S. Department of Health and Human Services (DHHS). (2005). National strategy for pandemic influenza. Retrieved from http://www.flu.gov/professional/federal/pandemic-influenza.pdf

U.S. Department of Health and Human Services (DHHS). (2010). Pandemic planning assumptions. Retrieved from http://www.flu.gov/professional/pandplan.html

U.S. Department of Homeland Security. (2006). *Pandemic influenza preparedness, response, and recovery guide for critical infrastructure and key resources.* Washington, DC: U.S. Department of Homeland Security.

U.S. Government Accounting Office (GAO). (2008). *Influenza pandemic: HHS Needs to continue its actions and finalize guidance for pharmaceutical interventions.* Washington, DC: U.S. Government Accounting Office.

Varki, A., Cummings, R. D., Esko, J., Freeze, H. H., Stanley, P., Bertozzi, C. R., et al. (2009). Essentials of glycobiology. In *Essentials of Glycobiology.* La Jolla, CA: The Consortium of Glycobiology Editors.

Webster, R. G. (2002). The importance of animal influenza for human disease. *Vaccine, 20*, S16–S20.

World Health Organization (WHO). (2005a). H_5N_1 avian influenza: Timeline. Retrieved from http://www.who.int/csr/disease/avian_influenza/Timeline_28_10a.pdf

World Health Organization (WHO). (2005b). Checklist for influenza pandemic preparedness planning. Retrieved from http://www.who.int/csr/resources/publications/influenza/WHO_CDS_CSR_GIP_2005_4/end/

World Health Organization (WHO). (2007). Recommendation for national measures before and during pandemics. Retrieved from http://www.flu.gov/professional/community/commitigation.html#XIV

World Health Organization (WHO). (2009, April). Pandemic influenza preparedness and response: A WHO document. Retrieved http://www.who.int/csr/disease/influenza/pipguidance2009/en/

World Health Organization (WHO). (2010a). Global alert and response. Retrieved from http://www.who.int/csr/disease/avian_influenza/phase/en/

World Health Organization (WHO). (2010b). Clinical aspects of pandemic 2009 influenza: A H_1N_1 virus infection. *New England Journal of Medicine, 362*, 1708–1719.

CHAPTER 12

Ethical and Legal Issues in Epidemiology

"Earth provides enough to satisfy every man's need, but not every man's greed."
—Mahatma Gandhi

Kiran Macha
John P. McDonough

OBJECTIVES

- Describe the history behind the international formulation of ethical guidelines.
- Explain the reasons that fuel unethical research in developing countries.
- Discuss the ethical standards you would use in your epidemiological research.
- Describe the role of epidemiologists in legal issues.

INTRODUCTION

In this chapter advanced practice nurses will learn about the origin of ethics as a subject and ethical principles in general. Facts shared in this chapter apply to every field. Ethical principles should be applied in our clinical practice and research to refine the difference that we intend to make in others life.

The question of ethics arises when our conscience and thoughts fail to agree. The greatest unethical disasters have happened in this world because of discrimination based on race, gender, color, accent, religion, and citizenship. The slave stories of Kingsley Plantation in Florida are no different from modern-day intellectual slavery. Every religion offers unbiased truths to educate its followers in certain ethical principles. The Ten Commandants received by Moses could not stop unethical disasters. Hippocrates' approach in conducting research was to "do no harm." The lives of Gautama Buddha and Mahatma Gandhi (**Figure 12-1**) were founded on Ahimsa (teachings of nonviolence). Yet, the most powerful proven ethical teaching has yet to inhibit humans from unethical acts.

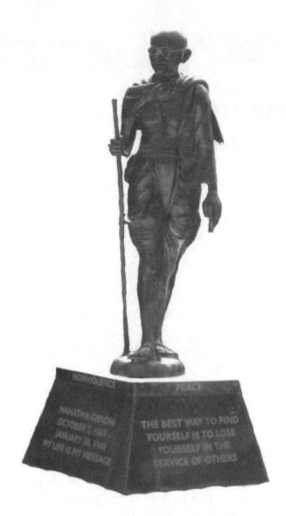

FIGURE 12-1   Mahatma Gandhi. Simplicity is the truth of life.
Source: Picture courtesy of Dr. Kiran Macha.

With conscience and morality being masked, unethical incidences continue to oc-cur throughout the world. World wars have divided nations, and the arrogance of self-declaration of racial superiority by some leaders has breached the respect of hu-manity's own species. The lessons learned from injustices of the past are still not ap-parently adequate to prevent human actions that threaten our own existence. For example, there is a lack of transparency in the secret programs carried out in the quest of creating the deadliest weapon. The mind, considered a divine gift to humans on this earth, has often been mentored along the wrong path.

UNFORGIVABLE HISTORY OF HUMANS _____

Wars create great energy, which is for the most part uncontrollable. After World War II numerous incidences of human torture and experimentation were unearthed. Events beyond human imagination happened under the rule of Nazis. The Nuremberg trial, conducted after the war, included a doctors' trial involving physicians who conducted experiments on civilians, prisoners, and those in concentration camps. The research experiments (such as on the effects of freezing, poisonous gases, epidemic jaundice, sterilization, transplantation, and seawater) were conducted against the will and without obtaining informed consent of the participants. All those found and tried who participated in conducting these crimes were executed. The bioethical response after learning the incidences of these experiments against the voluntary will of the subjects led to the development of the "Nuremberg Code."

What if a nation's health system discriminates against its own citizens? In 1932 the U.S. Public Health Service along with the Tuskegee Institute began conducting a gender-specific study in the American African community in Macon County, Alabama. Black men who either suffered from syphilis or did not were recruited into the study group. Even though subjects were diagnosed with syphilis, they were not informed about it. Local physicians were hired to conduct free medical examinations, and meals were provided to the subjects for participating in the study. In 1945 the antibiotic penicillin became available, but subjects were not treated. Unfortunately, medical associations in the United States supported continuation of the study. In 1972, after 40 years, the Tuskegee study was stopped after its existence was publicized and federal inquiries were made. The participants were later compensated. The outcome of such unethical study by the nation's largest health agency was the creation of the President's Council on Bioethics; in addition, the Centers for Disease Control and Prevention now supports research on such bioethical issues. The National Research Act was enacted in 1974 to address bioethical issues, and the National Commission for the Protection of Human Subjects of Biomedical and Behavioral Research was formed.

The profits of the drug industry are driven by new drug innovations. Previously, new drugs were released into the market without going through trials. As a result, members of the general populace became the scapegoats of new, untested drug innovations, with adverse effects identified from the user's feedback or complaints. Thalidomide was one such drug that was released into the market in 1950 to alleviate pregnancy-related symptoms such as morning sickness. Later, thalidomide was identified as a teratogenic drug, and 12,000 children were born with birth defects. In 1962 thalidomide was withdrawn from the international community. The Food, Drug, and Cosmetic Act as amended mandates that drug manufacturers must prove the safety and effectiveness of a drug before they market it in the United States. Today, the U.S. Food and Drug Administration has tightened the testing and safety of the drugs used in pregnancy. Even though thalidomide was proven to cause birth defects, ethical research was conducted to explore the possibility of its use for other conditions. This research has shown that the angiogenic properties of thalidomide, in combination with dexamethasone, can help multiple myeloma patients.

Other unethical practices of drug companies include the development of drugs in one country and testing in another country without sharing the benefits in the country where the testing was done. The international community is actively monitoring the unethical practices of testing, although it is challenging to control the activities of drug company giants.

Just as the world started thinking the Nuremberg Code of 1948 would restore the confidence of people in the integrity of research experiments, the cold war fueled secret deadly experiments. Humans believed they controlled the atom, but the bombing of Hiroshima and Nagasaki in 1945 taught us the lesson of how the atom can control and impact our lives. A reporter published an investigative report in 1993 regarding secret radiation experiments carried out by federal agencies on U.S. citizens between 1940 and 1960. The Plutonium Experiment was carried out by injecting plutonium into human subjects to study the effects on the body. Another experiment involved giving iron-59 to pregnant women to obtain nutritional information. U.S military personnel were deliberately exposed to radiation and radioactive material. A military manned aircraft was flown through radioactive clouds in the Marshall Islands in 1955. The subjects in these experiments were not informed about the research experiments and the radiation to which they would be exposed. The truth was hidden for years by federal agencies, ignoring the Nuremberg Code. After an inquiry was ordered by former President Clinton, he officially apologized after learning that the American government had acted against the welfare of its own people.

In 1964 the World Health Association developed bioethical principles for conducting medical research involving humans as subjects, principles known as the "Declaration of Helsinki." The principles protect the rights of humans involved in medical research, which must be conducted for either diagnostic or therapeutic benefits. The World Health Association meets regularly to review and update these principles. The Declaration, as amended in 2008, follows:

WORLD MEDICAL ASSOCIATION DECLARATION OF HELSINKI
Ethical Principles for Medical Research Involving Human Subjects

Adopted by the 18th WMA General Assembly, Helsinki, Finland, June 1964, and amended by the:

29th WMA General Assembly, Tokyo, Japan, October 1975

35th WMA General Assembly, Venice, Italy, October 1983

41st WMA General Assembly, Hong Kong, September 1989

48th WMA General Assembly, Somerset West, Republic of South Africa, October 1996

52nd WMA General Assembly, Edinburgh, Scotland, October 2000

53rd WMA General Assembly, Washington, 2002 (Note of Clarification on paragraph 29 added)

55th WMA General Assembly, Tokyo 2004, (Note of Clarification on Paragraph 30 added)

59th WMA General Assembly, Seoul, October 2008

A. INTRODUCTION

1. The World Medical Association (WMA) has developed the Declaration of Helsinki as a statement of ethical principles for medical research involving human subjects, including research on identifiable human material and data.

   The Declaration is intended to be read as a whole and each of its constituent paragraphs should not be applied without consideration of all other relevant paragraphs.

2. Although the Declaration is addressed primarily to physicians, the WMA encourages other participants in medical research involving human subjects to adopt these principles.

3. It is the duty of the physician to promote and safeguard the health of patients, including those who are involved in medical research. The physician's knowledge and conscience are dedicated to the fulfillment of this duty.

4. The Declaration of Geneva of the WMA binds the physician with the words, "The health of my patient will be my first consideration," and the International Code of Medical Ethics declares that, "A physician shall act in the patient's best interest when providing medical care."

5. Medical progress is based on research that ultimately must include studies involving human subjects. Populations that are underrepresented in medical research should be provided appropriate access to participation in research.

6. In medical research involving human subjects, the well-being of the individual research subject must take precedence over all other interests.

7. The primary purpose of medical research involving human subjects is to understand the causes, development and effects of diseases and improve preventive, diagnostic and therapeutic interventions (methods, procedures and treatments). Even the best current interventions must be evaluated continually through research for their safety, effectiveness, efficiency, accessibility and quality.

8. In medical practice and in medical research, most interventions involve risks and burdens.

9. Medical research is subject to ethical standards that promote respect for all human subjects and protect their health and rights. Some research populations are particularly vulnerable and need special protection. These include those who cannot give or refuse consent for themselves and those who may be vulnerable to coercion or undue influence.

10. Physicians should consider the ethical, legal and regulatory norms and standards for research involving human subjects in their own countries as well as applicable international norms and standards. No national or international ethical, legal or regulatory requirement should reduce or eliminate any of the protections for research subjects set forth in this Declaration.

B. PRINCIPLES FOR ALL MEDICAL RESEARCH

11. It is the duty of physicians who participate in medical research to protect the life, health, dignity, integrity, right to self-determination, privacy, and confidentiality of personal information of research subjects.

12. Medical research involving human subjects must conform to generally accepted scientific principles, be based on a thorough knowledge of the scientific literature, other relevant sources of information, and adequate laboratory and, as appropriate, animal experimentation. The welfare of animals used for research must be respected.

13. Appropriate caution must be exercised in the conduct of medical research that may harm the environment.

14. The design and performance of each research study involving human subjects must be clearly described in a research protocol. The protocol should contain a statement of the ethical considerations involved and should indicate how the principles in this Declaration have been addressed. The protocol should include information regarding funding, sponsors, institutional affiliations, other potential conflicts of interest, incentives for subjects and provisions for treating and/or compensating subjects who are harmed as a consequence of participation in the research study. The protocol should describe arrangements for post-study access by study subjects to interventions identified as beneficial in the study or access to other appropriate care or benefits.

15. The research protocol must be submitted for consideration, comment, guidance and approval to a research ethics committee before the study begins. This committee must be independent of the researcher, the sponsor and any other undue influence. It must take into consideration the laws and regulations of the country or countries in which the research is to be performed as well as applicable international norms and standards but these must not be allowed to reduce or eliminate any of the protections for research subjects set forth in this Declaration. The committee must have the right to monitor ongoing studies. The researcher must

provide monitoring information to the committee, especially information about any serious adverse events. No change to the protocol may be made without consideration and approval by the committee.

16. Medical research involving human subjects must be conducted only by individuals with the appropriate scientific training and qualifications. Research on patients or healthy volunteers requires the supervision of a competent and appropriately qualified physician or other health care professional. The responsibility for the protection of research subjects must always rest with the physician or other health care professional and never the research subjects, even though they have given consent.

17. Medical research involving a disadvantaged or vulnerable population or community is only justified if the research is responsive to the health needs and priorities of this population or community and if there is a reasonable likelihood that this population or community stands to benefit from the results of the research.

18. Every medical research study involving human subjects must be preceded by careful assessment of predictable risks and burdens to the individuals and communities involved in the research in comparison with foreseeable benefits to them and to other individuals or communities affected by the condition under investigation.

19. Every clinical trial must be registered in a publicly accessible database before recruitment of the first subject.

20. Physicians may not participate in a research study involving human subjects unless they are confident that the risks involved have been adequately assessed and can be satisfactorily managed. Physicians must immediately stop a study when the risks are found to outweigh the potential benefits or when there is conclusive proof of positive and beneficial results.

21. Medical research involving human subjects may only be conducted if the importance of the objective outweighs the inherent risks and burdens to the research subjects.

22. Participation by competent individuals as subjects in medical research must be voluntary. Although it may be appropriate to consult family members or community leaders, no competent individual may be enrolled in a research study unless he or she freely agrees.

23. Every precaution must be taken to protect the privacy of research subjects and the confidentiality of their personal information and to minimize the impact of the study on their physical, mental and social integrity.

24. In medical research involving competent human subjects, each potential subject must be adequately informed of the aims, methods, sources of funding, any possible conflicts of interest, institutional affiliations of the researcher, the anticipated benefits and potential risks of the study and the discomfort it may entail, and any other relevant aspects of the study. The potential subject must be

informed of the right to refuse to participate in the study or to withdraw consent to participate at any time without reprisal. Special attention should be given to the specific information needs of individual potential subjects as well as to the methods used to deliver the information. After ensuring that the potential subject has understood the information, the physician or another appropriately qualified individual must then seek the potential subject's freely-given informed consent, preferably in writing. If the consent cannot be expressed in writing, the non-written consent must be formally documented and witnessed.

25. For medical research using identifiable human material or data, physicians must normally seek consent for the collection, analysis, storage and/or reuse. There may be situations where consent would be impossible or impractical to obtain for such research or would pose a threat to the validity of the research. In such situations the research may be done only after consideration and approval of a research ethics committee.

26. When seeking informed consent for participation in a research study the physician should be particularly cautious if the potential subject is in a dependent relationship with the physician or may consent under duress. In such situations the informed consent should be sought by an appropriately qualified individual who is completely independent of this relationship.

27. For a potential research subject who is incompetent, the physician must seek informed consent from the legally authorized representative. These individuals must not be included in a research study that has no likelihood of benefit for them unless it is intended to promote the health of the population represented by the potential subject, the research cannot instead be performed with competent persons, and the research entails only minimal risk and minimal burden.

28. When a potential research subject who is deemed incompetent is able to give assent to decisions about participation in research, the physician must seek that assent in addition to the consent of the legally authorized representative. The potential subject's dissent should be respected.

29. Research involving subjects who are physically or mentally incapable of giving consent, for example, unconscious patients, may be done only if the physical or mental condition that prevents giving informed consent is a necessary characteristic of the research population. In such circumstances the physician should seek informed consent from the legally authorized representative. If no such representative is available and if the research cannot be delayed, the study may proceed without informed consent provided that the specific reasons for involving subjects with a condition that renders them unable to give informed consent have been stated in the research protocol and the study has been approved by a research ethics committee. Consent to remain in the research should be obtained as soon as possible from the subject or a legally authorized representative.

30. Authors, editors and publishers all have ethical obligations with regard to the publication of the results of research. Authors have a duty to make publicly available the results of their research on human subjects and are accountable for the completeness and accuracy of their reports. They should adhere to accepted guidelines for ethical reporting. Negative and inconclusive as well as positive results should be published or otherwise made publicly available. Sources of funding, institutional affiliations and conflicts of interest should be declared in the publication. Reports of research not in accordance with the principles of this Declaration should not be accepted for publication.

C. ADDITIONAL PRINCIPLES FOR MEDICAL RESEARCH COMBINED WITH MEDICAL CARE

31. The physician may combine medical research with medical care only to the extent that the research is justified by its potential preventive, diagnostic or therapeutic value and if the physician has good reason to believe that participation in the research study will not adversely affect the health of the patients who serve as research subjects.

32. The benefits, risks, burdens and effectiveness of a new intervention must be tested against those of the best current proven intervention, except in the following circumstances:
    * The use of placebo, or no treatment, is acceptable in studies where no current proven intervention exists; or
    * Where for compelling and scientifically sound methodological reasons the use of placebo is necessary to determine the efficacy or safety of an intervention and the patients who receive placebo or no treatment will not be subject to any risk of serious or irreversible harm. Extreme care must be taken to avoid abuse of this option.

33. At the conclusion of the study, patients entered into the study are entitled to be informed about the outcome of the study and to share any benefits that result from it, for example, access to interventions identified as beneficial in the study or to other appropriate care or benefits.

34. The physician must fully inform the patient which aspects of the care are related to the research. The refusal of a patient to participate in a study or the patient's decision to withdraw from the study must never interfere with the patient–physician relationship.

35. In the treatment of a patient, where proven interventions do not exist or have been ineffective, the physician, after seeking expert advice, with informed consent from the patient or a legally authorized representative, may use an unproven intervention if in the physician's judgement it offers hope of saving life, reestablishing health or alleviating suffering. Where possible, this intervention

should be made the object of research, designed to evaluate its safety and efficacy. In all cases, new information should be recorded and, where appropriate, made publicly available.

Courtesy: World Medical Association, www.wma.net. Web link: http://www.wma. net/en/20activities/10ethics/10helsinki/index.html

Permission granted for publication on May 24, 2010.

BELMONT REPORT

In the Belmont Report (DHHS, 2008), the fundamental ethical principles that apply to all human subjects involved in research were identified as *respect for persons*, *beneficence*, and *justice*.

Respect for Persons

This principle includes the concepts of *autonomy* and *protection to diminished autonomy*. The participation of human subjects in research studies should be voluntary, and the subjects should be provided with adequate information, including the benefits and risks of the study. Informed consent is a vital step to protect the interests of the participants. The subjects should be protected from harmful activities; risk to the subjects should not be ignored based on the benefits. Subjects suffering from conditions that affect judgment, such as illness, emotions, and other conditions making them vulnerable, should be protected. The individual's judgment capacity should be reevaluated regularly because the subject's physical and mental status may change with time. If a subject decides to leave at any point of time during the study, his or her decision must be respected. Language barriers should also be minimized in research studies.

Beneficence

This principle includes the concepts of *do not harm* and *maximize the benefits*. Benefits to subjects in any research study should be maximized, and the risk to subjects should be minimized. An ethical approach that reduces harm to the subjects is through learning from past research and also by improving knowledge about specific interventions. If an intervention or a procedure is already known to cause harm, it should be avoided. Any research involving children and elderly should be carefully evaluated.

Justice

This principle includes the concept of *fairness*. The subjects are to be treated equally, and fairness in decisions made by the investigator is encouraged. Benefits and risks should be equally distributed across participants. The benefit to a subject should never be denied, and at the same time risk should not be imposed on a particular group. The benefits derived from the study should help the community if the study has been paid for by the public. Discrimination factors such as race, gender, ethnicity, and economic status should not play any role in the selection of participants, inclusion and exclusion criteria, intervention methods, or the distribution of benefits.

THIRD WORLD AS A SCAPEGOAT

Many studies conducted in the African countries by international drug companies and health organizations are most unethical and breach the Declaration of Helsinki. The high incidence of human immunodeficiency virus (HIV) and poverty in the African continent attracts many organizations to conduct studies. The poorer governments cannot afford to provide antiretroviral drugs to their HIV-infected people. Drug companies are generally not willing to share the benefits of the research studies conducted in these poor nations, believing they cannot afford the price of the drug after the companies have spent millions of dollars on research. We are aware that antiretroviral drugs given to pregnant HIV-infected women can reduce the incidence of HIV transmission to infants. Observational studies are conducted on these HIV-infected women to learn more about the long-term effects of HIV using methods similar to the Tuskegee study (Angell, 1997). The treatment regime is often downgraded to monotherapy in developing countries, overlooking the fact that the virus can develop resistance to the drug. Even though some of the HIV drugs can be prepared at affordable costs in developing countries, finalizing international trade contracts become barriers to treatment (Thomas, 1998). No law, declaration, oath, or coalition seems capable of addressing this human rights issue. The global inequalities caused by unethical research have resulted in the incidence of HIV climbing to pandemic levels. The only way past this legal discrimination was medical pluralism, exploring avenues other than Western medicine such as Ayurvedic, homeopathic, and Unani medicine. The law now mandates that HIV-positive findings are to be communicated to the spouse and family members.

Studies have shown that the long-term exposure to chlorine can cause bladder cancer (Villanueva et al., 2007). Water is chlorinated in many developing and developed countries to contain the spread of cholera disease. Water in swimming pools contains high levels of chlorine, which is absorbed through the skin. The policies in these countries have not changed even though today we know chlorine exposure can cause bladder cancer. Outbreaks of cholera no longer occur frequently, and the chlorination process is carried out without any legitimate need. Similarly, pesticides and insecticides are sprayed on water bodies to control the *Anopheles* mosquito, the malaria vector that breeds in stagnant water. Local people drink water that is available and are exposed to many toxic chemicals. The effects of such actions are seen in pregnant women and children. More advanced ways of dealing with public health issues cost money; even though the governments can afford changes in practice, they are not generally willing to recognize the need for and implement changes in policy.

- How can we stop human rights violations by the countries that advocate them?
- Research is done on humans, and the benefits should be enjoyed by them. What factors do you believe play a role in creating barriers?

ETHICAL ISSUES ASSOCIATED WITH GENETIC TESTING

Advances in genetic testing methods have enabled us to predict the likely occurrence of the diseases in a person's lifetime. This awareness can be beneficial to individuals, but it can also be emotionally challenging. Infants are not mature enough to give consent for genetic testing. Some religions may not favor the idea of disclosure of God's will. Also, medical insurance companies may take advantage of a subject's genetic history and may not provide coverage if an identified disease is not treatable. Genetic testing kits available in the market can be misused by testing the blood that is given for some other reasons.

Genetic testing is not generally cost-effective, and false-positives and false-negatives are another concern. Pharmacogenetics has changed the way one gets treated based on a person's genetic composition. The benefits and risks of genetic testing depend on each individual situation and cannot be easily justified if an emotional or discriminatory event occurs. Informed consent, confidentiality, privacy, and discrimination are some of the ethical issues associated with genetic testing.

- What if genetic testing is made mandatory by healthcare organizations?
- How can one counter the beliefs of religious groups on genetic testing?

ETHICAL ISSUES ASSOCIATED WITH PUBLIC HEALTH DATA

Hospitals and clinics continually collect patient demographic and health information. With recent technological advancements, patient information is now stored in the form of electronic medical records. A patient's health information is reportable in certain situations to local public health departments. Because of legal challenges, the courts may order public health departments to disclose patient information. This is a tricky situation, because nondisclosure of the information can affect millions and, if disclosed, the privacy of the patients is breached. In the hospital setting, many health-care professionals can access sensitive information such as drugs, fertility, and emotional conditions and can take advantage of them.

Some photocopy machines are equipped with hard drives that store all information from the scanned or photocopied documents. When these machines break down, they are sometimes sold to companies that repair them. The information stored in the hard drives is not erased, and cases have been reported where the confidential information was leaked out.

Health care in countries such as the United Kingdom and Denmark is controlled by the government. Any research conducted using patients' electronic medical records is supported by public tax dollars. Many ethical issues are involved in research done on public citizens that is paid for by them.

- Is it ethical to compromise the health of millions when a well-identified problem exists in our community (but the public is not fully advised)?
- How can we balance the rights of an individual and public safety?

HONORARY COAUTHORSHIP

Honorary coauthorship is not an uncommon practice because some department heads in academia and healthcare facilities press junior faculty and researchers to do this. These issues are difficult to deal with, because continued presence of this practice in a system for years can create dependency even as sharing of opportunities and knowledge occurs. Maintaining balance in relationships at the workplace can be challenging if this type of invasive practice is frequent. Research on honorary coauthorship has shown that encouraging such activities can dilute the quality of a research paper and is not beneficial in the long run (O'Brien, 2009). Discussing such issues with higher administration and defining the role of researchers in the study may solve some of the issues.

- What measure will you take to protect your epidemiological research work from the day you start?

CYBERSPACE RESEARCH AND ETHICAL DILEMMAS

The Internet has revolutionized the ways of reaching people for various purposes. Universities across the world are encouraging research through the Internet, and students are conducting online surveys. Ethical issues associated with online-based research include informed consent without face-to-face contact, accuracy of the information gathered, technological issues, access to e-mail identifications, and biases associated with qualitative research.

Public websites are encouraging people to be connected every minute of the day. Public websites offer an opportunity to feed brains with all kinds of updates, whether one needs these or not. The personal information of users is often available on these websites, with many issues of poor privacy protection reported. At times, the availability of data and the intentions of research using these raise serious concerns regarding confidentiality, consent, and privacy issues. Negative outcomes such as emotional reactions associated with online research are not yet studied, and a cautious approach is recommended.

- The response of the chief executive officer of a famous public website to compromised privacy settings is that the website is for sharing information. Is it ethical to use private information without educating users as to this possibility?
- With the modern-day technology we use, are we encouraging stalking?

ETHICAL ISSUES WITH RESEARCH INVOLVING THE ELDERLY

The elderly population is an interesting group to research because the aging process multiplies many medical conditions. The most common conditions that interfere with the informed consent process are confusion and dementia. With growing cultural diversity in the United States, cultural issues may also arise. The elderly are at risk for violation of privacy, and yet researchers may continue doing their research on these participants for extended periods of time. Any research involving technology may be challenging to the elderly, and they may not welcome this change. Institutional review boards should carefully review any research involving the elderly and take care to protect them from harm or abuse.

- Is it ethical to involve elderly persons with cognitive problems in research?

CONTROVERSIAL PUBLIC HEALTH ISSUES

With the rise in the incidence of autism in children, numerous studies have been designed. Numerous publications have flooded the medical journals linking autism to vaccinations. Andrew Wakefield, a British surgeon and researcher, held in 1998 that there was a link between the measles, mumps, and rubella (MMR) vaccine and autism. The causal relationship between the MMR vaccine and autism was disproved by studies done in Japan and Denmark. However, many parents feared and did not want their children to receive the MMR vaccine based on information they had heard. Wakefield's research was sponsored by solicitors, and he performed procedures on children based on his own perceptions—not an accepted scientific or ethical approach to research. After several years of inquiry, the General Medical Council (a medical licensing body in the United Kingdom) took Wakefield off the medical register for his professional misconduct. Although doing research can be a worthwhile undertaking, the actions of this researcher in boosting his ideas with the support of mercenary sponsors impacted autistic children's health by increasing their susceptibility to deadly viruses and led to the misuse of public health resources.

In the past, quarantine was often considered the best preventive method. In the modern world this practice is still applied for some diseases. Those who were suffering from scarlet fever were quarantined, and there are many similar practices worldwide. Advanced practice nurses should understand the limits and consequences of implementing such options and the repercussions of decisions that may affect millions.

- What is the best approach to controversial public health issues?

TRAUMATIC EXPERIENCE OF NATURAL DISASTERS

Hurricanes Katrina and Rita blasted the eastern and western parts of Louisiana so badly that more than 1,800 people lost their lives. Many complained that the government response was poor and inadequate. The evacuation process, provision of basic needs and health services, and future planning was a huge burden to state governments. Many people lost everything they owned, were at risk of exposure to the environment and diseases, and were not sure of any long-term support from the government. Resources were compromised as hurricanes hit the state one after another and in different parts of the state.

In 1994, in the western parts of India, outbreaks of plague were reported in many villages after three decades of silence. More than 10 million tablets of tetracycline and thousands of tons of insecticides were used to counter the situation. The number of cases started decreasing after 2 months. Some family members were not prepared to bury the dead. In some cases officials had to bury the dead even before family members could see them. Lack of surveillance was one of the causes of resurgence of outbreaks; increased, continual surveillance was able to suppress similar outbreaks that later occurred. Effective communication, training of public health professionals, immediate prophylaxis, and dissemination of information eventually contained the plague.

Decisions made by public health professionals during disasters should be based on the principles of autonomy, beneficence, and justice. The local community should be involved in the planning process. Communication, transparency, and resource management are very important in the management of disasters to protect the public health.

- How can we monitor the application of ethical principles in decisions made during disasters?

2010 GULF OF MEXICO OIL SPILL

Never before have we seen impacts on such a large scale as that experienced with the BP oil spill in the Gulf of Mexico. Even with the experience gained from the Exxon *Valdez* spill in Alaska, we have not had such a similar unfortunate opportunity to study the effects of a disaster of this magnitude on the environment and on humans. Predictions of impacts associated with the human error leading to this catastrophe are beyond calculation. The warm-water habitats of plankton, corals, shrimp, dolphins, pelicans, and countless other life forms have been contaminated beyond short-term restoration. Millions of gallons of dispersants were also sprayed into the region. Not only were beaches spoiled and islands of oil plumes identified in deep water, the mixture of water, chemicals, oil, and warm temperatures in the region present an unknown phenomenon that threatens the regional health and economy. The companies that manage these oil fields were not prepared to deal with such leaks in deep water. With the hurricane season approaching, threatening weather made an impact on plans to stop the oil leak. The federal government was attempting to manage the cleanup by overseeing operations of the oil company but had little equipment or skills to deal with this untenable situation. The government temporarily blocked all future plans for deep water oil drilling, reeling from lessons learned. For all living things in the Gulf, another paradise on Earth has been destroyed, with impacts on public health and the environment years into the future.

- What do you think about this environmental catastrophe?
- Is it ethical that the oil industry makes profits in the billions while ignoring safety?

RESOURCES FOR PUBLIC HEALTH ETHICS

Advanced practice nurses who identify potential in gathering health data should first understand the global impacts of their research question. One should anticipate and answer ethical and legal questions associated with his or her research study. Most solutions come from studying very similar situations that happened in the past. Health beliefs are strengthened from facts revealed from analyzing health data. In conducting research, one must remember that the public trust is in you, and you must not fail to honor this trust. Evidence-based facts in action fuel public health advocacy and health policy changes.

Some of the following resources may help you as you meditate on ethical issues:

- Journal
  Public Health Ethics
    http://phe.oxfordjournals.org/
- Websites
  Ethics in Medicine
    http://depts.washington.edu/bioethx/topics/index.html
  Centers for Disease Control and Prevention: Public Health Ethics
    http://www.cdc.gov/od/science/phethics/
  American Public Health Association
    http://www.apha.org/programs/education/progeduethicalguidelines.htm
  Public Health Leadership Society
    http://www.phls.org/home/section/3-26/
- Books
  An Autobiography: The Story of My Experiments with Truth
    Author: Mohandas K. Gandhi
  International Ethical Guidelines for Epidemiological Studies
    Author: Council for International Organizations of Medical Sciences, Switzerland. http://www.cioms.ch/

LEGAL EPIDEMIOLOGY

Epidemiologists play an important role in identifying the evidence of causation in legal issues. The statistically significant conclusions of clinical studies conducted to explore causation may help the legal decision-making process. In some cases the conclusions of an epidemiological study can be misused. Previous correlational studies on an issue, the volume of positive evidence of association of a risk factor with the disease/conditions, and the acceptance or rejection of causation in peer-reviewed journals may affect legal decisions. Advance practice nurses should read following court cases to understand the importance of exploration of evidence and legal action.

- *Daubert v. Merrell Dow Pharmaceuticals,* 509 U.S. 579 (1993)
- *Canavan v. Brigham and Women's Hospital,* 48 Mass. App. Ct. 297 (1999)
- *Weisgram v. Marley Co.,* 528 U.S. 440 (2000)

- *Soldo v. Sandoz Pharmaceuticals Corp.*, 244 F. Supp. 2d 434, 532 (W.D. Pa. 2003)
- *General Electric Co. v. Joiner*, 522 U.S. 136, 144 n.2 (1997)
- *Perry v. Novartis Pharmaceuticals Corp.*, 564 F. Supp. 2d 452 (E.D. Pa. 2008)

KEY POINTS

- Public health ethics is an emerging subject, because complex and challenging questions can impede progress in epidemiological research.
- The Nuremberg Code was a first step in the establishment of ethical standards in the international community. The Declaration of Helsinki and the Belmont Report have strengthened the foundations of ethics.
- Even though the international community agrees on ethical standards, unethical research conducted on human subjects in the Third World is still continuing.
- The ethical questions that one should answer in any public health disaster situation are autonomy, beneficence, and justice.
- When in doubt, the ideal way to confirm whether our ethical decisions are right or wrong is by learning about similar cases that happened in the past.

CRITICAL QUESTIONS

1. How can the international community strictly monitor research conducted in the Third World?
2. How will you make sure ethical standards are met in your research projects?
3. How will you address ethical issues that arise during your research?

REFERENCES

Angell, M. M. (1997). The ethics of clinical research in the third world. *New England Journal of Medicine, 337*(12), 847–849.

O'Brien, J. (2009). Honorary coauthorship: Does it matter? *Canadian Association of Radiologists Journal, 60*(5), 231.

Thomas, J. (1998). Ethical challenges of HIV clinical trials in developing countries. *Bioethics, 12*(4), 320–327.

U.S. Department of Health and Human Services (2008). Belmont Report. Retrieved from http://www.hhs.gov/ohrp/belmontArchive.html

Villanueva, C. M., Cantor, K. P., Grimalt, J. O., Malats, N., Silverman, D., Tardon, A. et al. (2007). Bladder cancer and exposure to water disinfection by-products through ingestion, bathing, showering, and swimming in pools. *American Journal of Epidemiology, 165*(2), 148–156.

CHAPTER 13

Epidemiological Applications in Clinical Nursing Science

"You will never do anything in this world without courage. It is the greatest quality of the mind next to honor."

—Aristotle

Kiran Macha
John P. McDonough

OBJECTIVES

- Describe the harmony that exists between epidemiology and nursing science.
- Discuss the outcomes of the application of epidemiological concepts in evidence-based nursing practice.
- Describe the role played by advanced practice nurses as part of an interdisciplinary team during public health emergencies.

EPIDEMIOLOGY AND NURSING SCIENCE

Epidemiology contributes an invaluable role to the process involving healthcare decisions. The investigation and evaluation of a public health emergency and the enforcement of public health policy can materialize in a short period of time. In recent years advances in epidemiology have helped to dispel a perception among some healthcare professionals that this field of specialization is limited to the study of epidemics. Epidemiology has branched out to include various subdisciplines, and an effective communication system has been built in the community to coordinate various activities to promote public health. Even though epidemiology as a branch of science did not exist in the time of Aristotle, early work done in communities is comparable with many modern epidemiological approaches. French and British nurses were the first to conduct epidemiological studies in the nursing community to identify causes of diseases in soldiers on the frontlines. Florence Nightingale was interested in opportunities for nurses in the field of preventive sciences. Pierre Charles Alexandre Louis was among the first to conduct statistical inquiries to challenge treatments such as bloodletting, popularized by Broussais. The foundations for many evidence-based practices had already been laid in the 18th century (Earl, 2009).

Epidemiology as a discipline integrates ideas and perspectives, so that health may be viewed as a global concern rather than an individual one. Political borders are becoming less important, because neither health nor disease, nor the global impacts of natural events, can be contained by national borders. The health effects associated with the melting of glaciers in the south and north poles as a result of global warming have yet to be studied. Humans are threatening their own existence by accumulating nuclear fuel and biological weapons, polluting water and air, overindustrializing, conducting deforestation, and extensively using pesticides. Nature is only reacting in trying to restore the balance of the five elements of earth in the form of hurricanes, earthquakes, tsunamis, volcanic eruptions, and tornados. There is no answer to the question of how to stop these natural and human-made disasters. The same issue divides world leaders, recognizing that keeping the Earth healthy and balanced is a collective responsibility. Because of the intermixing of races, dynamic changes occurring in the gene pool will have an impact on health. Holistic and clinical concepts of nursing science combined with preventive aspects of epidemiology may play a major role in the coming years to address some of the above issues.

From the inception of nursing as a profession, nursing leaders have continued to explore new avenues to address public health needs. The research opportunities in the field of epidemiology are an interesting area for nurses. Health data are available in hospitals and clinics, and nurses also have access to the community to collect and analyze data and identify health trends. A competent healthcare professional designs and implements an action plan from his or her observations in the community, and the outcomes of such actions can be effectively disseminated by professionals such as advanced practice nurses.

INTEGRATION OF PREVENTION AND NURSING SCIENCE

In 2000 the Quad Council of Public Health Nursing Organizations was formed to address the need to develop public health competencies in nurses. As part of its recommendations relative to the doctor of nursing practice curriculum, the American Association of Colleges of Nursing formulated prevention practices as one of its objectives, making up "Essential #7 - Clinical Prevention and Population Health for Improving the Nation's Health." These collective recommendations from various nursing and public health organizations working together are positively impacting the community participation of advanced practice nurses and their nursing practices.

Graduate education in nursing that was previously focused only on the clinical role of nurses is at present more grounded in the concept of evidence-based practice. The best evidence can be found in the community. To explore evidence, the best approach is to apply basic concepts of epidemiology in nursing practice.

CHANGING FACE OF EPIDEMIOLOGY THROUGH NURSING SCIENCE

Community health nursing is a potential channel for the advanced practice nurse to effectively learn about the complex health challenges prevalent in the community. Nursing schools throughout the country have been instrumental in the establishment of partnerships with community organizations. The redesigned nursing curriculum prepares students for leadership roles by encouraging application of public health competencies while participating in the delivery of essential public health services in their communities (Ouzts, Brown, & Diaz Swearingen, 2006). The environmental, economic, social, and cultural barriers specific to a community are today well understood by advanced practice nurses. In the formulation of health policy and to gain public and political commitment to a health issue, the contribution of unbiased information from professionals such as advanced practice nurses is encouraged.

A complex web of health conditions suffered by the uninsured and underinsured, the range of healthcare services offered in the community, socioeconomic conditions, and access to health care are some of the factors that may influence growing healthcare costs. Community health education interventions conducted by nurses can have significant positive impacts on health disparities. Assessing community needs is essential in focusing efforts on a specific area of health education. Advanced practice nurses can effectively fulfill such roles, and the community programs they have helped to plan and implement around identified needs have been very successful.

Many civilizations have collapsed as a result of the deadly work of microbes. Microorganisms are continually mutating, and failure to effectively counter their activity can be disastrous. Every habitat on Earth can be a breeding place for microbes, and we now know that hospital facilities are places where bacteria can take hold, multiply, and quickly spread. The resurgence of influenza viruses is causing great concern, because the outcome is more deaths before vaccines can be prepared. Hand washing and use of alcohol-based hand sanitizers seem to be effective ways to prevent transmission of diseases. Advanced practice nurses in healthcare settings perform many skilled invasive procedures. Nurses share the same responsibility as other healthcare professionals in precluding the evolution of microbes by teaching and practicing preventive methods.

Breast cancer is most prevalent in women and is a primary cause of mortality. In 2006, 191,410 women were diagnosed with breast cancer in the United States, of which 40,820 died (Centers for Disease Control and Prevention, 2010). Breast self-examination is a cost-effective method for detecting breast cancer. Breast cancer awareness is essential given its aggressive nature and extraordinarily high incidence, affecting both the young and old. Advanced practice nurses are in a good position to identify changes in breast from the history and examination of patients. As one of the largest groups of healthcare professionals with mostly women serving in this profession, nurses (especially women) can promote trust and communication, and a better understanding of the breast self-examination procedure has been shown to promote confidence in women. Education and promotion of preventive health behaviors in women help to detect cancers early, leading to a better prognosis.

Prenatal programs implemented in the community, especially those targeting vulnerable populations including immigrants, are effective in reducing health risks to pregnant women and in reducing infant mortality. These efforts are also improving access to health care. Nurses have an opportunity to encourage breastfeeding, and at the same time breast self-examination can be promoted. As a large population, nurses have themselves been participants in numerous health studies. Studies conducted on nurses working for the National Health Service in the United Kingdom revealed no association between breastfeeding and breast cancer (Michels, 2001).

The current prevalence of hypertension, stroke, diabetes, and obesity in the community is far greater than expected. The Framingham study determined the risk factors for cardiovascular disease to include a lack of physical activity, high cholesterol, excess alcohol intake, smoking, and excess salt consumption. Almost one-third of deaths in the United States are associated with heart disease. The prevalence of obesity in children is growing every year, and the incidence of juvenile diabetes is also on the rise. The fact that children know more about French fries than what they are made from is a great concern. School-based nurses can promote healthy nutrition, healthy behaviors, and resources to overcome children's addictions to fatty and sugary foods. Encouraging healthy behaviors in children will indirectly have long-term positive effects on the prevalence of chronic diseases. The education of patients suffering from chronic diseases by advanced practice nurses may help prevent disability and longer lives for many, with fewer episodes of hospitalization.

Preventive home visits conducted by nurses in the community to assess the functional status of the elderly population are extremely beneficial. Making changes at home in association with home visit recommendations can prevent injuries caused by falls. Nursing home and hospital admissions can be greatly reduced, and a healthier environment can be created as a result of home visit assessments. Nurses can also help elderly people recover from emotional experiences.

Advanced practice nurses are actively conducting health screening in the community. Screening for cervical cancer is important to detect human papilloma virus and cervical cancer, which is treatable at early stages. Even though the Papanicolau test may not identify endocervical changes, it has been widely used as a screening test for early identification of changes in the cervical epithelium. The human papilloma virus vaccine may prevent changes in the cervical epithelium. Early identification of cancer leads to less invasive interventions, better prognosis, and more effective follow-up care. Advanced practice nurses play an important role at each and every stage to reduce the impact of cancer and incidence of disease in the community.

"Culture" is a complex issue in the United States, because the country has become so culturally diverse. Graduate nursing education curricula have been modified to teach cultural values to nurses to help them develop cultural competency. Research on cultural issues related to practice conducted by nurses in the community has shown improvements in health outcomes (McGrath & Ka'ili, 2010). Because the nursing profession is founded on holistic care, cultural competency complements practice toward establishing better communication with patients in the diagnosis and treatment process.

The code of ethics for nurses mandates collaboration with other public health professionals to meet the health needs of a community. Pandemics caused by influenza can be prevented through vaccination. Voluntarily, hundreds of nurses participate in these vaccination programs to stop the spread of disease. Experiences gained by nurses during their participation in disasters are essential to the emergency preparedness planning process, where an interdisciplinary approach lessens communication errors and encourages cooperation in the community in times of disaster.

Technology in health care is expanding its role with continuing inventions. Telemedicine, online offerings of health programs, chat rooms for specific health topics, centralized patient information software in hospitals, and online counseling with dedicated teams have revolutionized the handling of and access to health information, also reducing the burden on healthcare professionals. For example, Nurses QuitNet is an online program with multidimensional online resources offered to nurses who want to participate in a smoking cessation program (Bialous et al., 2009). These types of evidence-based online programs have been proven to result in positive behavioral change for most participants. Integration of informatics in curricula designed to develop the technological competency of nurses is a financial challenge. Electronic medical records and other technological software programs can help with screening to identify high-risk patients and alert health professionals. Geographical information systems help advanced practice nurses to identify, assess, and analyze environmental exposures. Many graduate nursing projects are designed to evaluate and explore the possibilities of technological applications in the field of nursing. The outcomes of this research are providing future insight and encouragement.

The application of epidemiological and nursing concepts continues to impact the changing architecture of community health. Epidemiology is a constructive science that can be used for balancing the energies both within us and in the environment in which we live. The many opportunities in epidemiology interest nurses; without nursing science, the field of epidemiology would be significantly handicapped.

KEY POINTS

- For many decades nursing leaders have been practicing holistic science combined with prevention practices.
- Advanced practice nurses have an important role to play in the field of epidemiology related to emergency preparedness.
- An interdisciplinary approach to any public health emergency is essential, and advanced practice nurses have the potential to make independent decisions to protect the public health.
- A major change in the epidemiological architecture of a community can be brought about through the dedicated efforts of advanced practice nurses.

CRITICAL QUESTIONS

1. List five outcomes of the applications of epidemiological concepts in nursing practices.
2. Why do you believe communication is important between interdisciplinary professionals during a public health emergency?
3. Why do you believe advanced nurses should be involved in epidemiological research?

REFERENCES

Bialous, S. A., Sarna, L., Wells, M., Elashoff, D., Wewers, M. E., & Froelicher, E. S. (2009). Characteristics of nurses who used the internet-based nurses QuitNet for smoking cessation. *Public Health Nursing, 26*(4), 329–338.

Centers for Disease Control and Prevention. (2010). Breast Cancer. Retrieved from http://www.cdc.gov/cancer/breast

Earl, C. E. (2009). Medical history and epidemiology: Their contribution to the development of public health nursing. *Nursing Outlook*, *57*(5), 257.

McGrath, B. B., & Ka'ili, T. O. (2010). Creating project talanoa: A culturally based community health program for U.S. Pacific Islander adolescents. *Public Health Nursing*, *27*(1), 17–24.

Michels, K. K. B. (2001). Being breastfed in infancy and breast cancer incidence in adult life: Results from the two nurses' health studies. *American Journal of Epidemiology*, *153*(3), 275–283.

Ouzts, K. N., Brown, J. W., & Diaz Swearingen, C. A. (2006). Developing public health competence among RN-to-BSN students in a rural community. *Public Health Nursing*, *23*(2), 178–182.

INDEX

Page numbers followed by *f* or *t* indicate figures or tables, respectively. Photographic figures or illustrations are indicated by *italics*.